T0263926

Pediatric Hematology

Editor

CATHERINE S. MANNO

PEDIATRIC CLINICS
OF NORTH AMERICA

www.pediatric.theclinics.com

December 2013 • Volume 60 • Number 6

ELSEVIER

1600 John F. Kennedy Boulevard • Suite 1800 • Philadelphia, Pennsylvania, 19103-2899

http://www.theclinics.com

THE PEDIATRIC CLINICS OF NORTH AMERICA Volume 60, Number 6
December 2013 ISSN 0031-3955, ISBN-13: 978-0-323-26118-0

Editor: Kerry Holland
Developmental Editor: Yonah Korngold

The Pediatric Clinics of North America (ISSN 0031-3955) is published bimonthly by Elsevier Inc., 360 Park Avenue South, New York, NY 10010-1710. Months of issue are February, April, June, August, October, and December. Periodicals postage paid at New York, NY and additional mailing offices. Subscription prices are $191.00 per year (US individuals), $462.00 per year (US institutions), $259.00 per year (Canadian individuals), $614.00 per year (Canadian institutions), $308.00 per year (international individuals), $614.00 per year (international institutions), $93.00 per year (US students and residents), and $159.00 per year (international and Canadian residents and students). To receive students/resident rare, orders must be accompanied by name of affiliated institution, date of term, and the signature of program/residency coordinator on institution letterhead. Orders will be billed at individual rate until proof of status is received. Foreign air speed delivery is included in all Clinics subscription prices. All prices are subject to change without notice. **POSTMASTER:** Send address changes to The Pediatric Clinics of North America, Elsevier Health Sciences Division, Subscription Customer Service, 3251 Riverport Lane, Maryland Heights, MO 63043. **Customer Service: 1-800-654-2452 (US and Canada). From outside of the US and Canada: 1-314-447-8871. Fax: 1-314-447-8029. For print support, E-mail: JournalsCustomerService-usa@elsevier.com. For online support, E-mail: JournalsOnlineSupport-usa@elsevier.com.**

Reprints. For copies of 100 or more, of articles in this publication, please contact the Commercial Reprints Department, Elsevier Inc., 360 Park Avenue South, New York, NY 10010-1710. Tel.: 212-633-3874; Fax: 212-633-3820; E-mail: reprints@elsevier.com.

The Pediatric Clinics of North America is also published in Spanish by McGraw-Hill Inter-americana Editores S.A., Mexico City, Mexico; in Portuguese by Riechmann and Affonso Editores, Rua Comandante Coelho 1085, CEP 21250, Rio de Janeiro, Brazil; and in Greek by Althayia SA, Athens, Greece.

The Pediatric Clinics of North America is covered in MEDLINE/PubMed (Index Medicus), Excerpta Medica, Current Contents, Current Contents/Clinical Medicine, Science Citation Index, ASCA, ISI/BIOMED, and BIOSIS.

Printed and bound by CPI Group (UK) Ltd, Croydon, CR0 4YY

Transferred to digital print 2012

PROGRAM OBJECTIVE
The goal of the *Pediatric Clinics of North America* is to keep practicing physicians and residents up to date with current clinical practice in pediatrics by providing timely articles reviewing the state-of-the-art in patient care.

TARGET AUDIENCE
All practicing pediatricians, physicians and healthcare professionals who provide patient care to pediatric patients.

LEARNING OBJECTIVES
Upon completion of this activity, participants will be able to:
1. Discuss the rationale and indications for pediatric therapeutic apheresis.
2. Recognize the special relevance of bloodbanking/immunohematology to the pediatric patient.
3. Review inherited abnormalities including bone marrow failure syndromes, inherited abnormalities of coagulation, and inherited platelet function disorder.

ACCREDITATION
The Elsevier Office of Continuing Medical Education (EOCME) is accredited by the Accreditation Council for Continuing Medical Education (ACCME) to provide continuing medical education for physicians.

The EOCME designates this enduring material for a maximum of 15 *AMA PRA Category 1 Credit*(s)™. Physicians should claim only the credit commensurate with the extent of their participation in the activity.

All other health care professionals requesting continuing education credit for this enduring material will be issued a certificate of participation.

DISCLOSURE OF CONFLICTS OF INTEREST
The EOCME assesses conflict of interest with its instructors, faculty, planners, and other individuals who are in a position to control the content of CME activities. All relevant conflicts of interest that are identified are thoroughly vetted by EOCME for fair balance, scientific objectivity, and patient care recommendations. EOCME is committed to providing its learners with CME activities that promote improvements or quality in healthcare and not a specific proprietary business or a commercial interest.

The planning committee, staff, authors and editors listed below have identified no financial relationships or relationships to products or devices they or their spouse/life partner have with commercial interest related to the content of this CME activity:
Monica Bessler, MD, PhD; Paula H.B. Bolton-Maggs, DM, FRCP, FRCPath, FRCPCH; Anthony K.C. Chan, MBBS, FRCPC, FRCPCH, FRCPI, FRCP (Glas), FRCPath; S. Deborah Chirnomas, MD, MPH; Pedro A. de Alarcón, MD; Karen S. Fernandez, MD; Patrick G. Gallagher, MD; Ruchika Goel, MD, MPH; Neil Goldenberg, MD, PhD; Helge D. Hartung, MD; Kerry Holland; Brynne Hunter; Julie Jaffray, MD; Riten Kumar, MD, MSc; Indu Kumari; Gary M. Kupfer, MD; Sandy Lavery; Jill McNair; Alissa Martin, MD; Dana C, Matthews, MD; Timothy S. Olson, MD, PhD; Lindsay Parnell; Charles Quinn, MD, MS; Steven Sloan, MD, PhD; David Teachey, MD; Alexis A. Thompson, MD, MPH; Howard Trachtman, MD; Suresh Vedantham, MD; Hannah M. Ware, Char M. Witmer, MD, MSCE; Edward C.C. Wong, MD; Janet Y.K. Yang, MBBS (HKU), MRCPCH, FHKAM(Pediatrics), FHKC.Paed; Guy Young, MD.

The planning committee, staff, authors and editors listed below have identified financial relationships or relationships to products or devices they or their spouse/life partner have with commercial interest related to the content of this CME activity:
Manuel Carcao, MD, MSc, FRCPC is on speakers bureau for Pfizer, Octapharma, Baxter, CSL Behring, Biogen Idec, Inc. and Novo Nordisk; is a consultant/advisor for Pfizer, Octapharma, Baxter, Novo Nordisk, CSL Behring and Biogen Idec, Inc.; has research grants from Pfizer, Novo Nordisk, and Biogen Idec, Inc.
Yeowon A. Kim, MD, MHS has an employment affiliation with Biogen Idec, Inc.
Janet L. Kwiatkowski, MD, MSCE is a consultant/advisor for Shire Pharmaceuticals and has a research grant from Resonance Health.
Michele P. Lambert, MD is a consultant/advisor for GlaxoSmithKline and Nestle, and has research grants from GlaxoSmithKline and Amgen.
Catherine S. Manno, MD is a consultant/advisor for Bayer HealthCare Pharmaceuticals, Inc. (International Network for Pediatric Hemophilia), and is a consultant/advisor for NOVO Nordisk (National Hemophilia Advisory Board).

UNAPPROVED/OFF-LABEL USE DISCLOSURE

The EOCME requires CME faculty to disclose to the participants:

1. When products or procedures being discussed are off-label, unlabelled, experimental, and/or investigational (not US Food and Drug Administration (FDA) approved); and
2. Any limitations on the information presented, such as data that are preliminary or that represent ongoing research, interim analyses, and/or unsupported opinions. Faculty may discuss information about pharmaceutical agents that is outside of FDA-approved labelling. This information is intended solely for CME and is not intended to promote off-label use of these medications. If you have any questions, contact the medical affairs department of the manufacturer for the most recent prescribing information.

TO ENROLL

To enroll in the *Pediatric Clinics of North America* Continuing Medical Education program, call customer service at 1-800-654-2452 or sign up online at http://www.theclinics.com/home/cme. The CME program is available to subscribers for an additional annual fee of USD 261.

METHOD OF PARTICIPATION

In order to claim credit, participants must complete the following:

1. Complete enrolment as indicated above.
2. Read the activity.
3. Complete the CME Test and Evaluation. Participants must achieve a score of 70% on the test. All CME Tests and Evaluations must be completed online.

CME INQUIRIES/SPECIAL NEEDS

For all CME inquiries or special needs, please contact elsevierCME@elsevier.com.

Contributors

EDITOR

CATHERINE S. MANNO, MD
Pat and John Rosenwald Professor of Pediatrics, Chair, Department of Pediatrics, NYU Langone Medical Center, New York, New York

AUTHORS

MONICA BESSLER, MD, PhD
Comprehensive Bone Marrow Failure Center, Division of Hematology, Department of Pediatrics, The Children's Hospital of Philadelphia; Division of Hemato-Oncology, Department of Medicine, Hospital of the University of Pennsylvania, Perlman School of Medicine, University of Pennsylvania, Philadelphia, Pennsylvania

PAULA H.B. BOLTON-MAGGS, DM, FRCP, FRCPath
Consultant Hematologist, Medical Director, Serious Hazards of Transfusion (SHOT), Manchester Blood Centre, Honorary Senior Lecturer, University of Manchester, Manchester, United Kingdom

MANUEL CARCAO, MD, MSc, FRCP(C)
Division of Haematology/Oncology, Department of Paediatrics; Child Health Evaluative Sciences, Research Institute, Hospital for Sick Children, University of Toronto, Toronto, Ontario, Canada

ANTHONY K.C. CHAN, MBBS, FRCPC, FRCPCH, FRCPI, FRCP (Glas), FRCPath
Division of Hematology and Oncology, Department of Pediatrics, McMaster University, Hamilton, Ontario, Canada

S. DEBORAH CHIRNOMAS, MD, MPH
Director, Assistant Professor of Pediatrics, Pediatric Stem Cell Transplant Program, Section of Pediatric Hematology-Oncology, Yale School of Medicine, New Haven, Connecticut

PEDRO A. DE ALARCÓN, MD
William H. Albers Professor and Chair, Department of Pediatrics, University of Illinois College of Medicine at Peoria and Children's Hospital of Illinois, Peoria, Illinois

KAREN S. FERNÁNDEZ, MD
Jim and Katie Owens Assistant Professor of Pediatrics, Division of Hematology/Oncology, Department of Pediatrics, University of Illinois College of Medicine at Peoria and Children's Hospital of Illinois, Peoria, Illinois

PATRICK G. GALLAGHER, MD
Professor of Pediatrics, Pathology and Genetics, Department of Pediatrics, Yale University School of Medicine, New Haven, Connecticut

RUCHIKA GOEL, MD
Division of Hematology and Oncology, Department of Pediatrics, Johns Hopkins School of Medicine, Baltimore, Maryland

NEIL A. GOLDENBERG, MD, PhD
Associate Professor of Pediatrics and Medicine, Divisions of Hematology, Departments of Pediatrics and Medicine, Johns Hopkins School of Medicine, Baltimore, Maryland; Pediatric Thrombosis and Stroke Programs, All Children's Hospital Johns Hopkins Medicine, St. Petersburg, Florida

HELGE D. HARTUNG, MD
Comprehensive Bone Marrow Failure Center, Division of Hematology, Department of Pediatrics, The Children's Hospital of Philadelphia, Philadelphia, Pennsylvania

JULIE JAFFRAY, MD
Coagulation Fellow, Department of Hematology/Oncology, Children's Hospital of Los Angeles, University of Southern California Keck School of Medicine, Los Angeles, California

YEOWON A. KIM, MD, MHS
Joint Program in Transfusion Medicine, Department of Laboratory Medicine, Boston Children's Hospital, Harvard Medical School, Boston, Massachusetts

RITEN KUMAR, MD, MSc
Division of Haematology/Oncology, Department of Paediatrics, Hospital for Sick Children, University of Toronto, Toronto, Ontario, Canada

GARY M. KUPFER, MD
Chief, Professor of Pediatrics and Pathology, Section of Pediatric Hematology-Oncology, Yale School of Medicine, New Haven, Connecticut

JANET L. KWIATKOWSKI, MD, MSCE
Director, Thalassemia Program, Division of Hematology, Department of Pediatrics, Children's Hospital of Philadelphia; Associate Professor of Pediatrics, Perelman School of Medicine, University of Pennsylvania, Philadelphia, Pennsylvania

MICHELE P. LAMBERT, MD
Assistant Professor of Pediatrics, Pediatric Hematology, Children's Hospital of Philadelphia, University of Pennsylvania School of Medicine, Philadelphia, Pennsylvania

ALISSA MARTIN, MD
Division of Hematology/Oncology, Ann and Robert H. Lurie Children's Hospital of Chicago, Chicago, Illinois

DANA C. MATTHEWS, MD
Associate Professor, Division of Hematology/Oncology, Department of Pediatrics, University of Washington School of Medicine; Director, Clinical Hematology, Cancer and Blood Disorders Center, Seattle Children's Hospital, Seattle, Washington

TIMOTHY S. OLSON, MD, PhD
Comprehensive Bone Marrow Failure Center, Division of Oncology, Department of Pediatrics, The Children's Hospital of Philadelphia, Philadelphia, Pennsylvania

CHARLES T. QUINN, MD, MS
Director of Hematology Clinical and Translational Research, Division of Hematology, Cincinnati Children's Hospital Medical Center; Associate Professor, Department of Pediatrics, University of Cincinnati College of Medicine, Cincinnati, Ohio

STEVEN R. SLOAN, MD, PhD
Associate Professor of Pathology, Joint Program in Transfusion Medicine, Department of Laboratory Medicine, Boston Children's Hospital, Harvard Medical School, Boston, Massachusetts

DAVID T. TEACHEY, MD
Assistant Professor of Pediatrics, Pediatric Hematology, Children's Hospital of Philadelphia, University of Pennsylvania School of Medicine, Philadelphia, Pennsylvania

ALEXIS A. THOMPSON, MD, MPH
Hematology Section Head, Division of Hematology/Oncology, Ann and Robert H. Lurie Children's Hospital of Chicago, Chicago, Illinois

HOWARD TRACHTMAN, MD
Professor of Clinical Pediatrics, Division of Nephrology, Department of Pediatrics, CTSI, NYU Langone Medical Center, New York, New York

SURESH VEDANTHAM, MD
Professor of Radiology and Surgery, Mallinckrodt Institute of Radiology, Washington University School of Medicine, St Louis, Missouri

HANNAH M. WARE
Division of Hematology, Department of Pediatrics, Children's Hospital of Philadelphia, University of Pennsylvania, Philadelphia, Pennsylvania

CHAR M. WITMER, MD, MSCE
Assistant Professor, Division of Hematology, Department of Pediatrics, Children's Hospital of Philadelphia, Perelman School of Medicine, University of Pennsylvania, Philadelphia, Pennsylvania

EDWARD C.C. WONG, MD
Director of Hematology, Associate Director of Transfusion Medicine, Division of Laboratory Medicine, Center for Cancer and Blood Disorders, Children's National Medical Center, Sheikh Zayed Campus for Advanced Children's Medicine; Associate Professor, Departments of Pediatrics and Pathology, George Washington University School of Medicine and Health Sciences, Washington, DC

JANET Y.K. YANG, MBBS, MRCPCH, FHKAM(Pediatrics), FHKC.Paed
Division of Hematology and Oncology, Department of Pediatrics, McMaster University, Hamilton, Ontario, Canada

GUY YOUNG, MD
Associate Professor of Pediatrics, Department of Hematology/Oncology, Director, Hemostasis and Thrombosis Center, Children's Hospital of Los Angeles, University of Southern California Keck School of Medicine, Los Angeles, California

Contents

The coagulation system involves a dynamic group of procoagulation and anticoagulation proteins that appear early in fetal life and whose levels change throughout childhood and into the teenage years. This process is called *developmental hemostasis*. Developmental hemostasis creates unique challenges for clinicians affecting the diagnosis and treatment of coagulation disorders during early childhood. The objective of this review is to assist pediatricians in understanding the coagulation system in fetal life and childhood and to provide guidance for interpreting basic coagulation testing, which will result in an improved ability to diagnose and treat patients with hemostatic and thrombotic disorders.

Bleeding disorders are broadly classified into primary and secondary hemostatic defects. Primary hemostatic disorders (disorders of platelets and von Willebrand factor) mainly result in mucocutaneous bleeding symptoms such as epistaxis, menorrhagia, petechiae, easy bruising, and bleeding after dental and surgical interventions. Secondary hemostatic disorders (congenital or acquired deficiencies of coagulation factors) typically manifest with delayed, deep bleeding into muscles and joints. This article provides a generalized overview of the pathophysiology, clinical manifestations, laboratory abnormalities, and molecular basis of inherited abnormalities of coagulation with a focus on hemophilia, von Willebrand disease, and rare inherited coagulation disorders.

Pediatric thrombosis and thrombophilia are increasingly recognized and studied. In this article, both the inherited and acquired factors for the development of thrombosis in neonates and children are categorized using the elements of Virchow's triad: stasis, hypercoagulable state, and vascular injury. The indications and rationale for performing thrombophilia testing are described. Also included are discussions on who, how, when, and why to test. Finally, recommendations for the use of contraceptives for adolescent females with a family history of thrombosis are outlined.

Pediatric deep vein thrombosis is an increasingly recognized phenomenon, especially with advances in treatment and supportive care of critically ill children and with better diagnostic capabilities. High-quality evidence and uniform management guidelines for antithrombotic treatment, particularly thrombolytic therapy, remain limited. Optimal dosing, intensity and duration strategies for anticoagulation as well as thrombolytic regimens that maximize efficacy and safety need to be determined through well-designed clinical trials using use of a risk-stratified approach.

PEDIATRIC CLINICS OF NORTH AMERICA

RELATED INTEREST

Hematology/Oncology Clinics June 2013 (Volume 27:2)
Disorders of the Platelets
A. Koneti Rao, MD, *Editor*

DOWNLOAD
Free App!

Review Articles
THE CLINICS

NOW AVAILABLE FOR YOUR iPhone and iPad

Preface

Pediatric Hematology

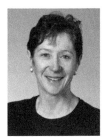

Catherine S. Manno, MD
Editor

Tremendous progress has been made over the past decade in the field of hematology, providing not only enhanced accuracy in the diagnosis of inherited and acquired nonmalignant blood disorders but also new therapeutic strategies that have resulted in improved patient outcomes. This volume of *The Pediatric Clinics of North America* provides a comprehensive view of pediatric hematology for the practicing pediatrician—from developmental hematopoiesis and developmental coagulation to inherited and acquired bone marrow failure syndromes, hemoglobin disorders, bleeding disorders, and immune cytopenias. New approaches to the treatment of children with relatively familiar diseases like sickle cell disease, ITP, and hemophilia are explored in depth. With the alarming increase of infants and children presenting with venous thrombosis over the past generation, an enhanced understanding of pediatric thrombophilia and optimized treatment algorithms for affected young patients are necessary tools for the pediatric practitioner. Transfusion medicine continues to play an essential role in the care of many patients with hematological diseases; thus, descriptions of blood component therapy, methods for improving blood safety, expanded use of pheresis in children, and treatment of transfusional iron overload are essential to principles of modern management.

A group of prominent experts from the field of Pediatric Hematology have contributed to this volume. Each author has distilled the essential developments from his or her specific area of expertise in order that the practicing general pediatrician can readily find relevant, up-to-date information for the diagnosis of these disorders, some of which are exceedingly rare. Also included are recommendations for supporting individual patient management. Several authors direct the reader to more in-depth discussions of background information. We hope that our readers find the information contained herein useful in their understanding of the best approaches to the patients they might evaluate and manage. I also hope these articles serve as a tantalizing

Pediatr Clin N Am 60 (2013) xv–xvi
http://dx.doi.org/10.1016/j.pcl.2013.10.002
0031-3955/13/$ – see front matter © 2013 Elsevier Inc. All rights reserved.

pediatric.theclinics.com

introduction to the important scientific developments in pediatric hematology that have been made through the familiar but critical avenues of discovery—basic, translational, and clinical investigations.

Catherine S. Manno, MD
Department of Pediatrics
NYU Langone Medical Center
145 East 32nd Street
14th Floor Penthouse, Room 1410
New York, NY 10016, USA

E-mail address:
catherine.manno@nyumc.org

Development of the Hematopoietic System and Disorders of Hematopoiesis that Present During Infancy and Early Childhood

Karen S. Fernández, MD[a], Pedro A. de Alarcón, MD[b],*

KEYWORDS

- Hematopoietic system • Hematopoiesis • Infancy • Early childhood

KEY POINTS

- The sequential site of hematopoiesis includes the yolk sac, the aorta-gonad mesonephros region, the fetal liver, and, finally, the bone marrow.
- Formation of the hematopoietic tissues begins with pluripotent stem cells capable of both self-renewal and clonal maturation into blood cell lineages.
- Hematopoietic stem cells require a combination of transcription factors (intrinsic determinants of cellular phenotype) for the survival and proliferation of hematopoietic stem cells (HSC). In addition, adjacent cells and local cytokines (the microenvironment) are necessary for optimal HSC growth and differentiation.
- A review of the development of the hematopoietic system provides a basic understanding of the pathophysiology of many inherited diseases, including bone marrow disorders, immunodeficiency, and alterations of hemoglobin.

INTRODUCTION

"The blood has always fascinated humanity. Blood has been regarded as a living substance, the very essence of life. Poets have written of thick blood and thin, pale blood, red blood and blue blood, royal blood, and pure and eloquent blood."[1]

Hematopoiesis refers to the continuous process of blood cell formation. Because mature blood cells are predominantly short lived, the establishment and maintenance

---

Funding Sources: None.
Conflict of Interest: None.
[a] Division of Hematology/Oncology, Department of Pediatrics, University of Illinois College of Medicine at Peoria, Children's Hospital of Illinois, 530 Northeast Glen Oak Avenue, Peoria, IL 61637, USA; [b] Department of Pediatrics, University of Illinois College of Medicine at Peoria, Children's Hospital of Illinois, 530 Northeast Glen Oak Avenue, Peoria, IL 61637, USA
* Corresponding author.
E-mail address: pdealarc@uic.edu

Pediatr Clin N Am 60 (2013) 1273–1289
http://dx.doi.org/10.1016/j.pcl.2013.08.002
0031-3955/13/$ – see front matter © 2013 Elsevier Inc. All rights reserved.

of the blood system requires self-renewing hematopoietic stem cells (HSC) throughout life to replenish multilineage progenitors and precursors committed to individual hematopoietic lineages. The ceaseless hematopoietic process replenishes the senescent cells that leave the circulation and produces nearly 200 billion red blood cells, 10 billion white blood cells, and 400 billion platelets every day. Blood cell production is closely regulated and responds to challenges to the host, like infection, hemorrhage, allergy, or inflammation.

Current understanding of hematopoiesis is based on the hypothesis that there is an HSC capable of self-renewal and differentiation into all hematopoietic cell lines.[2-6] HSC transplantation has confirmed the remarkable regenerative properties of the HSCs for a variety of human disorders.

DEVELOPMENT OF THE HEMATOPOIETIC SYSTEM

Hematopoiesis comprises a continuum of functionally distinct hematopoietic cell compartments during the embryonic period that starts with the presence of the HSC. In mammals, hematopoiesis occurs as a sequential process that moves to different anatomic sites during embryonic and fetal development. The sites of hematopoiesis include the yolk sac; the aorta-gonad-mesonephros region (AGM) (a sheet of lateral mesoderm that migrates medially, touches the endoderm, and then forms a single aorta tube where clusters of HSC appear); the fetal liver; and, finally, the bone marrow.

HSCs can divide to give rise to a daughter cell that retains all of the pluripotentiality of the parent (self-renewal) or it can proliferate into daughter cells that have lost some multipotentiality and have become committed to produce multipotential progenitor (MPP) cells.[7] Pluripotent HSCs generate cells with the capacity for long-term engraftment and are, therefore, also called LT-HSCs. As illustrated in **Fig. 1**, once committed, the MPP cell gives rise to progressively more lineage-committed hematopoietic progenitor cells and eventually to mature cells. HSCs require a combination of transcription factors (intrinsic determinants of cellular phenotype) for their survival and proliferation. In addition, adjacent cells and local cytokines (microenvironment) are necessary for optimal HSC growth and differentiation. Lineage-committed progenitor cells are dependent on lineage-specific factors to undergo final differentiation. **Fig. 1** provides a general overview of the interactions between cytokines, transcription factors, and growth factors in the proliferation and differentiation of hematopoietic cells.[8,9] **Table 1** summarizes the function of the interleukins in hematopoiesis.

The initial phase of hematopoiesis occurs in the yolk sac (**Fig. 2**A). The first wave of blood production, termed *primitive*, is red blood cell production to facilitate tissue oxygenation and allow for the rapid growth of the embryo. Although this initial phase of blood production is largely erythropoietic, megakaryocytes and macrophages are also included. Primitive progenitors can be found from embryonic day (E) 7.25 in the mouse and within 3 to 4 weeks of human gestation.

The second hematopoietic wave also begins in the yolk sac and demonstrates definitive progenitors around embryonic day (E) 8.25 in the mouse and by week 4 in humans. The second wave contains erythroid and myeloid lineages. During this phase, definitive progenitors migrate from the yolk sac to the fetal liver where they expand and mature.

The third wave of hematopoiesis is more complex and arises from HSCs produced in the AGM, major blood vessels, and the placenta. Whether these stem cells are endogenous to the AGM or arise from the yolk sac is controversial.

From the fetal liver, hematopoietic progenitors migrate and colonize the thymus, spleen, and ultimately the bone marrow. None of these sites are characterized by

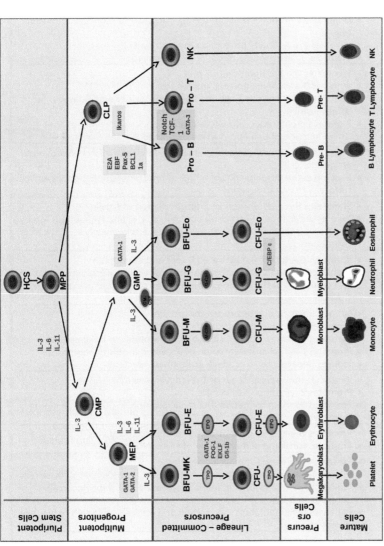

Fig. 1. Schematic Representation of Hematopoiesis. Early–acting hematopoietic growth factors are in green box. Growth factors are represented in colored circles. BFU-E, burst-forming unit-Erythrocyte; BFU-Eo, burst-forming unit-Eosinophil; BFU-G, burst-forming unit-Granulocyte; BFU-M, burst-forming unit-Monocyte/Macrophage; BFU-MK, burst-forming unit-Mekagaryocyte; CFU-E, colony-forming unit-Erythrocyte; CFU-Eo, colony-forming unit-Eosinophil; CFU-G, colony-forming unit-Granulocyte; CFU-M, colony-forming unit-Monocyte/Macrophage; CFU-MK, colony-forming unit-Megakaryocytes; CLP, common lymphoid progenitors; CMP, common myeloid progenitors; EPO, erythropoietin; G-CSF, granulocyte colony stimulating factor; GM-CSF, granulocyte/(Monocyte/Macrophage) colony stimulating factor; GMP, granulocyte/macrophage progenitors; HSC, hematopoietic stem cells; M-CSF, Monocyte/Macrophage colony stimulating factor; MEP, megakaryocyte/erythroid progenitors; MPP, multipotent progenitors; TPO, thrombopoietin.

Table 1
Cytokines involved in hematopoiesis

Interleukin	Function
IL-1	• Increases the proliferative responses of fetal thymocyte progenitors to IL-2 • Upregulates production of G-CSF by monocytes in human fetuses from 14–24 wk after conception • Upregulates production of GM-CSF by tracheal and bronchial epithelial cells • Increases the antibody production induced by IL-2 • Mediates an acute phase response in inflammation
IL-2	• Stimulates the proliferation of T cells • Activates T and B lymphocytes and NK cells • Stimulates CD8 positive T-cell–mediated cytotoxicity and delayed hypersensitivity • Promotes proliferation of mature B cells • Drives immunoglobulin production by primed B-1 and mature B cells
IL-3	• Promotes the differentiation of human basophils and other hematopoietic progenitor cells • Maximizes the development of BFU-E of fetal mouse liver cells grown in culture with erythropoietin
IL-4	• Stimulates the proliferation and differentiation of B cells • Induces production of immunoglobulin IgM, IgG, and IgE, but not IgA by pre-B cells from the liver, spleen, and bone marrow as early as 12 wk after conception
IL-5	• Promotes the growth of activated B cells and eosinophils • Mobilizes eosinophils from the bone marrow during allergic inflammation and regulation of the homing and migration of eosinophils in response to chemotactic stimuli
IL-6	• Supports hematopoietic progenitor growth • Promotes T- and B-cell function • Mediates the acute phase response of hepatocytes to inflammation • Promotes the final differentiation of activated B cells to plasma cells • Induces hepatocytes to produce acute phase reactants
Il-7	• Regulates the earliest stages of T-cell development • Promotes B lymphopoiesis in mice • Promotes γδ chain formation and the expression of CD8 in fetal mouse thymocytes
IL-8	• Promotes chemotaxis of neutrophils to inflammatory sites • Promotes softening and dilatation of the cervix in rabbits
IL-10	• Prevents antigen-specific T-cell activation • Inhibits T-cell expansion by directly inhibiting IL-2 production by these cells • Inhibits the lethal effects of lipopolysaccharide and staphylococcal enterotoxin B in mice • Enhances immunoglobulin production and causes plasma cells to increase in number
IL-11	• Stimulates megakaryopoiesis and production of macrophages
IL-12	• Stimulates CD8+ cells to become cytotoxic lymphocytes • Induces IFN-gamma production • Promotes antitumor immunity and influences antiviral responses

(continued on next page)

Table 1 (continued)	
Interleukin	**Function**
IL-13	• Inhibits production of proinflammatory cytokines and chemokines by monocytes • Promotes B-cell proliferation and differentiation • Induces expression of IgE by pre-B cells from the marrow and spleen
IL-14	• B-cell growth factor
IL-15	• Activates T cell and NK cells • Promotes immunoglobulin production from B cells
IL-16	• Activates helper T cells • Acts as a strong chemoattractant for lymphocytes and eosinophils
IL-17	• Induces IL-6 secretion from mouse stromal cells
IL-18	• Induces IFN-gamma production by helper T cells • Increases the production of GM-CSF • Decreases production of IL-10 • Activates NK cells and cytotoxic T lymphocytes

Abbreviations: BFU-E, burst-forming unit erythroid; G-CSF, granulocyte colony-stimulating factor; GM-CSF, granulocyte-macrophage colony-stimulating factor; IFN, interferon; Ig, immunoglobulin; IL, interleukin; NK, natural killer.

Reproduced from Rivers AE, Slayton W. Development of the immune system. In: de Alarcon PA, Werner EJ, Christensen RD, editors. Neonatal hematology: pathogenesis, diagnosis, and management of hematologic problems. 2nd edition. New York: Cambridge University Press; 2013; with permission.

de novo generation of HSCs, but rather these niches support the expansion of HSCs that migrated to these new sites (see **Fig. 2**B) from earlier sites. The production of all blood lineages is not achieved by intraembryonic HSC until colonization and development of the bone marrow.[10] Colonization of the bone marrow results in the production of a small pool of HSCs that are responsible for the maintenance of hematopoiesis throughout life.[11]

In humans, by week 10 to 12 of gestation, extraembryonic hematopoiesis has essentially ceased. The liver remains the predominant erythropoietic organ through 20 to 24 weeks of gestation. Hepatic hematopoietic production diminishes during the second trimester, whereas bone marrow hematopoiesis increases (see **Fig. 2**).

FETAL ERYTHROPOIESIS

After their initial development in yolk-sac blood islands (see **Fig. 2**), primitive erythroid progenitors (EryP) enter the newly formed vasculature of the embryo where they continue to divide for several days. EryP differentiate within the bloodstream, gradually accumulating increasing amounts of hemoglobin (Hb) and becoming progressively less basophilic. Hb synthesis, directed by stable globin transcripts, continues until cell replication ceases.[12]

In the mouse, EryP are large nucleated primitive erythroid cells that express both embryonic and adult globins while confined to the yolk sac. In contrast, burst-forming unit erythroid (BFU-E), which later differentiate into colony-forming unit erythroid (CFU-E), are definitive erythroid progenitors (EryD) that give rise to colonies in 7 to 10 days and 2 to 3 days, respectively. EryD are found in the yolk sac; they enter the newly formed bloodstream of the embryo and seed the liver primordium as soon as it begins to form. Once there, EryD rapidly generate mature erythrocytes to support the growing fetus. Yolk sac–derived EryD (BFU-E and CFU-E) cannot fully differentiate

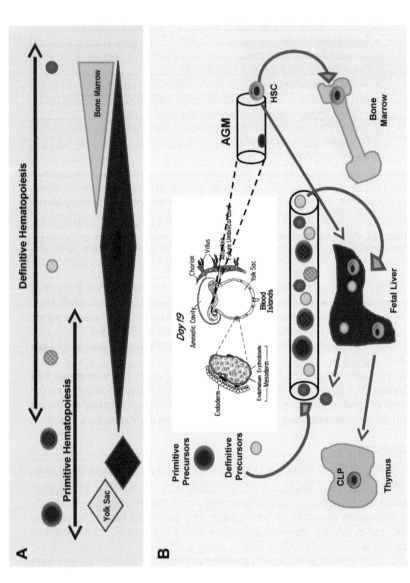

Fig. 2. (A) Sequential sites of hematopoiesis, showing the primitive and definitive waves of erythropoiesis as well as the hematopoietic stem cells arising from the AGM in (B). The first wave of blood production is termed *primitive* and occurs in the yolk sac. Large erythroid progenitors are produced to facilitate tissue oxygenation and allow the rapid growth of the embryo. The second hematopoietic wave called *definitive* also originates in the yolk sac. During this phase, definitive progenitors migrate to the fetal liver where they expand, mature and give origin to erythroid and meyloid cells. The third wave of hematopoiesis arises from *HSCs produced in AGM region*. These HSC seed the liver and the bone marrow. From the fetal liver, hematopoietic progenitors migrate and colonize the thymus, spleen, and ultimately the bone marrow. Crescendo/decrescendo figures illustrate the predominant sites of hematopoiesis during fetal life.

within the yolk-sac environment; they experience definitive differentiation as they exit to the fetal liver (see **Fig.** 2B). There are several features that distinguish primitive and definitive erythropoiesis: (1) EryP are 6-fold larger than EryD. (2) EryP express embryonic and adult globins. (3) EryD depend on erythropoietin (EPO) signaling for definitive EryD differentiation.[13,14]

In humans, the yolk sac serves as the initial site of erythropoiesis from weeks 3 to 6 of gestation. The liver functions as the primary site for hematopoiesis from weeks 6 to 22 of gestation, after which the bone marrow becomes the predominant and lifelong site of blood-cell production.

Fetal erythropoiesis is regulated by growth factors produced by the fetus not by the mother. The role of EPO during primitive erythropoiesis is controversial, but it facilitates differentiation of EryD. EPO is produced in the fetal liver during the first and second trimesters, principally by cells of monocytic and macrophage origin (**Table 2**). After birth, the anatomic site of EPO production shifts to the kidney. The specific stimulus for the shift is unknown but might involve the increase in arterial oxygen tension that occurs at birth. EPO mRNA and EPO protein can be found in fetal kidneys, but their relevance to fetal erythropoiesis is unclear because anephric fetuses have normal serum EPO concentrations and normal hematocrits.

EMBRYONIC AND FETAL HB

Hb is a tetrameric protein consisting of 4 iron-containing heme moieties and 4 protein (globin) chains. The erythroid cells of early human embryos contain Hb Gower-1, Hb Gower-2, and Hb Portland. The ζ chains of Hb Gower-1 and Hb Portland are structurally similar to α chains. Both Gower Hbs contain the β-like globin ϵ combined with either α or the α-like globin ζ (**Fig. 3**C). Gower Hbs predominate during weeks 4 to 8 of gestation, but they usually disappear by the end of the first trimester when fetal Hb (HbF) ($\alpha 2\gamma 2$) synthesis begins (see **Fig. 3**C). The major Hb from infancy through adult life is HbA, which consists of 2 α and 2 β chains and is represented symbolically as $\alpha 2\beta 2$. The genes for the globin chains reside in 2 clusters: an α-like family of genes (ζ and α) on chromosome 16 and a β-like family of genes (ϵ, γ, δ, β) on chromosome 11. The α-chain gene is duplicated, and both α genes ($\alpha 1$ and $\alpha 2$) on each chromosome 11 are active (see **Fig. 3**A). Throughout the embryonic and fetal life, globin chain production varies (see **Fig. 3**B). Certain embryonic Hbs are only expressed in yolk sac erythroblasts, whereas others predominate in the fetal liver and spleen; finally, HbA is expressed in the bone marrow. It is thought that embryonic and HbF facilitate the transplacental delivery of oxygen during intrauterine development because they both exhibit higher oxygen affinity than HbA. The role of HbF in the oxygen delivery system of the growing fetus has been extensively studied. The functional properties of embryonic Hbs, particularly Hb Gower-1, remain unclear. There are other significant differences between Hb Gower-1 and HbF beyond their increased oxygen affinity. The role of Hb Gower-1 in human development must likely entail other aspects of development beyond oxygen delivery; this is in need of further study.[15]

FETAL THROMBOPOIESIS

Platelet production occurs from 2 pools of cells: megakaryocyte progenitors and megakaryocytes. Megakaryocytes are present in the yolk sac of mouse embryos by E7.5 to 8.5.[16,17] The earliest primitive lineage-committed megakaryocyte progenitor is the BFU-megakaryocyte (BFU-MK).[18] This cell, in vitro, is capable of forming large multifocal colonies containing more than 50 megakaryocytes. It differentiates into the more mature progenitor, the CFU-megakaryocyte (CFU-MK), which is capable of generating in vitro

Table 2
Hematopoietic growth factors

Growth Factor	Action	Developmental Facts
EPO	Stimulates the production of red blood cells	• It is produced in fetal liver during the first and second trimesters, principally by cells of monocytes and macrophage origin. • After birth, the anatomic site of its production shifts to the kidney. • Its role in the fetus may not have biologic relevance for normal fetal erythropoiesis. • Fetal production is independent of maternal production.
TPO	Physiologic regulator of platelet production Acts as a stimulator of all stages of megakaryocyte growth and development Stimulates the proliferation and survival of other cell line progenitors	• As pluripotent cells become more committed to megakaryocyte differentiation, they become more dependent on its stimulation to lose their proliferative capacity and be able to differentiate and mature.
G-CSF	Promotes the differentiation of neutrophils	• It is present in the developing fetal bone as early as 6 wk after conception and in the fetal liver at least as early as 8 wk after conception. • It causes monocytes in the fetal liver to produce less G-CSF in response to IL-1 than monocytes in the marrow.
GM-CSF	Stimulates phagocytosis, chemotaxis, adhesion, and tumor lysis	• It is produced by endothelial cells, T lymphocytes, macrophages, endothelial cells, trophoblasts and decidua, and the epithelial lining of the bronchi, trachea, amnion; a large amount is produced in the fetal lungs.
M-CSF	Promotes the growth of monocytes and macrophages	• M-CSF is present in the human fetal liver and developing fetal bone as early as 6 wk after conception. • Mice that are deficient in M-CSF lack osteoclastic activity and consequently develop osteopetrosis.
SCF	Promotes the growth and differentiation of mast cells Plays a role in the early stages of lymphocyte development Plays a role in fetal development of gut-associated lymphoid tissue	• During embryogenesis, SCF and *c-kit* are expressed along the migratory pathways and destinations of primordial germ cells, melanocytes, hematopoietic cells, the gut, and the central nervous system. • Absence of either SCF in mice leads to intrauterine death or death shortly after birth from severe macrocytic anemia.

Abbreviations: G-CSF, granulocyte colony-stimulating factor; GM-CSF, granulocyte-macrophage colony-stimulating factor; M-CSF, macrophage colony-stimulating factor; SCF, stem cell factor; TPO, thrombopoietin.

Reproduced and modified from Rivers AE, Slayton W. Development of the immune system. In: de Alarcon PA, Werner EJ, Christensen RD, editors. Neonatal hematology: pathogenesis, diagnosis, and management of hematologic problems. 2nd edition. New York: Cambridge University Press; 2013; with permission.

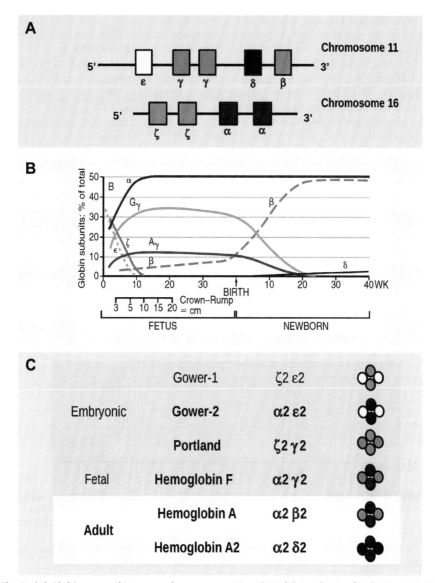

Fig. 3. (*A*) Globin gene Clusters on chromosome 16 and 11. (*B*) Synthesis of individual globin chains in prenatal and postnatal life. The different globin chains are produced independently depending on globin gene activation or suppression. (*C*) Globin chains combination to produce the different hemoglobins through embryonic, fetal and adult life.

mono-focal colonies containing 3 to 50 cells.[18–21] The bone marrow contains both CFU-MK and BFU-MK; peripheral blood has a relative increasing BFU-MK due mostly to a relative loss of circulating CFU-MK.[22,23] **Fig. 1** illustrates how the stem cell differentiates into multi-potential progenitor cells including megakaryocytic development.[24] As the cells commit to megakaryocyte differentiation, they become more dependent on thrombopoietin (TPO) stimulation and lose the proliferative capacity but become more able to differentiate and mature.[2,25] The megakaryocyte is a peculiar cell that, as it matures, undergoes nuclear duplication without undergoing cell division. This process is called *endoreduplication*. The cell becomes larger and increases the amount of DNA per cell or ploidy.[26–28] The process of platelet production is illustrated on **Fig. 4**.

Fully mature megakaryocytes develop elongated pseudopods known as *proplatelets*. The younger the megakaryocyte is, the thicker the pseudopod and the large the platelet. Thus, early platelet release from a megakaryocyte, as occurs during response to thrombocytopenia, leads to large platelet formation.[29]

The number of megakaryocyte progenitors circulating in the peripheral blood of neonates is higher than in children and adults.[22,23,27,30,31] They give rise to BFU-MK with a greater number of megakaryocytes and may be more sensitive to TPO stimulation when compared with those of children or adults.[23] The cell size of megakaryocytes in the fetus/newborn is smaller; megakaryocytes have lower ploidy, but their cytoplasm is that of a mature cell.[23,32,33] Neonates maintain normal platelet counts because of the increased proliferative potential of their megakaryocyte progenitors. Recent studies in murine models have begun to elucidate the molecular mechanisms responsible for these differences and, so far, have revealed a complex network of developmentally regulated pathways and transcription factors that simultaneously promote MK proliferation and maturation. Among those pathways are the insulinlike growth factor signaling and increased sensitivity to TPO that promotes proliferation and overexpression of GATA-1, contributing to increased cytoplasmic maturation.[34,35]

The receptors for TPO, c-Mpl, and CD4 are expressed on the surface of megakaryocyte progenitors, differentiated megakaryocytes, and platelets.[36] TPO is the physiologic regulator of platelet production and acts as a stimulator of all stages of megakaryocyte

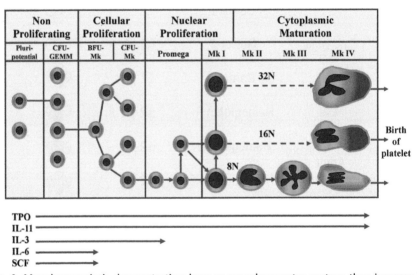

Fig. 4. Megakaryopoiesis demonstrating how as megakaryocytes mature they increase in size and lobulation and their content of DNA, or ploidy, increases. Megakaryocytes type I are small mononuclear cells with a lobulated nucleus and a deep blue cytoplasm; type II are larger cells with a lobulated nucleus but with a high nuclear to cytoplasm ratio; type III, a cell with abundant cytoplasm with a multilobulated nucleus, usually horse shoe shaped; type IV, a larger cell with abundant pink cytoplasm and a multi-lobulated nucleus in the periphery of the cytoplasm. (*Modified from* de Alarcon PA. Newborn platelet disorders. In: de Alarcon PA, Werner E, editors. Neonatal Hematology. 1st edition. New York: Cambridge University Press; 2005; with permission.)

growth and development. It is the primary, but not exclusive, regulator of platelet production and stimulates the proliferation and survival, not only of megakaryocytic progenitors but also of erythroid, myeloid, and multipotent progenitors. Recombinant TPO (rTPO) is able to support the growth of megakaryocytic colonies of neonates and children. Progenitors of preterm neonates are more sensitive to rTPO than are progenitors of term neonates (see **Table 2**).

FETAL MYELOPOIESIS

Multiple myeloid lineages originate and expand in the yolk sac. The first myeloid cells identified in the mouse embryo yolk sac are macrophages. Embryonic macrophages seem to directly differentiate from granulocyte/macrophage progenitors (GMP). In the liver, these macrophages are known as Kupffer cells; they line the sinusoidal spaces and initially account for approximately 70% of the HSC in the liver. Macrophages may be involved in remodeling the hepatic structure to make space for hematopoiesis, which will follow at 6 to 7 weeks after conception.[37]

Neutrophils are first observed in the human fetus about 5 weeks after conception as small clusters of cells around the aorta. The fetal bone marrow space begins to develop around the eighth week after conception; from weeks 8 to 10, the marrow space enlarges, but no neutrophils appear there until 10.5 weeks. From 14 weeks through term, the most common granulocytic cell type in the fetal bone marrow space is the neutrophil.

Granulocyte colony-stimulating factor (G-CSF) and macrophage CSF are expressed in developing fetal bone as early as 6 weeks after conception, and both are expressed in the fetal liver as early as 8 weeks (see **Table 2**).

Fetal blood contains few neutrophils until the third trimester. At 20 weeks of gestation, the blood neutrophil count is 0 to 500/mm^3. Although mature neutrophils are scarce, progenitor cells with the capacity to generate neutrophil clones are abundant in fetal blood. The fetal production of G-CSF is low; however, G-CSF receptors on the surface of neutrophils of newborn infants are equal in number and affinity to those on adult neutrophils.[38]

FETAL LYMPHOPOIESIS

Lymphoid cells normally mature during the second half of gestation within the fetal liver and thymus of the human embryo. The developmental origin of the lymphoid progenitors that seed these organs remains controversial. The fetal liver contains precursor cells that produce the full repertoire of immune cells. The current theory of fetal lymphopoiesis derives from murine models. MPP give rise to a common myeloid progenitor (CMP) and a common lymphoid progenitor (CLP) (see **Fig. 1**).

The CLP can generate all lymphoid cells, T-, B-, and natural killer (NK) cells. The CLP has an upregulated receptor for interleukin-7 that is critical for T- and B-cell survival.

The thymus appears approximately 8 weeks after conception at roughly the same time that hematopoiesis is established in the bone marrow. The function of the thymus is to support the differentiation of T lymphocytes. Progenitors of T cells originating in the fetal liver, and later from the bone marrow, migrate to the thymus beginning 8 to 9 weeks after conception.[39] Lymphocytes constitute 95% of the cells present in the thymus by week 10. Once in the thymus, T-cell lymphocytes mature and differentiate into antigen-responsive lymphocytes and acquire the ability to distinguish self from nonself proteins and to express T-cell receptors and other cell-surface proteins. The differentiation of T-cell lymphocytes in the thymus is a highly complex process.

B-cell precursors appear simultaneously in the omentum and fetal liver at 8 weeks after conception. Three weeks later, lymphocytes begin to appear in the spleen. By week 22, 70% of splenocytes are lymphocytes. Lymph nodes first appear around 11 weeks after conception, and lymphocytes appear within the lymph nodes approximately 1 week later.[40]

NK cells appear in the human fetal liver 5 weeks after conception. As early as 6 weeks, 5% to 8% of cells in the fetal liver are NK cells; by 18 weeks, these increase to 15% to 25% of cells. Approximately10% to 15% of cord blood lymphocytes are NK cells. Little is known about the function of NK during the developmental and neonatal period.

DISORDERS OF HEMATOPOIESIS THAT MANIFEST DURING INFANCY AND EARLY CHILDHOOD

Some of the more common, well-described disorders of hematopoiesis in newborns are summarized in **Table 3**. Several examples of bone marrow disorders that present in the newborn period, which illustrate how derangement of normal hematopoiesis can lead to disease, are presented. More extensive discussions of blood diseases of the newborn are covered in detail in other articles of this issue and in other references.[41]

Congenital amegakaryocytic thrombocytopenia (CAMT) is a rare disease, presenting with isolated thrombocytopenia during the first year of life, with development of pancytopenia in later childhood, suggesting a general defect in hematopoiesis. The bone marrow of patients with CAMT shows decreased to absent megakaryocytes with normal erythroid and myeloid precursors. Most affected infants have petechiae or other evidence of bleeding and physical anomalies. Highly elevated serum levels of TPO in patients with CAMT suggested a lack of response to the regulator of thrombopoiesis or an intrinsic stem cell defect rather than an abnormality of the bone marrow microenvironment. Ballmaier and colleagues[42] reported a lack of expression of the TPO receptor c-Mpl corresponding with the finding of point mutations and nonsense mutations in the c-Mpl gene that resulted in defective c-Mpl expression and loss of function of the TPO receptor, causing thrombocytopenia and progressive pancytopenia in patients with CAMT. Multiple investigators have confirmed that most patients with CAMT have mutations in c-Mpl.[43]

Kostmann syndrome (severe congenital neutropenia, autosomal recessive type 3 or SCN3) is a condition characterized by severe neutropenia with a bone marrow maturation block in myelopoiesis at the promyelocytic/myelocytic stage. Kostmann syndrome is predominantly inherited as autosomal recessive disorder. In the absence of treatment, affected children have recurrent fevers, skin infections, oral ulcers and gingivitis, and early life-threatening infections. Administration of recombinant human G-CSF normalizes neutrophil numbers, and most patients have an improved quality of life. Recently, Carlsson and colleagues[44] studied bone marrow progenitor cells of 4 surviving members of the original Kostmann family and one patient with severe congenital neutropenia of unknown inheritance. He and his associates showed that the defect in this disorder is not a defect in the production of hematopoiesis but rather a defect in premature cell death of the myeloid bone marrow precursors. He found excessive apoptosis in CD34 (early progenitor) as well as CD33 (myeloid progenitor) and CD15 (granulocyte precursor) subpopulations of bone marrow cells. Their data indicate that myeloid progenitors were particularly prone to apoptosis, in line with the arrest of myelopoiesis at the myelocytic/promyelocytic stage in these patients. Those patients had an unbalanced proportion of antiapoptotic and apoptotic molecules (Bcl-2/Bax ratio) that normalized after receiving treatment with G-CSF. It is thought that G-CSF protects mature neutrophils from spontaneous apoptosis. The clinical benefit of G-CSF in Kostmann syndrome resides in an increased absolute

Table 3
Disorders of hematopoiesis that present during infancy and early childhood

Erythrocytes	Platelets	Granulocytes	Lymphocytes
1. Failure of red cell production	1. Disorders of platelet production	1. Disorders of neutrophil production	1. Disorders of antibody production
Congenital	• Congenital amegakaryocytic thrombocytopenia	• Kostmann syndrome	• X-linked agammaglobulinemia
• Diamond-Blackfan anemia	• Amegakaryocytic thrombocytopenia with radioulnar synostosis	• Shwachman-Diamond syndrome	• Hyper-IgM syndrome
• Dyskeratosis congenita	• Thrombocytopenia absent radius syndrome	2. Antibody mediated	• Transient hypogammaglobulinemia of infancy
• Fanconi anemia	• X-linked thrombocytopenia with dyserythropoiesis	• Autoimmune neutropenia of infancy	2. Disorders of cellular function
• Aase syndrome	• May-Hegglin anomaly	• Alloimmune neonatal neutropenia	• Chromosome 22q11.2 deletion syndrome
• Pearson syndrome	• Sebastian syndrome	• Neonatal neutropenia owing to autoimmune disease in mother	• Wiskott-Aldrich syndrome
• Sideroblastic anemia	• Fechtner syndrome	• Chronic benign neutropenia	3. Severe combined immunodeficiency
• Congenital dyserythropoietic anemia	• Epstein syndrome		T⁻B⁻NK⁻
Acquired	2. Disorders of platelet function		• Adenosine deaminase deficiency
• Viral infection	• Wiskott-Aldrich syndrome		• Purine nucleotide phosphorylase deficiency
• Malaria	• Glanzmann thrombasthenia		T⁻B⁻NK⁺
• Anemia of prematurity	• Bernard-Soulier syndrome		• Ommen syndrome
2. Membrane defects	3. Disorders of platelet granules		T⁻B⁺NK⁻
• Hereditary spherocytosis	• Idiopathic dense-granule disorders (δ-storage pool disease)		• X-linked SCID
• Hereditary elliptocytosis	• Hermansky-Pudlak syndrome		T⁻B⁺NK⁺
• Hereditary stomatocytosis	• Chediak-Higashi syndrome		• Defect in IL-7 receptor α chain
• Hereditary xerocytosis	• Gray platelet syndrome		• CD4 deficiency
• Infantile pyknocytosis	• Paris-Trousseau/Jacobsen syndrome		• MHC class II deficiency
• Pyropoikilocytosis			• CD8 deficiency
3. Hb defects			• Zap-70 deficiency
• α-thalassemia syndromes			
• γβ-thalassemia			
• εγδβ-thalassemia			
• β-thalassemia			
• Unstable Hb			
4. Enzyme defects			
• Pyruvate kinase deficiency			
• G6PD deficiency			

Abbreviation: IgM, immunoglobulin M.

number of neutrophils owing to the protection against apoptosis of neutrophil precursors.[44] Several genes have now been shown to be associated with severe congenital neutropenia.[45]

Physiologic and pathologic alterations of HbF are common during infancy. In general, HbF levels decline during the first year of life. However, postnatal HbF levels may be influenced by various factors; for instance, in β-thalassemia trait (heterozygous), HbF decline is delayed, and about 50% of such patients have elevated HbF (>2%) later in life. In homozygous β-thalassemia major, large amounts of HbF are found. In patients with β-chain hemoglobinopathies, such as sickle cell hemoglobinopathy (HbSS) and sickle-C hemoglobinopathy (HbSC), HbF is usually increased. Moderate elevations of HbF can occur in many diseases accompanied by hematologic stress, such as hemolytic anemias, leukemia, and aplastic anemia. Tetramers of γ chains (γ4 or Hb Barts) or β chains (β4 or HbH) may be found in α-thalassemia syndromes. The normal adult level of HbA2 (2.0%–3.5%) is rarely altered. However, higher levels are found in patients with β-thalassemia trait and megaloblastic anemia. Low HbA2 levels are found in patients with iron-deficiency anemia and α-thalassemia.

Severe combined immunodeficiency (SCID) constitutes a heterogeneous group of genetic disorders characterized by profound defects in cellular and humoral immunity. Infants with SCID often have fatal opportunistic infections caused by bacteria, pneumocystis jiroveci pneumonia, cytomegalovirus, mycobacteria, or fungi. Patients may also have noninfectious clinical manifestations, such as graft-versus-host disease, caused by maternal lymphocyte engraftment, or nonirradiated blood product transfusion. Patients can be subclassified at the initial evaluation according to peripheral lymphocyte subsets: $T^-B^-NK^-$, $T^-B^-NK^+$, $T^-B^+NK^-$, and $T^-B^+NK^+$. Patients with SCID with adenosine deaminase deficiency accumulate toxic amounts of deoxyadenosine in progenitors of lymphocytes, which ultimately kills the precursors of T cells, B cells, and NK cells. Other genetic mutations responsible for the differentiation of embryologic mature T cells within the thymus are also responsible for various SCID phenotypes. For the interested reader, details of the ontogeny of mature T lymphocyte and the genetic mutations responsible for SCID and the clinical presentation for SCID are available in the recently published reviews by Lee and colleagues[46] and Fischer.[47]

SUMMARY

The sequential sites of hematopoiesis include the yolk sac, the AGM, the fetal liver, and, finally, the bone marrow. Formation of the hematopoietic tissues begins with pluripotent stem cells capable of both self-renewal and clonal maturation into blood cell lineages. Once HSCs seed the fetal liver and the bone marrow, they evolve into MPP that soon differentiate into a colony-forming unit of each particular hematopoietic lineage to ultimately produce mature erythrocytes, granulocytes, and platelets. HSCs require a combination of transcription factors (intrinsic determinants of cellular phenotype) for the survival and proliferation of HSCs. In addition, adjacent cells and local cytokines, such as growth factors (microenvironment), are also necessary for optimal HSC growth and differentiation. Within the context of hematopoietic development, the authors outline the pathophysiology of some illustrative bone marrow disorders, immunodeficiencies, and alterations of hemoglobin.

REFERENCES

1. Wintrobe WW. A story of discovery, of people, and of ideas. New York: McGraw-Hill Book, co; 1980.

2. Metcalf D. Stem cells, pre-progenitor cells and lineage-committed cells: are our dogmas correct? Ann N Y Acad Sci 1999;872:289–303 [discussion: 303–4].

3. Nakahata T, Tsuji K, Ishiguro A, et al. Single-cell origin of human mixed hemopoietic colonies expressing various combinations of cell lineages. Blood 1985;65(4): 1010–6.

4. Suda T, Suda J, Ogawa M. Single-cell origin of mouse hemopoietic colonies expressing multiple lineages in variable combinations. Proc Natl Acad Sci U S A 1983;80(21):6689–93.

5. Morrison SJ, Uchida N, Weissman IL. The biology of hematopoietic stem cells. Annu Rev Cell Dev Biol 1995;11:35–71.

6. McCulloch EA. Stem cells in normal and leukemic hemopoiesis (Henry Stratton lecture, 1982). Blood 1983;62(1):1–13.

7. Ogawa M. Differentiation and proliferation of hematopoietic stem cells. Blood 1993;81(11):2844–53.

8. Orkin SH, Zon LI. Hematopoiesis: an evolving paradigm for stem cell biology. Cell 2008;132(4):631–44.

9. Zhu J, Emerson SG. Hematopoietic cytokines, transcription factors and lineage commitment. Oncogene 2002;21(21):3295–313.

10. Ciriza J, Thompson H, Petrosian R, et al. The migration of hematopoietic progenitors from the fetal liver to the fetal bone marrow: lessons learned and possible clinical applications. Exp Hematol 2013;41(5):411–23.

11. Godin I, Cumano A. Of birds and mice: hematopoietic stem cell development. Int J Dev Biol 2005;49(2–3):251–7.

12. Fantoni A, De la Chapelle A, Rifkind RA, et al. Erythroid cell-development in fetal mice: synthetic capacity for different proteins. J Mol Biol 1968;33(1):79–91.

13. Baron MH. Concise review: early embryonic erythropoiesis: not so primitive after all. Stem Cells 2013;31(5):849–56.

14. Baron MH, Isern J, Fraser ST. The embryonic origins of erythropoiesis in mammals. Blood 2012;119(21):4828–37.

15. He Z, Russell JE. Expression, purification, and characterization of human hemoglobins Gower-1 (zeta(2)epsilon(2)), Gower-2 (alpha(2)epsilon(2)), and Portland-2 (zeta(2)beta(2)) assembled in complex transgenic-knockout mice. Blood 2001; 97(4):1099–105.

16. Xie X, Chan RJ, Johnson SA, et al. Thrombopoietin promotes mixed lineage and megakaryocytic colony-forming cell growth but inhibits primitive and definitive erythropoiesis in cells isolated from early murine yolk sacs. Blood 2003;101(4): 1329–35.

17. Xu MJ, Matsuoka S, Yang FC, et al. Evidence for the presence of murine primitive megakaryocytopoiesis in the early yolk sac. Blood 2001;97(7):2016–22.

18. Briddell RA, Brandt JE, Straneva JE, et al. Characterization of the human burst-forming unit-megakaryocyte. Blood 1989;74(1):145–51.

19. Mazur EM, Hoffman R, Chasis J, et al. Immunofluorescent identification of human megakaryocyte colonies using an antiplatelet glycoprotein antiserum. Blood 1981;57(2):277–86.

20. Mouthon MA, Freund M, Titeux M, et al. Growth and differentiation of the human megakaryoblastic cell line (ELF-153): a model for early stages of megakaryocytopoiesis. Blood 1994;84(4):1085–97.

21. Vainchenker W, Kieffer N. Human megakaryocytopoiesis: in vitro regulation and characterization of megakaryocytic precursor cells by differentiation markers. Blood Rev 1988;2(2):102–7.

22. Drygalski A, Xu G, Constantinescu D, et al. The frequency and proliferative potential of megakaryocytic colony-forming cells (Meg-CFC) in cord blood, cytokine-mobilized peripheral blood and bone marrow, and their correlation with total CFC numbers: implications for the quantitation of Meg-CFC to predict platelet engraftment following cord blood transplantation. Bone Marrow Transplant 2000;25(10):1029–34.
23. Hoffman R, Murrav LJ, Young JC, et al. Hierarchical structure of human megakaryocyte progenitor cells. Stem Cells 1996;14(Suppl 1):75–81.
24. Debili N, Coulombel L, Croisille L, et al. Characterization of a bipotent erythro-megakaryocytic progenitor in human bone marrow. Blood 1996;88(4):1284–96.
25. Arriaga M, South K, Cohen JL, et al. Interrelationship between mitosis and endomitosis in cultures of human megakaryocyte progenitor cells. Blood 1987;69(2):486–92.
26. Ebbe S, Yee T, Carpenter D, et al. Megakaryocytes increase in size within ploidy groups in response to the stimulus of thrombocytopenia. Exp Hematol 1988;16(1):55–61.
27. Kobayashi Y, Kondo M. Human megakaryocyte ploidy. Histol Histopathol 1999;14(4):1223–9.
28. Zimmet J, Ravid K. Polyploidy: occurrence in nature, mechanisms, and significance for the megakaryocyte-platelet system. Exp Hematol 2000;28(1):3–16.
29. Choi ES, Nichol JL, Hokom MM, et al. Platelets generated in vitro from proplatelet-displaying human megakaryocytes are functional. Blood 1995;85(2):402–13.
30. Campagnoli C, Fisk N, Overton T, et al. Circulating hematopoietic progenitor cells in first trimester fetal blood. Blood 2000;95(6):1967–72.
31. Wyrsch A, dalle Carbonare V, Jansen W, et al. Umbilical cord blood from preterm human fetuses is rich in committed and primitive hematopoietic progenitors with high proliferative and self-renewal capacity. Exp Hematol 1999;27(8):1338–45.
32. Olson TA, Levine RF, Mazur EM, et al. Megakaryocytes and megakaryocyte progenitors in human cord blood. Am J Pediatr Hematol Oncol 1992;14(3):241–7.
33. Mattia G, Vulcano F, Milazzo L, et al. Different ploidy levels of megakaryocytes generated from peripheral or cord blood CD34+ cells are correlated with different levels of platelet release. Blood 2002;99(3):888–97.
34. Sola-Visner M. Platelets in the neonatal period: developmental differences in platelet production, function, and hemostasis and the potential impact of therapies. Hematology Am Soc Hematol Educ Program 2012;2012:506–11.
35. Liu ZJ, Sola-Visner M. Neonatal and adult megakaryopoiesis. Curr Opin Hematol 2011;18(5):330–7.
36. Debili N, Wendling F, Cosman D, et al. The Mpl receptor is expressed in the megakaryocytic lineage from late progenitors to platelets. Blood 1995;85(2):391–401.
37. Kelemen E, Janossa M. Macrophages are the first differentiated blood cells formed in human embryonic liver. Exp Hematol 1980;8(8):996–1000.
38. Palis J, Yoder MC. Yolk-sac hematopoiesis: the first blood cells of mouse and man. Exp Hematol 2001;29(8):927–36.
39. Haynes BF, Denning SM, Singer KH, et al. Ontogeny of T-cell precursors: a model for the initial stages of human T-cell development. Immunol Today 1989;10(3):87–91.
40. Kelemen E, Carlo W, Fliedner TM. Atlas of human hemopoietic development. New York: Springer-Verlag; 1979.

41. de Alarcon P, Werner EJ, Christensen RD. Neonatal hematology: pathogenesis, diagnosis, and management of hematologic problems. 2nd edition. New York: Cambridge University Press; 2013.
42. Ballmaier M, Germeshausen M, Schulze H, et al. c-mpl mutations are the cause of congenital amegakaryocytic thrombocytopenia. Blood 2001;97(1):139–46.
43. Geddis AE. Congenital amegakaryocytic thrombocytopenia. Pediatr Blood Cancer 2011;57(2):199–203.
44. Carlsson G, Aprikyan AA, Tehranchi R, et al. Kostmann syndrome: severe congenital neutropenia associated with defective expression of Bcl-2, constitutive mitochondrial release of cytochrome c, and excessive apoptosis of myeloid progenitor cells. Blood 2004;103(9):3355–61.
45. Klein C. Molecular basis of congenital neutropenia. Haematologica 2009;94(10): 1333–6.
46. Lee PP, Chan KW, Chen TX, et al. Molecular diagnosis of severe combined immunodeficiency-identification of IL2RG, JAK3, IL7R, DCLRE1C, RAG1, and RAG2 mutations in a cohort of Chinese and Southeast Asian Children. J Clin Immunol 2011;31(2):281–96.
47. Fischer A. Have we seen the last variant of severe combined immunodeficiency? N Engl J Med 2003;349(19):1789–92.

The Inherited Bone Marrow Failure Syndromes

S. Deborah Chirnomas, MD, MPH, Gary M. Kupfer, MD*

KEYWORDS

- Ribosomopathies • Fanconi anemia • Diamond-Blackfan anemia
- Dyseratosis congenita • Shwachman-Diamond • Bone marrow failure • DNA repair
- Cancer susceptibility

KEY POINTS

- Despite the rarity of inherited bone marrow failure syndromes (IBMFS), they represent diseases for which the molecular pathogenesis may be elucidated.
- The study and presentation of the details of their molecular biology and biochemistry are warranted not only for appropriate diagnosis and management of afflicted patients but also because they lend clues to the normal physiology of the normal hematopoiesis and, in many cases, mechanisms of carcinogenesis.
- Several themes have emerged within each subsection of IBMFS, including the ribosomopathies, which include both ribosome assembly as well as ribosomal RNA processing.
- The Fanconi anemia pathway itself has become interdigitated with the familial breast cancer syndromes.

Despite the rarity of inherited bone marrow failure syndromes (IBMFS), careful studies of the molecular pathogenesis of these disorders has led to a deeper understanding of normal and aberrant bone marrow function. Understanding the molecular biology and biochemistry of IBMFS helps in the appropriate diagnosis and management of afflicted patients and also lends clues to the physiology of normal hematopoiesis and, in many cases, elucidates mechanisms of carcinogenesis. Several themes have emerged within each subsection of IBMFS, including the ribosomopathies, which include both ribosome assembly as well as ribosomal RNA processing. The Fanconi anemia (FA) pathway itself has become interdigitated with the familial breast cancer syndromes. This article analyses the diseases that account for most IBMFS diagnoses.

Section of Pediatric Hematology-Oncology, LMP 2073, Yale School of Medicine, 333 Cedar Street, New Haven, CT 06520, USA
* Corresponding author.
E-mail address: Gary.Kupfer@yale.edu

Pediatr Clin N Am 60 (2013) 1291–1310
http://dx.doi.org/10.1016/j.pcl.2013.09.007
0031-3955/13/$ – see front matter © 2013 Elsevier Inc. All rights reserved.

THE RIBOSOMOPATHIES

In recent years, the subset of patients affected with Diamond-Blackfan anemia (DBA), Shwachman-Diamond-Bodian syndrome (SDBS), dyskeratosis congenita (DC), and cartilage hair hypoplasia (CHH) have all been shown to have mutations in ribosomal proteins and in proteins responsible for processing of ribosomal RNA.[1] The reports of amelioration of a DBA-like phenotype in the p53-deficient mouse and zebrafish imply that defects in the ribosome assembly pathway and imbalances in protein synthesis lead to cell stress that can activate the p53 pathway and cause subsequent apoptosis, resulting in a depletion of sensitive cell populations, such as the hematopoietic stem cell pool.[2,3] Even although the biology of these syndromes does not completely overlap (ie, DC involves biology directly at the telomere), several investigators have organized these diseases into a linear or cooperative pathway, in which ribosomal RNA is assembled in a multistep process.[4]

DBA

The most common disease of isolated inherited red cell production failure is DBA, with an incidence of approximately 5 to 7 cases per million live births in North America. Presentation of the disease can be at any age, but most patients are diagnosed in the first year of life, with at least 10% in 1 series presenting at birth and 25% within the first month of life.[5–9]

DBA is a genetic disease with evidence of mixed inheritance, although most cases are sporadic. Many inherited cases are autosomal dominant, with equal sex frequency. This group of patients seem to have fewer physical anomalies. Some cases are autosomal recessive, with disproportionately more males than females, implying an X-linked form of the disease.[10–12] Approximately 50% of patients with DBA have physical abnormalities, including dysmorphic facies, short stature, eye, kidney, and hand abnormalities.[13–15] Patients first present typically with macrocytic anemia and reticulocytopenia and associated pallor, often in the setting of failure to thrive. In the neonatal period, diagnosis can be uncertain, because the normal newborn proceeds through the physiologic nadir of erythropoiesis over the first 4 to 8 weeks and the normal newborn red blood cells are macrocytic at birth. Thus, most commonly, patients present between 2 and 4 months of age. The confirming finding is reticulocytopenia and decreased erythroid activity in the bone marrow.[16,17]

In addition, some patients present with neutropenia, thrombocytosis, or thrombocytopenia, even although DBA is thought of as a pure red cell aplasia.[18] Other nonspecific abnormalities include increases of fetal hemoglobin, red cell antigen, iron, folate, and vitamin B_{12} levels.[16,17] An increased erythrocyte adenosine deaminase level has been proposed as a good diagnostic test for DBA, with a sensitivity of 84% and specificity of 95%. However, 16% of affected people have a normal erythrocyte adenosine deaminase level.[19]

The 2 most common therapeutic options are corticosteroids or transfusion therapy for patients who are symptomatic from their anemia. Corticosteroids may be initiated with anemia that causes cardiovascular and developmental compromise. Prednisone is usually the first-line agent, at a dose of 2 mg/kg/d. If the child has a response to steroids, the goal is to reach a hemoglobin level of 10 g/dL and sustained reticulocytosis, after which the steroids can be slowly tapered off. Slightly more than half of patients with DBA are steroid responders; within this group, many can be weaned to a very low dose or off prednisone completely.[15,20,21] Corticosteroids may become problematic with chronic use, leading to growth retardation, weight gain, gastritis, and decreased bone mineralization. Those who are positive responders show a distinctive gene expression signature that may characterize the underlying difference in response as host related.

For patients who do not respond to steroids or cannot tolerate them, transfusion therapy is an effective option. As is the case with chronic transfusion therapy for any disease, iron overload becomes the chief difficulty, resulting in cardiac, endocrine, and pulmonary disease. Chronic iron chelation using subcutaneous desferoxamine has been poorly tolerated and adherence limited. Since 2006, deferasirox, a daily oral chelator, has been available for treatment of iron overload, and more recently, deferiprone, an oral agent given 3 times a day, was approved by the US Food and Drug Administration for use in this setting.[22]

Any discussion of transfusion and iron overload must be balanced against the role of bone marrow transplantation (BMT) as a curative modality, with its associated side effects. The side effects of BMT include graft-versus-host disease (GVHD), infections, and chemotherapeutic toxicity involved with conditioning. With matched sibling donors, the risk of GVHD has become markedly lower, with long-term survival of more than 80%. The optimal timing of BMT in DBA is not known. The younger patient is more likely to show less GVHD and better long-term survival but have more late effects, leading some to argue for waiting for additional time to allow for late remissions.[23,24]

Growth factors have also been used in DBA. Erythropoietin has been the logical choice, without any evidence of efficacy.[25] Interleukin 3 has shown some modest benefit amongst transfusion-dependent patients, along with side effects of deep venous thromboses and constitutional symptoms.[26,27] In recent years, additional agents have been shown to be at least anecdotally beneficial, including leucine and metaclopropamide.

Patients with DBA have a reduced life expectancy from causes largely related to treatment side effects and long-term risks of malignancy. In addition, hematologic malignancy is a major cause of death because patients with DBA have a risk of acute myelogenous leukemia (AML) with a lifelong risk of up to 25%.[28] Anecdotally, acute lymphoblastic leukemia (ALL), Hodgkin disease, and myelodysplastic syndrome (MDS) have all been reported in DBA.[29–32] Reports of osteogenic sarcoma and hepatocellular carcinoma, which are likely associated with concomitant viral hepatitis infection, have also been published.[33,34] An overall risk of 5.4 odds ratio for developing cancer in DBA has been calculated, with predominance in MDS, AML, colon cancer, osteogenic sarcoma, and genital cancer.

Often mentioned in the differential diagnosis of DBA are transient erythrocytopenia of childhood (TEC) and infection with parvovirus. TEC and parvovirus-induced aplasia should resolve within a month, and both are unusual in the newborn period.

The science of DBA has exploded in the last decade. The first gene identified as mutated in DBA, ribosomal protein RPS19, was cloned positionally by analyzing a patient with DBA who had a translocation interrupting the RPS19 locus. Twenty-five percent of patients with DBA have RPS19 mutations in the heterozygous state, which implies that the allele acts in a dominant negative fashion or that a dosage effect exists and that the presence of 2 mutated alleles may be lethal.[35,36] As many as 8 additional mutations in ribosomal genes have been identified, both in the large as well as the small subunit of the ribosome (RPL5, RPL11, RPL15, RPL35, RPS7, RPS10, RPS17, RPS24, RPS26), leaving almost 50% of DBA cases having no identified mutation.[37] A recent report[38] detailed the first nonribosomal mutation found in a patient with DBA, showing a GATA splice site mutation.

The cloning of these genes alone does not answer the basic question of why DBA occurs. In general, reduced colony-forming activity in patients with DBA has been observed, but this has not proved to be a reliable predictor of DBA.[39–42] Progenitors have been marked by accelerated apoptosis.[43] Defects in the microenvironment of the marrow have also been proposed as contributors to pathogenesis because of inhibition of erythropoiesis by bone fragments from a patient with DBA. Other affected functions include growth factors, their receptors, and transcription factors.[44]

A mouse with an RPS19 knockout showing the DBA phenotype has been created and is being studied. As noted earlier, increased understanding of DBA came through amelioration of its phenotype in a p53 knockout background in both the mouse and the zebrafish, leading to a lower rate of apoptosis and suggesting that the imbalance of ribosome synthesis or inefficiency of protein translation leads to cell stress. In addition, RPS26 has been shown through an RPL11-mediated pathway to stabilize p53 via interaction in an inhibitory fashion with MDM2, which is the E3 ubiquitin ligase for p53, thus leading to the stabilization of p53.[45]

An interesting overlap with adult MDS has been characterized in the identification of the cause of the 5q- syndrome, which arises as a result of deletion of the RPS14 gene. This acquired defect leads to a lower-risk MDS, which has been treated with lenalidomide.[46,47]

DC

DC is a genetically heterogeneous disorder related to defects in telomere maintenance. The classic X-linked recessive form in particular seems to be associated with the classic DC findings of hyperpigmented reticular lacy pigmented skin, dystrophic nails, and leukoplakia. Up to 90% of patients develop bone marrow failure, although the time to recognition of classic findings is variable. The inheritance pattern can also be autosomal dominant or autosomal recessive. Two particularly severe variants are Hoyeraal-Hreidarsson (HH), presenting as systemic DC with cerebellar hypoplasia and developmental dysfunction, and Revesz syndrome, similar to HH coupled with exudative retinopathy. Reported cases have included probands with intrauterine growth retardation and microcephaly. In addition, these patients have a predisposition to myelodysplasia, myeloid leukemia, and an assortment of solid tumors, including squamous cell cancers of the head, neck, and anogenital region.[20,48–50] As in numerous genetic cancer predisposition syndromes, sporadic mutations have been found in DC genes in cancers, suggesting the importance of the telomere broadly in cancer outside DC.

On a cellular level, DC cells are characterized by progressive telomere shortening that accumulates in an age-dependent fashion, thus leading to variability in the phenotype. The age of presentation has been reported to be as high as 75 years. When a patient with bone marrow failure does present, given the clinical heterogeneity of many of these disorders in question, telomere analysis should be a part of the workup for all bone marrow failure. Although some variability exists in telomere length analysis, overall, it is a sensitive test for DC, and combination analysis with flow cytometry to measure telomeres in multiple cell subsets can enhance its usefulness.[51]

The first identified gene, DKC, is X linked (and the most common form of DC), encoding the dyskerin protein that resides in ribonucleoprotein (RNP) complexes at the telomere as well as in ribosomal RNA. This finding implies a duality in mechanism of the proteins involved in DC. Dyskerin binds to the RNA that serves as the template for the TTAGGG repeats found at telomeres. Other members of the telomerase RNP found to be causative when mutant in DC include NOP10, NHP2, TCAB1, TERC, and TERT (telomerase reverse transcriptase), all of which are autosomal-recessive inheritance.[51–53] Dyskerin also seems to be involved in the pseudouridylation of ribosomal RNA (rRNA), but the specific function in the ribosome of this modification is unclear.[54]

The other genes responsible for DC reside in the shelterin complex, which protects telomeres from degradation. Shelterin is a 6-member protein complex, which includes the DC causative gene TIN2. The function of the shelterin complex is to protect telomeres from exonuclease activity, thus enabling the integrity of telomere length.[52]

The classic presentation of DC includes 2 of the 3 following findings: dystrophic nails, a reticular lacy rash, leukoplakia. Other features recognized to be part of the DC spectrum include premature graying hair, pulmonary fibrosis, liver disease, leukemia or MDS, esophageal stenosis, urethral stenosis, short stature, and developmental delay. Recently described is the high prevalence of neuropsychiatric disorders in this population, which have previously been reported as 25% in children but in a recent small prospective study performed by the National Cancer Institute, the lifetime risk for children with DC was 83% for disorders including attention-deficit/hyperactivity disorder, pervasive developmental disorder, anxiety, and mood disorders.[55]

The diagnosis of DC can be difficult, with still close to 50% of patients lacking a known mutation in the DC pathway. The measurement of telomere lengths in lymphocyte subsets has become an important element that supports a diagnosis of DC. Patients with DC have very short telomeres, well below the normal range, in contrast to patients with other IBMFS, who often have short telomeres compared with the general population but that are not significantly shorter than the first percentile. Clinicians must use a combination of physical examination findings, family history, and features of leukemia or bone marrow failure or very short telomere lengths. Often, the family history can be particularly useful in anticipating new patients, who may have worse disease than their forebears, perhaps because the telomere inheritance becomes shorter with each generation.

Management of DC generally centers around treating the symptoms of marrow failure. Because the treatment options have significant morbidity, a watch-and-wait approach is often used. When cytopenias cause symptoms, androgens can be used to good effect, despite masculinizing side effects and the need for careful monitoring for liver tumors later in life. The use of growth factors has achieved some temporary improvement in counts and related symptoms, but worry of malignant transformation in the resultant stressed marrow remains a concern.[56,57]

If those therapies do not help, BMT can be considered. Outcomes for BMT have been poor based both on patients' sensitivities to conditioning regimens as well as the underlying disease. Patients with DC are unique in having very late pulmonary and liver complications, likely caused by their underlying disease, which may be worsened or accelerated by the transplant process. Recent data from 2013 looking at 34 patients treated from 1981 to 2009 reported a 10-year survival probability of 30%. Unrelated donors or mismatched related donors and regimen intensity were independent risk factors for early mortality.[58–60]

Shwachman-Diamond Syndrome

Shwachman-Diamond syndrome (SDS) is a syndrome of neutropenia, pancreatic exocrine function insufficiency, and metaphyseal dysostosis. Anemia and thrombocytopenia can accompany the neutropenia. Patients with SDS can also have a wide array of physical findings, including short stature, failure to thrive, skin rashes and macules, teeth and palatal defects, and syndactyly.[7,61,62]

The putative gene that when mutated leads to SDS is the SBDS gene, encoding a 250 amino acid protein with predicted functions in RNA metabolism. Its widespread expression may be the basis of the multiple organ involvement of SDS.[63] A recent model[64] using induced pluripotent stem cells as a model for SDS manifests exocrine and hematopoietic cell dysfunction, which phenocopies SDS. A recent study[65] has reported the defective processing of rRNA into ribosome assembly, suggesting that SDS is closely associated with the molecular pathogenesis of DBA. Most patients with SDS do not show a mutation in the SBDS gene, suggesting additional genes underlying the pathogenesis of SDS.

The diagnosis of SDS can be difficult, because many patients do not have an identifiable mutation in the SBDS gene. Clues can be found by examining trypsinogen, isoamylase, and obtaining an ultrasound scan of the pancreas. Family history may provide a clue but is less useful than in DC.

No definitive therapy exists for SDS neutropenia, except for BMT, whereas pancreatic insufficiency is managed by administration of exogenous pancreatic enzymes. Supportive care is indicated, with transfusions in the 20% of patients with SDS who develop pancytopenia. Some efficacy has been reported with the use of granulocyte-stimulating growth factors (G-CSF), with 6 of 7 responding to G-CSF in 1 series. Like other IBMFS, the diagnosis of SDS confers a 5% risk of leukemia, including ALL, chronic myelogenous leukemia, and AML, making the use of growth factors a difficult decision for fear of stimulating a clonal expansion, despite minimal data to support this concern.[66–68]

CHH

CHH is a recessive disease with a constellation of skeletal abnormalities consisting of short stature, lordosis, scoliosis, and chest wall deformities. The disorder was first described amongst the Old Order Amish. Sparse, fine hair is the other consistent feature.[69,70] Growth failure occurs prenatally with shortness of limbs or stature noted on fetal ultrasonography or perinatally. Patients with CHH also have increased risk of Hirschsprung disease.[71] Mutations in the RNA component of RNA mannose-6-phosphatereceptor endoribonuclease involved in mitochondrial and nucleolar RNA processing have been reported to be responsible for CHH.[72] Together with TERT, RMRP forms a complex that produces double-strand RNA, which participates in small interfering RNAs.[73] RMRP works in parallel with DBA defects, upstream of Shwachman-Diamond, and downstream of DC, in the processing of the 80S unit of the ribosome.[74]

Anemia and macrocytosis occur in the variable context of pancytopenia.[75] Lymphopenia is reported, along with defective cellular immunity.[76] Corticosteroids and transfusion have been used temporarily with some patients outgrowing marrow failure.[77] However, increased malignancy risk was also reported throughout infancy, childhood, and adulthood.[69,78] T-cell lymphoproliferative disease has been seen as a consequence of immunodeficiency.[79]

FA/BRCA PATHWAY

FA is an autosomal and X-linked recessive disorder characterized by bone marrow failure, AML, solid tumors, and developmental abnormalities. At the molecular level, cells derived from patients with FA show hypersensitivity to DNA cross-linking agents, resulting in increased numbers of chromosomal abnormalities, including translocations and radial chromosomes. This hypersensitivity has made successful treatment of patients with FA a challenge in the past because traditional treatments of symptoms resulted in more harm than good. In recent years, care of the patient with FA has improved with modern blood banking, antibiotics, and hematopoietic stem cell transplantation (SCT), which has been used in patients with FA for almost 30 years.[80]

Despite greater survival of children into adulthood as a result of SCT, the specter of the potential for solid tumors, such as squamous cell carcinomas (SCC) of the head, neck, and genitourinary track, remains a serious problem.[81,82]

Even although the classic features of thumb abnormalities and radius absence generally characterize these patients, children with FA typically present in the first decade of life on recognition of aplastic anemia.[83–85] A sizable subset of patients with FA have no discernible abnormalities at all. As a result, the index of suspicion of the clinician must be high to recognize the diagnosis of FA in the differential diagnosis of aplastic anemia.

The gold standard tests for FA quantify chromosomal breakage in cells exposed to cross-linking agents to which FA cells are hypersensitive, typically diepoxybutane (DEB).[80,85] On occasion, despite the strong suspicion of FA being present in a patient, the chromosome fragility test can be negative because of somatic reversion.[86,87] In the face of this possibility, if a negative DEB or mitomycin C result has been obtained in the setting of strong suspicion of an FA diagnosis, then a skin biopsy should be obtained for culture and subsequent DEB testing.

Ninety percent of patients with FA first present with bone marrow failure, but a percentage nonetheless first present with AML. These cases of AML are typically M1 to M4 FAB subtype and display no characteristic cytogenetic or molecular abnormality, although numerous translocations, deletions, and other aneuploidogenic changes can be found.[88] Some report distinctly different clones in FA-associated AML versus sporadic AML.[89] Patients treated in a fashion similar to other patients with AML experience intolerance to standard doses of alkylating agents. Thus, morbidity precludes an aggressive approach. In addition, analysis of cells derived from these AML cases suggests that some are paradoxically resistant, perhaps a result of the underlying genomic instability of FA cells that could allow acquisition of resistance.[90]

Patients with FA are at markedly increased risk of SCC of the head and neck and genitourinary tract. These tumors have been only sporadically positive for human papilloma virus (HPV), although vaccination for HPV is strongly encouraged in the population with FA. In addition, routine laryngoscopy and ear, nose, and throat follow-up is considered standard of care for patients with FA.[81,82,91] Breast cancer is also typical of adult patients with FA, which is in line with the fact that 5 FA genes are familial breast cancer genes: BRCA2, PALB2, RAD51C, SLX4, and BACH1.[92–96]

FA genes have also been implicated in sporadic cancers by virtue of detection of non–germ-line mutations in tumors such as lung, pancreatic, ovarian, and breast. It has been proposed that such tumors can be targeted by using agents specifically inducing hypersensitivity in FA-mutant cells.[97]

Because the patient with FA is at increased risk of toxicity from SCT regimens, clinicians must time the procedure before the onset of leukemia, avoiding the long-term effects of blood product provision or unaffected by serious infections from invasive organisms like *Aspergillus*. The complementation group and gene mutation should be identified in order to assess the suitability of a family member stem cell donor, averting the possibility that a matched donor has a subclinical case of FA. It has become clear from the experience of FA clinicians that patients with FA-D1 and those with the Ashkenazi FANCC mutation are at significant and early risk of progression to AML, often before the presentation of aplastic anemia.[98] In general terms, it is believed that such a risk of early AML progression is coincident with a more severe FA phenotype.[99–101]

Historically, the challenges of SCT in patients with FA have been numerous. The issue of graft failure has a prevalence of 10%, but use of fludarabine has reduced this risk to less than 1%. As a result, efforts at reduction of conditioning have been steady and the use of total body irradiation has been diminished down to doses of 400 to 600 cGy. In addition, the use of cyclophosphamide has also been decreased in recent years. With an allogenic-related transplant, the long-term survival is often greater than 80%.[101,102]

Matched-unrelated transplants have posed a greater challenge, with a greater incidence of GVHD. Toxicity-associated GVHD occurs with greater intensity in the patient with FA, perhaps because of the greater degree of toxicity caused by conditioning. Such toxicity is synergistic with the increased GVHD risk. With diminished toxicity has come greater GVHD control and subsequent increased survival for patients with FA undergoing matched-unrelated transplants.[101,103]

Secondary effects of SCT have important consequences for patients with FA presumably because of their underlying issues of growth delay, endocrine dysfunction, and increased risk of malignancy, all of which are associated with long-term consequences of undergoing SCT. A markedly increased risk of acquisition of SCC is seen after transplantation beyond that observed in untransplanted patients with FA; these SCC are only weakly linked to human papillomavirus.[82] GVHD greatly increases the risk of SCC in patients with FA and patients undergoing unrelated stem cell transplant.

The idea that FA cells are hypersensitive to endogenous and exogenous stimuli suggests that FA stem cells in the bone marrow are susceptible to a sort of natural selection. Probably for this reason, somatic reversion is observed in some patients with FA. As a result, it has been postulated that gene therapy is an ideal approach to treatment of FA. Clinical trials targeting the most common complementation group, FA-A, have been instituted using a lentiviral transduction system of hematopoietic stem cells from patients with FA, manipulated ex vivo. In vitro data suggest that hematopoietic stem cells can be transduced with subsequent colony-forming assays, suggesting increased growth and reconstitution. However, such trails have been disappointing, because lack of permanent transduction of progenitors has led to failure to establish long-term hematopoiesis.[104,105]

Traditionally, androgens have proved to be an efficacious treatment in some patients with bone marrow failure, patients with FA included. Androgens can stimulate more effective hematopoiesis, resulting in an increase in peripheral blood counts. The use of androgens has been marked by their limitations in females, given the masculinizing side effects. In addition, their use has been associated with increased risk of liver adenomas.[106,107]

The FA pathway is composed of at least 16 genes.[108] Each of these genes, when biallelically mutated, causes FA, except for the X-linked FANCB. The encoded proteins (**Table 1**) can be subdivided within the FA pathway into 3 groups: (1) proteins that make up the core complex; (2) the FANCD2 and FANCI proteins, which compose the ID complex; and (3) 5 downstream effector proteins, FANCD1/BRCA2, FANCJ/BRIP1/BACH1, FANCN/PALB2, FANCO/SLX4, and FANCP/RAD51C. Many of the FA proteins contain no recognizable motifs, which has made discovering their contributions to the FA pathway and the main function of the FA pathway more challenging.[108–111]

Teleologically, the involvement of specific developmental abnormalities in patients with FA implies that the FA proteins have the potential for other functions aside from those that they perform in protecting the genome. Some have argued that the main function of the FA pathway is to regulate oxidative stress, because reactive oxygen species have been documented to be involved in bone marrow failure,[112,113] cancer,[114] endocrinopathies,[115] abnormalities in skin pigmentation,[116] and malformations.[117] This explanation becomes even more plausible when considering the redox-related functions of some FA proteins.[118,119] Recent provocative work has supported

Table 1
A summary of IBMFS and their genetics, physical findings, and testing

Syndrome	Inheritance Pattern	Genes		Physical Findings	Laboratory Testing
FA	AR, XLR	FA-A—FA-P Breast cancer genes		Short stature, radial limb, thumb	DEB chromosome breakage Mitomycin C breakage assay Gene testing
DC	AR, AD, XLR	TERT, TERC, DKC, TINF2, NOP10, TCAB1, NHP2		Nails, skin, leukoplakia	Telomere lengths lymph subsets Gene testing
Shwachman-Diamond	AR	SBDS		Pancreatic insufficiency, skeletal abnormalities	Serum trypsinogen, isoamylase, fecal elastase, pancreatic imaging Gene testing
DBA	AD	RPS7 RPS17 RPS19 RPS24 RPS26	RPL5 RPL11 RPL15 RPL35a	Short stature, head, upper limbs, urogenital	Erythrocyte adenosine deaminase Gene testing
Congenital amegakaryocytic thrombocytopenia	AR	C-MPL		—	Gene testing

the idea that acid aldehydes are the toxic metabolite in vivo, because mouse models knocking out enzymes that detoxify such chemicals phenocopy FA.[120]

Several lines of evidence have shown that excessive apoptosis and consequent malfunction of the hematopoietic stem cell compartment lead to progressive bone marrow failure in patients with FA. The FANCC protein functions independently of the FA core complex to suppress apoptosis in hematopoietic cells in response to environmental cues, which induce expression or secretion of certain cytokines.[121] Patients with FA show altered expression levels of some growth factors and cytokines, including unusually high levels of intracellular tumor necrosis factor α (TNF-α), a cytokine capable of initiating the apoptotic pathway. However, neoplastic stem cell clones, which are resistant to these cytokines, frequently evolve in patients with FA and result in leukemia. Cells from TNF-α–treated fancc–/– mice also showed increased levels of chromosomal aberrations and decreased levels of repair of DNA damage caused by reactive oxygen species, indicating that FANCC may also play a role in the cellular response to oxidative DNA damage.[122–124]

MITOCHONDRIAL DISEASES
Pearson Syndrome

Pearson syndrome is a rare sideroblastic anemia with associated exocrine pancreatic dysfunction, liver dysfunction, and renal tubule defects.[125,126] Often, patients are diagnosed in the neonatal period, and Pearson syndrome has been reported as a cause of hydrops. Rarely, these patients can have physical abnormalities such as retinopathy, ataxia, or muscle weakness but often present with failure to thrive or poor growth along with persistent, macrocytic anemia.[127] These cases, numbering no more than 40 reported in the literature, have been diagnosed histologically with vacuolization of bone marrow precursors.[20,128] In the 1990s, the molecular defect of Pearson syndrome was characterized, involving deletions and duplications of regions of mitochondrial DNA.[129,130] As a result of the mitochondrial defect, the enzymes of the oxidative respiration cascade are compromised, and thus acidosis is the major component of the disease. In patients with the disease who survive the neonatal period, the anemia improves, and increases in hemoglobin level have been observed. Recently, induced pluripotent stem cells have been produced, which serve as a new primary cell model for Pearson syndrome.[131] Growth factors have been used in the therapy for Pearson syndrome but have not proved effective. Transfusions remain the mainstay of therapy, but mortality is high in early childhood, from acidosis, sepsis, or liver and kidney failure. Malignancy has not been associated with this disease.

RETICULAR DYSGENESIS

This extremely rare disease almost exclusively presents in the neonatal period with leukopenia and lymphopenia and no myeloid and lymphoid precursors but usually not complete marrow aplasia.[132–135] Lymphoid tissue is generally absent. Early progenitors are probably the defective cells, because 2 distinct lineages are affected. However, a subset of patients has anemia and thrombocytopenia. Genetic analysis has shown that reticular dysgenesis (RD) is of mitochondrial origin, with mutations found in the adenylate kinase 2 gene.[136] The action of this gene has been postulated to be involved with the unfolded protein response, the absence of which may lend to imbalance in secretory protein load.

BMT has been curative in patients with RD who clinically act like patients with severe combined immune deficiency. Mixed results occur because of the difficulty of infant BMT, and the resulting mortality is high.[137,138]

CONGENITAL THROMBOCYTOPENIAS
Amegakaryocytic Thrombocytopenia

A few cases with isolated thrombocytopenia have been reported in patients who show none of the classic findings of FA or thrombocytopenia/absent radii syndrome (TAR). These patients have a range of developmental defects, including microcephaly, low birth weight, delay, cardiac defects, central nervous system defects, and orthopedic anomalies. The presentation of most patients includes thrombocytopenia without megakaryocytes on marrow examination. Progressively, an increasingly hypocellular picture emerges over time, suggesting that pancytopenia is a bigger issue than at initial presentation. A familial pattern has emerged in these patients, which fits both autosomal-recessive and X-linked inheritance. Several candidates have been identified as the causative gene, including MPL, RUNX1, ANKRD26, MYH9, and PTPN1, but most cases of mutations have been in MPL, the thrombopoietin receptor. Forty percent of patients develop pancytopenia along a variable timeline and are at risk of leukemia. Corticosteroids have been used with limited success, and little BMT experience exists in this disease.[7,20,139,140]

TAR Syndrome

TAR is an autosomal-recessive disease with preserved thumbs. Thrombocytopenia is usually evident from birth and almost certainly by 4 months of age and is accompanied by significant hemorrhagic events. Megakaryocytes are absent, classifying it as a progenitor disease affecting only the platelet lineage. Some patients have a leukemoid reaction, but this subsides in infancy. Because of the lack of malignancy, genomic instability, and no reports of FA mutations, this disease entity is likely not an overlap with FA nor a premalignant syndrome, although sporadic cases of leukemia associated with TAR exist. Platelet counts improve after infancy; thus, afflicted patients do well after the first year of life, requiring platelet transfusions only during infancy. Other modalities have not been shown to be effective.[20,141,142]

CONGENITAL DYSERYTHROPOIETIC ANEMIA

The congenital dyserythropoietic anemias (CDAs) are a group of isolated red cell production disorders characterized by morphologic abnormalities of erythroid precursors in the bone marrow, a consequence of dyserythropoiesis and ineffective erythropoiesis.[143,144] In addition, distal limb malformations, including syndactyly, absence of phalanges and nails, an additional phalanx, and duplication or hypoplasia of the metatarsals, have been reported in several cases of CDA I.[145] Other congenital abnormalities found include café au lait spots, short stature, flattened vertebral bodies, hypoplastic rib, Madelung deformity, deafness, and retinal angioid streaks.[146,147]

From morphologic abnormalities of the bone marrow, CDAs have been classified into 3 different types: type I, type II, and type III, but additional variants requiring further characterization have also been identified. Approximately 600 cases of CDA have been reported worldwide, CDA II being the most common.[148] CDA II in particular has been associated with the HEMPAS phenotype (hereditary erythroid multinuclearity with positive acidified serum). CDA I and II are inherited in an autosomal-recessive pattern, and CDA III shows autosomal-dominant inheritance and a sporadic form.[143] The disease-related genes for CDA I, II, and III have been localized by linkage analysis, and the disease- causing genes have been identified for CDA I, II, and III. Additional reports suggest other distinct forms of CDA. Most of these have been tentatively assigned to 4 phenotype-based groups designated CDA group IV, V, VI, and VII, with varying degrees of anemia and erythroid dysplasia. They have been designated as groups rather than types, because there is evidence of phenotypic or genetic heterogeneity within each group. In addition to these groups, each of which includes 3 or more families, there are cases with unique features reported in only 1 or 2 families.

The ineffective erythropoiesis of CDA leads to intermittent jaundice, splenomegaly, hepatomegaly, and iron overload, also a result of blood transfusion therapy.[144,149,150] Dyserythropoiesis results in abnormal features of marrow erythroblasts, such as internuclear chromatin bridges, multinuclearity, vacuolization, and duplication of the plasma membrane.

CDA I is an autosomal-recessive disease marked by mutations in cdan1, the encoded protein of which has no obvious function.[151] Additional variants of CDA I have shown mutations in the erythroid transcription factor KLF1 in a dominant fashion.[152] CDA I is marked by spongy heterochromatin, suggesting a role for cdan1 in chromatin, and a link to the chromatin-binding protein HP1 has been made.[153] CDA II is also autosomal recessive, with mutations reported in the secretory pathway gene SEC23B.[154] CDA III is an autosomal-dominant disease, with reported mutations in the KIF23 gene, a kinesin.[155] Given the lack of a cancer phenotype and the involvement of these gene products in chromatin and in the secretory pathway, these genes suggest a pathway for regulation of nuclear extrusion and red cell maturation and the lack of involvement in early erythropoiesis.

Treatment varies amongst groups of CDA, although generally, attention to gallstones and iron overload is warranted. Splenectomy is often indicated for CDA II, less so for other groups. Interferon α has been shown to be efficacious, especially in CDA I.[148]

WORKUP OF A PATIENT WITH BONE MARROW FAILURE

The clinical signs of pancytopenia include infection, bruising, and pallor. A blood count, usually performed by the primary care physician or emergency department, then shows pancytopenia. Sepsis or viral suppression can result in neutropenia and thrombocytopenia, and thus, the clinical situation must be considered any time one considers the diagnosis of hypoplastic marrow. In the absence of sepsis, a complete blood count and manual examination of the peripheral smear are mandatory. In addition, a bone marrow aspiration and biopsy are crucial to determine a primary cause. Samples should be sent for.

Cytogenetics

Culturing of mononuclear cells and examination of chromosomes for cytogenetic abnormalities is required for aplastic presentation. An abnormality that indicates malignancy, myelodysplasia, genetic syndrome (eg, Down syndrome), or clonal process alters therapeutic interventions.

DEB Chromosome Fragility Assay

This assay involves the incubation of a mononuclear fraction of blood cells in the presence of a bifunctional alkylating agent, that is an agent which can cause an inter or intrastrand DNA crosslink. The cells are then treated with colchicine to arrest them in mitosis and are dropped onto a slide for a karyotypelike analysis. Increased chromosome breaks in this setting are pathognomonic for FA. The test is sensitive and specific. The DEB test is crucial, because many patients with FA bear none of the classic physical findings of FA.

Flow Cytometry

Delivery of mononuclear cells into the fluorescence-activated cell sorting machine after fluorescent detection of surface antigens shows the full panel of normal mature and precursor cells in bone marrow and peripheral blood. Detection of abnormal groups of cells shows potential clonality or malignant process. Flow for CD55, the paroxysmal nocturnal hemoglobinuria (PNH) clone, should be performed. It is common to find a clone at low percentage, but consensus is that more than approximately 15% clone would be concerning for PNH.

Genotype Analysis

Cases in which an inherited transmission is responsible and for which a gene has been likely cloned should be analyzed for presence of mutation. For example, 16 FA genes have been cloned, and retroviral gene correction is available that can establish the genetic complementation subgroup for FA as well as focus the search for mutations. Once the mutation is described, then effective genetic counseling may be provided for the family. Genetic sequencing panels that have been approved by Clinical Laboratory Improvement Amendments now exist, whereby genes in the FA, DC, DBA, and other syndromes may be interrogated for mutations, assuming some clinical suspicion.

Infectious Causes

Titers for suspected viral causes of aplasia may be sent for IgG and IgM so the source and status of infection can be determined and followed. In some cases, polymerase chain reaction may be used to directly test for presence of pathogens associated with marrow aplasia. Such viruses include hepatitis, parvovirus, cytomegalovirus, Epstein-Barr virus, and human herpesvirus 6.

Telomere Length Analysis

Similar to DEB testing, telomere length analysis is a functional assay to screen for DC. The test should be performed on lymphocyte subsets and not simply granulocytes or all white blood cells combined. If the results are well below the first percentile of the normal population for age, then there is a high likelihood that the patient has DC. Also, many patients with IBMFS have shorter telomere lengths, closer to the first percentile, and so it may also give some support to a clinical suspicion of an inherited process even if it is not DC.

Research

The physician should consider the collection of additional blood or marrow for research purposes per approved institutional protocol, given the rarity of marrow failure syndromes.

REFERENCES

1. Narla A, Ebert BL. Ribosomopathies: human disorders of ribosome dysfunction. Blood 2010;115(16):3196–205.
2. Danilova N, Sakamoto KM, Lin S. Ribosomal protein S19 deficiency in zebrafish leads to developmental abnormalities and defective erythropoiesis through activation of p53 protein family. Blood 2008;112(13):5228–37.
3. McGowan KA, Li JZ, Park CY, et al. Ribosomal mutations cause p53-mediated dark skin and pleiotropic effects. Nat Genet 2008;40(8):963–70.
4. Burwick N, Shimamura A, Liu JM. Non-Diamond Blackfan anemia disorders of ribosome function: Shwachman Diamond syndrome and 5q- syndrome. Semin Hematol 2011;48(2):136–43.
5. Diamond LK. Congenital hypoplastic anemia: Diamond-Blackfan syndrome. Historical and clinical aspects. Blood Cells 1978;4(1–2):209–13.
6. Alter BP, Nathan DG. Red cell aplasia in children. Arch Dis Child 1979;54(4): 263–7.
7. Slayton WB, Schibler KR. Congenital bone marrow failure syndromes associated with protean developmental defects and leukemia. Clin Perinatol 2000; 27(3):543–58.
8. Willig TN, Gazda H, Sieff CA. Diamond-Blackfan anemia. Curr Opin Hematol 2000;7(2):85–94.
9. Willig TN, Ball SE, Tchernia G. Current concepts and issues in Diamond-Blackfan anemia. Curr Opin Hematol 1998;5(2):109–15.
10. Gray PH. Pure red-cell aplasia. Occurrence in three generations. Med J Aust 1982;1(12):519–21.
11. Gojic V, van't Veer-Korthof ET, Bosch LJ, et al. Congenital hypoplastic anemia: another example of autosomal dominant transmission. Am J Med Genet 1994; 50(1):87–9.

12. Viskochil DH, Carey JC, Glader BE, et al. Congenital hypoplastic (Diamond-Blackfan) anemia in seven members of one kindred. Am J Med Genet 1990; 35(2):251–6.
13. Alter BP. Thumbs and anemia. Pediatrics 1978;62(4):613–4.
14. Sieff CA, Nisbet-Brown E, Nathan DG. Congenital bone marrow failure syndromes. Br J Haematol 2000;111(1):30–42.
15. Krijanovski OI, Sieff CA. Diamond-Blackfan anemia. Hematol Oncol Clin North Am 1997;11(6):1061–77.
16. Hammond D, Shore N, Movassaghi N. Production, utilization and excretion of erythropoietin. I. Chronic anemias. II. Aplastic crisis. 3. Erythropoietic effects of normal plasma. Ann N Y Acad Sci 1968;149(1):516–27.
17. Alter BP. Fetal erythropoiesis in stress hematopoiesis. Exp Hematol 1979; 7(Suppl 5):200–9.
18. Buchanan GR, Alter BP, Holtkamp CA, et al. Platelet number and function in Diamond-Blackfan anemia. Pediatrics 1981;68(2):238–41.
19. Giri N, Kang E, Tisdale JF, et al. Clinical and laboratory evidence for a trilineage haematopoietic defect in patients with refractory Diamond-Blackfan anaemia. Br J Haematol 2000;108(1):167–75.
20. Alter B, Young N. The bone marrow failure syndromes. In: Nathan D, Orkin S, editors. Hematology of infancy and childhood. Philadelphia: WB Saunders; 1998. p. 237–335.
21. Sjolin S, Wranne L. Treatment of congenital hypoplastic anemia with prednisone. Scand J Haematol 1970;7(1):63–72.
22. Vlachos A, Muir E. How I treat Diamond-Blackfan anemia. Blood 2010;116(19): 3715–23.
23. Greinix HT, Storb R, Sanders JE, et al. Long-term survival and cure after marrow transplantation for congenital hypoplastic anaemia (Diamond-Blackfan syndrome). Br J Haematol 1993;84(3):515–20.
24. Mugishima H, Gale RP, Rowlings PA, et al. Bone marrow transplantation for Diamond-Blackfan anemia. Bone Marrow Transplant 1995;15(1):55–8.
25. Niemeyer CM, Baumgarten E, Holldack J, et al. Treatment trial with recombinant human erythropoietin in children with congenital hypoplastic anemia. Contrib Nephrol 1991;88:276–80.
26. Gillio AP, Faulkner LB, Alter BP, et al. Treatment of Diamond-Blackfan anemia with recombinant human interleukin-3. Blood 1993;82(3):744–51.
27. Dunbar CE, Smith DA, Kimball J, et al. Treatment of Diamond-Blackfan anaemia with haematopoietic growth factors, granulocyte-macrophage colony stimulating factor and interleukin 3: sustained remissions following IL-3. Br J Haematol 1991; 79(2):316–21.
28. Janov AJ, Leong T, Nathan DG, et al. Diamond-Blackfan anemia. Natural history and sequelae of treatment. Medicine (Baltimore) 1996;75(2):77–8.
29. Basso G, Cocito MG, Rebuffi L, et al. Congenital hypoplastic anaemia developed in acute megakarioblastic leukaemia. A case report. Helv Paediatr Acta 1981;36(3):267–70.
30. Krishnan EU, Wegner K, Garg SK. Congenital hypoplastic anemia terminating in acute promyelocytic leukemia. Pediatrics 1978;61(6):898–901.
31. D'Oelsnitz M, Vincent L, De Swarte M, et al. Proceedings: acute lymphoblastic leukemia following treatment of Blackfan-Diamond's disease. Arch Fr Pediatr 1975;32(6):582 [in French].
32. van Dijken PJ, Verwijs W. Diamond-Blackfan anemia and malignancy. A case report and a review of the literature. Cancer 1995;76(3):517–20.

33. Seip M. Malignant tumors in two patients with Diamond-Blackfan anemia treated with corticosteroids and androgens. Pediatr Hematol Oncol 1994;11(4):423–6.
34. Aquino VM, Buchanan GR. Osteogenic sarcoma in a child with transfusion-dependent Diamond-Blackfan anemia. J Pediatr Hematol Oncol 1996;18(2):230–2.
35. Willig TN, Draptchinskaia N, Dianzani I, et al. Mutations in ribosomal protein S19 gene and Diamond Blackfan anemia: wide variations in phenotypic expression. Blood 1999;94(12):4294–306.
36. Draptchinskaia N, Gustavsson P, Andersson B, et al. The gene encoding ribosomal protein S19 is mutated in Diamond-Blackfan anaemia. Nat Genet 1999; 21(2):169–75.
37. Landowski M, O'Donohue MF, Buros C, et al. Novel deletion of RPL15 identified by array-comparative genomic hybridization in Diamond-Blackfan anemia. Hum Genet 2013. [Epub ahead of print].
38. Sankaran VG, Ghazvinian R, Do R, et al. Exome sequencing identifies GATA1 mutations resulting in Diamond-Blackfan anemia. J Clin Invest 2012;122(7): 2439–43.
39. Nathan DG, Clarke BJ, Hillman DG, et al. Erythroid precursors in congenital hypoplastic (Diamond-Blackfan) anemia. J Clin Invest 1978;61(2):489–98.
40. Freedman MH, Amato D, Saunders EF. Erythroid colony growth in congenital hypoplastic anemia. J Clin Invest 1976;57(3):673–7.
41. Lipton JM, Kudisch M, Gross R, et al. Defective erythroid progenitor differentiation system in congenital hypoplastic (Diamond-Blackfan) anemia. Blood 1986; 67(4):962–8.
42. McGuckin CP, Ball SE, Gordon-Smith EC. Diamond-Blackfan anaemia: three patterns of in vitro response to haemopoietic growth factors. Br J Haematol 1995;89(3):457–64.
43. Perdahl EB, Naprstek BL, Wallace WC, et al. Erythroid failure in Diamond-Blackfan anemia is characterized by apoptosis. Blood 1994;83(3):645–50.
44. Ershler WB, Ross J, Finlay JL, et al. Bone-marrow microenvironment defect in congenital hypoplastic anemia. N Engl J Med 1980;302(24):1321–7.
45. Cui D, Li L, Lou H, et al. The ribosomal protein S26 regulates p53 activity in response to DNA damage. Oncogene 2013. [Epub ahead of print].
46. Ellis SR. DBA, del(5q): a reciprocal relationship. Blood 2011;118(8):2032–3.
47. Payne EM, Virgilio M, Narla A, et al. L-Leucine improves the anemia and developmental defects associated with Diamond-Blackfan anemia and del(5q) MDS by activating the mTOR pathway. Blood 2012;120(11):2214–24.
48. Drachtman RA, Alter BP. Dyskeratosis congenita. Dermatol Clin 1995;13(1): 33–9.
49. Dokal I. Dyskeratosis congenita in all its forms. Br J Haematol 2000;110(4): 768–79.
50. Anil S, Beena VT, Raji MA, et al. Oral squamous cell carcinoma in a case of dyskeratosis congenita. Ann Dent 1994;53(1):15–8.
51. Dokal I. Dyskeratosis congenita. Hematology Am Soc Hematol Educ Program 2011;2011:480–6.
52. Mason PJ, Bessler M. The genetics of dyskeratosis congenita. Cancer Genet 2011;204(12):635–45.
53. Ballew BJ, Savage SA. Updates on the biology and management of dyskeratosis congenita and related telomere biology disorders. Expert Rev Hematol 2013; 6(3):327–37.
54. Liu JM, Ellis SR. Ribosomes and marrow failure: coincidental association or molecular paradigm? Blood 2006;107(12):4583–8.

55. Rackley S, Pao M, Seratti GF, et al. Neuropsychiatric conditions among patients with dyskeratosis congenita: a link with telomere biology? Psychosomatics 2012;53(3):230–5.

56. Pritchard SL, Junker AK. Positive response to granulocyte-colony-stimulating factor in dyskeratosis congenita before matched unrelated bone marrow transplantation. Am J Pediatr Hematol Oncol 1994;16(2):186–7.

57. Oehler L, Reiter E, Friedl J, et al. Effective stimulation of neutropoiesis with rh G-CSF in dyskeratosis congenita: a case report. Ann Hematol 1994;69(6):325–7.

58. Rocha V, Devergie A, Socie G, et al. Unusual complications after bone marrow transplantation for dyskeratosis congenita. Br J Haematol 1998;103(1):243–8.

59. Knight S, Vulliamy T, Copplestone A, et al. Dyskeratosis Congenita (DC) Registry: identification of new features of DC. Br J Haematol 1998;103(4):990–6.

60. Gadalla SM, Sales-Bonfim C, Carreras J, et al. Outcomes of allogeneic hematopoietic cell transplantation in patients with dyskeratosis congenita. Biol Blood Marrow Transplant 2013;19(8):1238–43.

61. Smith OP, Hann IM, Chessells JM, et al. Haematological abnormalities in Shwachman-Diamond syndrome. Br J Haematol 1996;94(2):279–84.

62. Smith OP. Shwachman-Diamond syndrome. Semin Hematol 2002;39(2):95–102.

63. Boocock GR, Morrison JA, Popovic M, et al. Mutations in SBDS are associated with Shwachman-Diamond syndrome. Nat Genet 2003;33(1):97–101.

64. Tulpule A, Kelley JM, Lensch MW, et al. Pluripotent stem cell models of Shwachman-Diamond syndrome reveal a common mechanism for pancreatic and hematopoietic dysfunction. Cell Stem Cell 2013;12(6):727–36.

65. Burwick N, Coats SA, Nakamura T, et al. Impaired ribosomal subunit association in Shwachman-Diamond syndrome. Blood 2012;120(26):5143–52.

66. Barrios N, Kirkpatrick D, Regueira O, et al. Bone marrow transplant in Shwachman Diamond syndrome. Br J Haematol 1991;79(2):337–8.

67. Adachi N, Tsuchiya H, Nunoi H, et al. rhG-CSF for Shwachman's syndrome. Lancet 1990;336(8723):1136.

68. Dale DC, Bonilla MA, Davis MW, et al. A randomized controlled phase III trial of recombinant human granulocyte colony-stimulating factor (filgrastim) for treatment of severe chronic neutropenia. Blood 1993;81(10):2496–502.

69. Makitie O, Kaitila I. Cartilage-hair hypoplasia–clinical manifestations in 108 Finnish patients. Eur J Pediatr 1993;152(3):211–7.

70. Makitie O, Sulisalo T, de la Chapelle A, et al. Cartilage-hair hypoplasia. J Med Genet 1995;32(1):39–43.

71. le Merrer M, Briard ML, Chauvet ML, et al. Autosomal recessive metaphyseal chondrodysplasia and Hirschsprung's disease. Ann Pediatr (Paris) 1991;38(1):27–30 [in French].

72. Ridanpaa M, van Eenennaam H, Pelin K, et al. Mutations in the RNA component of RNase MRP cause a pleiotropic human disease, cartilage-hair hypoplasia. Cell 2001;104(2):195–203.

73. Maida Y, Yasukawa M, Furuuchi M, et al. An RNA-dependent RNA polymerase formed by TERT and the RMRP RNA. Nature 2009;461(7261):230–5.

74. Ganapathi KA, Shimamura A. Ribosomal dysfunction and inherited marrow failure. Br J Haematol 2008;141(3):376–87.

75. Juvonen E, Makitie O, Makipernaa A, et al. Defective in-vitro colony formation of haematopoietic progenitors in patients with cartilage-hair hypoplasia and history of anaemia. Eur J Pediatr 1995;154(1):30–4.

76. Virolainen M, Savilahti E, Kaitila I, et al. Cellular and humoral immunity in cartilage-hair hypoplasia. Pediatr Res 1978;12(10):961–6.
77. Makitie O, Rajantie J, Kaitila I. Anaemia and macrocytosis–unrecognized features in cartilage-hair hypoplasia. Acta Paediatr 1992;81(12):1026–9.
78. Gorlin R. Cartilage-hair-hypoplasia and Hodgkin disease. Am J Med Genet 1992;44:539.
79. Taskinen M, Jeskanen L, Karjalainen-Lindsberg ML, et al. Combating cancer predisposition in association with idiopathic immune deficiency: a recurrent nodal and cutaneous T-cell lymphoproliferative disease in a patient with cartilage-hair hypoplasia. Clin Lymphoma Myeloma Leuk 2013;13(1):73–6.
80. Alter BP. Fanconi's anemia, transplantation, and cancer. Pediatr Transplant 2005;9(Suppl 7):81–6.
81. Lowy DR, Gillison ML. A new link between Fanconi anemia and human papillomavirus-associated malignancies. J Natl Cancer Inst 2003;95(22):1648–50.
82. Masserot C, Peffault de Latour R, Rocha V, et al. Head and neck squamous cell carcinoma in 13 patients with Fanconi anemia after hematopoietic stem cell transplantation. Cancer 2008;113(12):3315–22.
83. Bagby GC, Alter BP. Fanconi anemia. Semin Hematol 2006;43(3):147–56.
84. D'Andrea AD, Dahl N, Guinan EC, et al. Marrow failure. Hematology Am Soc Hematol Educ Program 2002;58–72.
85. Tischkowitz M, Dokal I. Fanconi anaemia and leukaemia–clinical and molecular aspects. Br J Haematol 2004;126(2):176–91.
86. Hirschhorn R. In vivo reversion to normal of inherited mutations in humans. J Med Genet 2003;40(10):721–8.
87. Soulier J, Leblanc T, Larghero J, et al. Detection of somatic mosaicism and classification of Fanconi anemia patients by analysis of the FA/BRCA pathway. Blood 2005;105(3):1329–36.
88. Velez-Ruelas MA, Martinez-Jaramillo G, Arana-Trejo RM, et al. Hematopoietic changes during progression from Fanconi anemia into acute myeloid leukemia: case report and brief review of the literature. Hematology 2006;11(5):331–4.
89. Rochowski A, Olson SB, Alonzo TA, et al. Patients with Fanconi anemia and AML have different cytogenetic clones than de novo cases of AML. Pediatr Blood Cancer 2012;59(5):922–4.
90. Mehta PA, Ileri T, Harris RE, et al. Chemotherapy for myeloid malignancy in children with Fanconi anemia. Pediatr Blood Cancer 2007;48(7):668–72.
91. Scheckenbach K, Wagenmann M, Freund M, et al. Squamous cell carcinomas of the head and neck in Fanconi anemia: risk, prevention, therapy, and the need for guidelines. Klin Padiatr 2012;224(3):132–8.
92. Somyajit K, Subramanya S, Nagaraju G. RAD51C: a novel cancer susceptibility gene is linked to Fanconi anemia and breast cancer. Carcinogenesis 2010; 31(12):2031–8.
93. Cantor SB, Guillemette S. Hereditary breast cancer and the BRCA1-associated FANCJ/BACH1/BRIP1. Future Oncol 2011;7(2):253–61.
94. Coulet F, Fajac A, Colas C, et al. Germline RAD51C mutations in ovarian cancer susceptibility. Clin Genet 2013;83(4):332–6.
95. Kobayashi H, Ohno S, Sasaki Y, et al. Hereditary breast and ovarian cancer susceptibility genes (Review). Oncol Rep 2013. [Epub ahead of print].
96. Tischkowitz M, Xia B. PALB2/FANCN: recombining cancer and Fanconi anemia. Cancer Res 2010;70(19):7353–9.
97. Do K, Chen AP. Molecular pathways: targeting PARP in cancer treatment. Clin Cancer Res 2013;19(5):977–84.

98. Meyer S, Fergusson WD, Whetton AD, et al. Amplification and translocation of 3q26 with overexpression of EVI1 in Fanconi anemia-derived childhood acute myeloid leukemia with biallelic FANCD1/BRCA2 disruption. Genes Chromosomes Cancer 2007;46(4):359–72.

99. Farzin A, Davies SM, Smith FO, et al. Matched sibling donor haematopoietic stem cell transplantation in Fanconi anaemia: an update of the Cincinnati Children's experience. Br J Haematol 2007;136(4):633–40.

100. Pasquini R, Carreras J, Pasquini MC, et al. HLA-matched sibling hematopoietic stem cell transplantation for Fanconi anemia: comparison of irradiation and non-irradiation containing conditioning regimens. Biol Blood Marrow Transplant 2008;14(10):1141–7.

101. Gluckman E, Wagner JE. Hematopoietic stem cell transplantation in childhood inherited bone marrow failure syndrome. Bone Marrow Transplant 2008;41(2): 127–32.

102. Chaudhury S, Auerbach AD, Kernan NA, et al. Fludarabine-based cytoreductive regimen and T-cell-depleted grafts from alternative donors for the treatment of high-risk patients with Fanconi anaemia. Br J Haematol 2008;140(6):644–55.

103. Balci YI, Akdemir Y, Gumruk F, et al. CD-34 selected hematopoetic stem cell transplantation from HLA identical family members for Fanconi anemia. Pediatr Blood Cancer 2008;50(5):1065–7.

104. Kelly PF, Radtke S, von Kalle C, et al. Stem cell collection and gene transfer in Fanconi anemia. Mol Ther 2007;15(1):211–9.

105. Croop JM. Gene therapy for Fanconi anemia. Curr Hematol Rep 2003;2(4): 335–40.

106. Velazquez I, Alter BP. Androgens and liver tumors: Fanconi's anemia and non-Fanconi's conditions. Am J Hematol 2004;77(3):257–67.

107. Ozenne V, Paradis V, Vullierme MP, et al. Liver tumours in patients with Fanconi anaemia: a report of three cases. Eur J Gastroenterol Hepatol 2008;20(10):1036–9.

108. Bogliolo M, Schuster B, Stoepker C, et al. Mutations in ERCC4, encoding the DNA-repair endonuclease XPF, cause Fanconi anemia. Am J Hum Genet 2013;92(5):800–6.

109. Kottemann MC, Smogorzewska A. Fanconi anaemia and the repair of Watson and Crick DNA crosslinks. Nature 2013;493(7432):356–63.

110. Green AM, Kupfer GM. Fanconi anemia. Hematol Oncol Clin North Am 2009; 23(2):193–214.

111. Kee Y, D'Andrea AD. Molecular pathogenesis and clinical management of Fanconi anemia. J Clin Invest 2012;122(11):3799–806.

112. Gordon-Smith EC, Rutherford TR. Fanconi anaemia–constitutional, familial aplastic anaemia. Baillieres Clin Haematol 1989;2(1):139–52.

113. Bornman L, Baladi S, Richard MJ, et al. Differential regulation and expression of stress proteins and ferritin in human monocytes. J Cell Physiol 1999;178(1):1–8.

114. Kovacic P, Jacintho JD. Mechanisms of carcinogenesis: focus on oxidative stress and electron transfer. Curr Med Chem 2001;8(7):773–96.

115. Evans LM, Davies JS, Anderson RA, et al. The effect of GH replacement therapy on endothelial function and oxidative stress in adult growth hormone deficiency. Eur J Endocrinol 2000;142(3):254–62.

116. Memoli S, Napolitano A, d'Ischia M, et al. Diffusible melanin-related metabolites are potent inhibitors of lipid peroxidation. Biochim Biophys Acta 1997;1346(1): 61–8.

117. Wells PG, Kim PM, Laposa RR, et al. Oxidative damage in chemical teratogenesis. Mutat Res 1997;396(1–2):65–78.

118. Cumming RC, Lightfoot J, Beard K, et al. Fanconi anemia group C protein prevents apoptosis in hematopoietic cells through redox regulation of GSTP1. Nat Med 2001;7(7):814–20.
119. Zanier R, Briot D, Dugas du Villard JA, et al. Fanconi anemia C gene product regulates expression of genes involved in differentiation and inflammation. Oncogene 2004;23(29):5004–13.
120. Langevin F, Crossan GP, Rosado IV, et al. Fancd2 counteracts the toxic effects of naturally produced aldehydes in mice. Nature 2011;475(7354):53–8.
121. Fagerlie SR, Koretsky T, Torok-Storb B, et al. Impaired type I IFN-induced Jak/STAT signaling in FA-C cells and abnormal CD4+ Th cell subsets in Fancc-/- mice. J Immunol 2004;173(6):3863–70.
122. Ceccaldi R, Parmar K, Mouly E, et al. Bone marrow failure in Fanconi anemia is triggered by an exacerbated p53/p21 DNA damage response that impairs hematopoietic stem and progenitor cells. Cell Stem Cell 2012;11(1):36–49.
123. Li J, Sejas DP, Zhang X, et al. TNF-alpha induces leukemic clonal evolution ex vivo in Fanconi anemia group C murine stem cells. J Clin Invest 2007; 117(11):3283–95.
124. Pang Q, Andreassen PR. Fanconi anemia proteins and endogenous stresses. Mutat Res 2009;668(1–2):42–53.
125. Pearson HA, Lobel JS, Kocoshis SA, et al. A new syndrome of refractory sideroblastic anemia with vacuolization of marrow precursors and exocrine pancreatic dysfunction. J Pediatr 1979;95(6):976–84.
126. Fellman V, Kotarsky H. Mitochondrial hepatopathies in the newborn period. Semin Fetal Neonatal Med 2011;16(4):222–8.
127. Finsterer J. Hematological manifestations of primary mitochondrial disorders. Acta Haematol 2007;118(2):88–98.
128. Bader-Meunier B, Rotig A, Mielot F, et al. Refractory anaemia and mitochondrial cytopathy in childhood. Br J Haematol 1994;87(2):381–5.
129. Rotig A, Cormier V, Blanche S, et al. Pearson's marrow-pancreas syndrome. A multisystem mitochondrial disorder in infancy. J Clin Invest 1990;86(5): 1601–8.
130. Casademont J, Barrientos A, Cardellach F, et al. Multiple deletions of mtDNA in two brothers with sideroblastic anemia and mitochondrial myopathy and in their asymptomatic mother. Hum Mol Genet 1994;3(11):1945–9.
131. Cherry AB, Gagne KE, McLoughlin EM, et al. Induced pluripotent stem cells with a pathological mitochondrial DNA deletion. Stem Cells 2013;31(7): 1287–97.
132. Vaal OD, Seynhaeve V. Reticular dysgenesia. Lancet 1959;2:1123.
133. Bujan W, Ferster A, Azzi N, et al. Use of recombinant human granulocyte colony stimulating factor in reticular dysgenesis. Br J Haematol 1992;81(1): 128–30.
134. Bujan W, Ferster A, Sariban E, et al. Effect of recombinant human granulocyte colony-stimulating factor in reticular dysgenesis. Blood 1993;82(5):1684.
135. Azcona C, Alzina V, Barona P, et al. Use of recombinant human granulocyte-macrophage colony stimulating factor in an infant with reticular dysgenesis. Eur J Pediatr 1994;153(3):164–6.
136. Pannicke U, Honig M, Hess I, et al. Reticular dysgenesis (aleukocytosis) is caused by mutations in the gene encoding mitochondrial adenylate kinase 2. Nat Genet 2009;41(1):101–5.
137. Levinsky RJ, Tiedeman K. Successful bone-marrow transplantation for reticular dysgenesis. Lancet 1983;1(8326 Pt 1):671–2.

138. Roper M, Parmley RT, Crist WM, et al. Severe congenital leukopenia (reticular dysgenesis). Immunologic and morphologic characterizations of leukocytes. Am J Dis Child 1985;139(8):832–5.

139. Ballmaier M, Germeshausen M. Congenital amegakaryocytic thrombocytopenia: clinical presentation, diagnosis, and treatment. Semin Thromb Hemost 2011;37(6):673–81.

140. Stoddart MT, Connor P, Germeshausen M, et al. Congenital amegakaryocytic thrombocytopenia (CAMT) presenting as severe pancytopenia in the first month of life. Pediatr Blood Cancer 2013;60(9):E94–6.

141. Fadoo Z, Naqvi SM. Acute myeloid leukemia in a patient with thrombocytopenia with absent radii syndrome. J Pediatr Hematol Oncol 2002;24(2):134–5.

142. Go RS, Johnston KL. Acute myelogenous leukemia in an adult with thrombocytopenia with absent radii syndrome. Eur J Haematol 2003;70(4):246–8.

143. Iolascon A, Esposito MR, Russo R. Clinical aspects and pathogenesis of congenital dyserythropoietic anemias: from morphology to molecular approach. Haematologica 2012;97(12):1786–94.

144. Wickramasinghe SN. Congenital dyserythropoietic anaemias: clinical features, haematological morphology and new biochemical data. Blood Rev 1998; 12(3):178–200.

145. Parez N, Dommergues M, Zupan V, et al. Severe congenital dyserythropoietic anaemia type I: prenatal management, transfusion support and alpha-interferon therapy. Br J Haematol 2000;110(2):420–3.

146. Halpern Z, Rahmani R, Levo Y. Severe hemochromatosis: the predominant clinical manifestation of congenital dyserythropoietic anemia type 2. Acta Haematol 1985;74(3):178–80.

147. Sandstrom H, Wahlin A, Eriksson M, et al. Intravascular haemolysis and increased prevalence of myeloma and monoclonal gammopathy in congenital dyserythropoietic anaemia, type III. Eur J Haematol 1994;52(1):42–6.

148. Wickramasinghe SN, Wood WG. Advances in the understanding of the congenital dyserythropoietic anaemias. Br J Haematol 2005;131(4):431–46.

149. Vainchenker W, Breton-Gorius J, Guichard J, et al. Congenital dyserythropoietic anemia type III. Studies on erythroid differentiation of blood erythroid progenitor cells (BFUE) in vitro. Exp Hematol 1980;8(8):1057–62.

150. Vainchenker W, Guichard J, Bouguet J, et al. Congenital dyserythropoietic anaemia type I: absence of clonal expression in the nuclear abnormalities of cultured erythroblasts. Br J Haematol 1980;46(1):33–7.

151. Dgany O, Avidan N, Delaunay J, et al. Congenital dyserythropoietic anemia type I is caused by mutations in codanin-1. Am J Hum Genet 2002;71(6):1467–74.

152. Arnaud L, Saison C, Helias V, et al. A dominant mutation in the gene encoding the erythroid transcription factor KLF1 causes a congenital dyserythropoietic anemia. Am J Hum Genet 2010;87(5):721–7.

153. Renella R, Roberts NA, Brown JM, et al. Codanin-1 mutations in congenital dyserythropoietic anemia type 1 affect HP1{alpha} localization in erythroblasts. Blood 2011;117(25):6928–38.

154. Schwarz K, Iolascon A, Verissimo F, et al. Mutations affecting the secretory CO-PII coat component SEC23B cause congenital dyserythropoietic anemia type II. Nat Genet 2009;41(8):936–40.

155. Liljeholm M, Irvine AF, Vikberg AL, et al. Congenital dyserythropoietic anemia type III (CDA III) is caused by a mutation in kinesin family member, KIF23. Blood 2013;121(23):4791–9.

Acquired Aplastic Anemia in Children

Helge D. Hartung, MD[a,1], Timothy S. Olson, MD, PhD[b,1],
Monica Bessler, MD, PhD[a,c],*

KEYWORDS

- Acquired aplastic anemia • Bone marrow failure • Immune-mediated aplastic anemia
- Immunosuppressive therapy for severe aplastic anemia in children
- Bone marrow transplant for severe aplastic anemia in children

KEY POINTS

- Acquired aplastic anemia (AA) is an acquired condition of bone marrow failure character-ized by peripheral pancytopenia and a hypoplastic bone marrow.
- There is increasing evidence that acquired AA is immune mediated.
- Bone marrow transplantation (BMT) is the recommended first-line therapy for patients with a human leukocyte antigen (HLA)-matched sibling donor, with 5-year survival rates exceeding 90%.
- Immunosuppressive therapy (IST) with horse antithymocyte globulin and cyclosporine is the recommended first-line therapy for patients without an HLA-matched sibling donor. Survival rates are similar to those for BMT with a matched sibling donor, but relapse, clonal hematopoiesis, leukemia, autoimmunity, and cancer remain concerns that require long-term follow-up.

Continued

Funding Sources: NCI NIH R01 CA105312 and Buck Family Endowed Chair in Hematology (M. Bessler); NHLBI K12 HL087064, The Canuso Foundation Innovation Grant, and The Chil-dren's Hospital of Philadelphia CTRC Junior Investigator Pilot Grant Program (Funded by NCATS NIH UL1TR000003) (T.S. Olson).
Conflict of Interest: None.

[a] Division of Hematology, Department of Pediatrics, Comprehensive Bone Marrow Failure Cen-ter, The Children's Hospital of Philadelphia, 3615 Civic Center Boulevard, ARC 302, Philadelphia, PA 19104, USA; [b] Division of Oncology, Department of Pediatrics, Comprehensive Bone Marrow Failure Center, The Children's Hospital of Philadelphia, 3615 Civic Center Boulevard, ARC 302, Philadelphia, PA 19104, USA; [c] Division of Hemato-Oncology, Department of Medicine, Hospi-tal of the University of Pennsylvania, Perelman School of Medicine, University of Pennsylvania, 3400 Spruce Street, 1218 Penn Tower, Philadelphia, PA 19104, USA
[1] H.D. Hartung and T.S. Olson contributed equally to this work.
* Corresponding author. Pediatric & Adult Comprehensive Bone Marrow Failure Center, The Children's Hospital of Philadelphia, University of Pennsylvania, Center Boulevard, ARC 302, Philadelphia, PA 19104.
E-mail address: besslerm@email.chop.edu

Continued

- BMT with an HLA-matched unrelated donor should be offered to all IST nonresponders early in the course of disease, and may be considered as a first-line treatment in selected cases and in countries where horse antithymocyte globulin is not available.

- A better understanding of underlying mechanisms that initiate and fuel immune dysregulation will help to develop targeted preventive strategies and more personalized and specific treatment options for patients with AA.

INTRODUCTION

Acquired aplastic anemia (AA) in childhood remains an uncommon, life-threatening disorder. Because of major advances in diagnosis and therapeutic approaches, AA in children is today a disease that results in long-term survival in more than 90% of cases. This article reviews current practices in the diagnosis and therapy for patients with acquired AA, discusses alternative approaches, and assesses the evidence base.

DEFINITIONS

AA is characterized by peripheral blood pancytopenia and a hypocellular bone marrow without dysplasia or fibrosis (**Fig. 1**). The degree or severity of AA is defined by peripheral blood cell counts in the presence of a hypocellular bone marrow (**Box 1**).[1,2] AA in children is distinct from that in adults; inherited AA is more frequently found in children

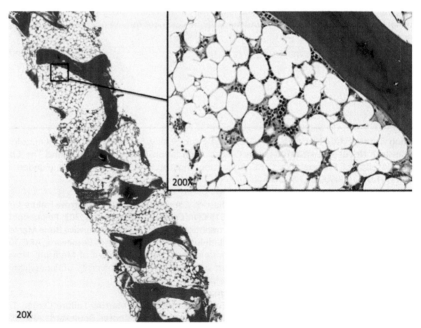

Fig. 1. Bone marrow aspirate and biopsy from a patient with acquired AA. Hematopoietic elements are greatly reduced, and there is replacement of marrow space with adipose tissue. Focal islands of left-shifted erythropoiesis (Fig 1: H&E stain, original magnification ×20; Inset: H&E stain, original magnification ×200). (*Courtesy of* Dr Michele E. Paessler, DO, Pathology, The Children's Hospital of Philadelphia.)

Box 1	
Definition of severity of aplastic anemia (AA)	
Moderate or nonsevere (NSAA)	Decreased bone marrow cellularity and peripheral blood cytopenia, NOT fulfilling criteria for SAA
Severe (SAA)[a]	Bone marrow cellularity <25%
	AND at least 2 of the following:
	a. Neutrophil count <500 $\times$ 10^6/L
	b. Platelet count <20,000 $\times$ 10^6/L
	c. Reticulocyte count[b] <60,000 $\times$ 10^6/L
Very severe (vSAA)[c]	Fulfilling criteria for SAA
	PLUS
	a. Neutrophil count <200 $\times 10^6$/L

[a] Camitta BM, Rappeport JM, Parkman R, et al. Selection of patients for bone marrow transplantation in severe aplastic anemia. Blood 1975;45:355–63.
[b] Automated reticulocyte counts (or manual counts of 20,000 $\times$ 10^6/L).
[c] Bacigalupo A, Hows J, Gluckman E, et al. Bone marrow transplantation (BMT) versus immunosuppression for the treatment of severe aplastic anemia (SAA): a report of the EBMT SAA working party. Br J Haematol 1988;70:177–82.

and the human leukocyte antigen (HLA) association differs, suggesting an age-specific immune pathogenesis. Moreover, there are age-specific differences in treatment, response to treatment, treatment outcome, and late manifestations.

Acquired AA must be distinguished from inherited bone marrow failure syndromes (IBMFS) and hypoplastic myelodysplastic syndrome (MDS). IBMFS are more frequent in the pediatric population and comprise roughly 25% to 30% of cases of bone marrow aplasia in children.[3] Distinguishing between acquired AA and IBMFS can be difficult in patients with inherited conditions lacking classic congenital anomalies or in patients without a supporting family history, which can be due to a de novo mutation or a mutation with low disease penetrance.[3] **Fig. 2** shows the interrelationship of acquired AA and IBMFS from a genetic viewpoint.

Similarly, hypoplastic MDS can be difficult to differentiate from acquired AA (and IBMFS), especially in children. The new World Health Organization (WHO) classification for myeloid neoplasms distinguishes refractory cytopenia of childhood (RCC) from AA and considers it as a provisional entity of childhood MDS (**Box 2**).[4] This new WHO classification is becoming increasingly established in Europe and Japan, but its application in North America is still limited. Of clinical importance is that RCC, though classified as a low-risk childhood MDS entity, differs from the current broader concept of MDS in older adults, which is associated with a poor prognosis. Current diagnosis, care, and treatment of AA and RCC are largely the same, so this review does not distinguish between AA and RCC. **Box 2** summarizes the histologic and morphologic criteria that differentiate AA from RCC.[5] Prospective future and ongoing studies will determine the clinical significance of the RCC MDS entity.

EPIDEMIOLOGY

Acquired AA is a rare disorder with an incidence of about 2 in 1 million children per year in North America and Europe and a 2- to 3-fold higher incidence in Asia.[6] The peak

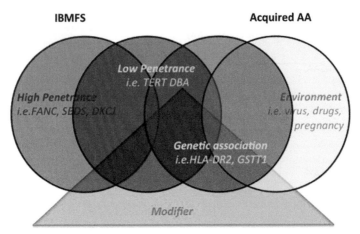

Fig. 2. Relationship between genetic mutations, disease penetrance, and gene-environment interaction in the pathogenesis of bone marrow failure. Mutations with a high disease penetrance almost always cause disease; that is, mutations in the Fanconi anemia genes (*FANC*), in the *SBDS* gene causing Shwachman-Diamond syndrome, or in *DKC1* causing X-linked dyskeratosis congenita. By contrast, mutations in genes with low disease penetrance may not manifest as clinically apparent bone marrow failure; examples include mutations in the *TERT* gene responsible for autosomal dominant dyskeratosis congenita or in certain *DBA* genes responsible for Diamond-Blackfan anemia.[3] Genetic polymorphisms associated with AA do not cause disease in the majority of carriers but, in combination with other modifier genes and the appropriate environmental insult, may contribute to the development of AA. Examples are HLA-DR2 in adult AA and HLA-B14 in pediatric AA or *GSTT1* gene deletions. (*Data from* Refs.[70,72,83,84])

incidence is in adolescents and young adults as well as in the elderly, with a roughly equal male to female ratio.[6] A classification of AA based on etiology is summarized in **Table 1**.

PATHOGENESIS

For many years, an immune-mediated pathogenesis has been postulated for AA because immunosuppressive therapy (IST) is often successful in the treatment of AA, and bone marrow lymphocytes from AA patients can suppress normal bone marrow in vitro.[7] Results from numerous laboratories have demonstrated increased cytokine expression, low CD4 T regulatory cells, oligoclonal CD8 cytotoxic T cells, and, to a lesser extent, expansion of specific CD4 cell populations in the bone marrow of AA patients.[8,9] Coupled with the recent finding of acquired copy number–neutral loss of heterozygosity of the short arm of chromosome 6 (6pLOH), representing a likely genetic signature of immune escape,[10] these findings have strengthened the belief that bone marrow aplasia in acquired AA is immune-mediated, replacing the conventional term "idiopathic AA" with "immune-mediated AA" (**Fig. 3**).

CLINICAL PRESENTATION

Most children with AA present with signs and symptoms resulting from advanced pancytopenia, with others being diagnosed by incidental laboratory findings. Thrombocytopenia may manifest as easy bruising or petechiae. Epistaxis and menorrhagia in postmenarchal girls are other common complaints at presentation. Anemia may

Box 2 Differentiation of aplastic anemia (AA) and refractory cytopenia of childhood (RCC)		
	AA	**RCC**
Erythropoiesis		
Bone marrow histology	Decreased	Decreased
	Possible single large loci with <10 cells	Left shifted, mitosis, clustered ± Dysplastic
Peripheral blood	Decreased reticulocytes	Increased MCV Increased fHb Increased reticulocytes
Granulopoiesis		
Bone marrow histology	Decreased	Decreased Left shifted ± Dysplastic
Megakaryopoiesis		
Bone marrow histology	Decreased or absent	Decreased Dysplastic Micromegakaryocytes
Dysplastic changes in bone marrow aspirate	None	<0% in 2 cell lineages >10% in 1 lineage
Reticulin in bone marrow biopsy	No increase	No increase
Cellularity of bone marrow biopsy	<25%	Hypocellular
Severity of cytopenia in peripheral blood	Frequently severe or very severe	Frequently severe or moderate
Lymphocytes		
Bone marrow histology	May be increased focally or dispersed	May be increased focally or dispersed
Blast in bone marrow aspirate and biopsy	Not increased	<5% (<2% peripheral blood)
Cytogenetics		
Numerical or structural chromosomal abnormality	Absent, transient	More prevalent than in AA

Abbreviations: fHb, fetal hemoglobin; MCV, mean corpuscular volume.

Data from Baumann I, Niemeyer C, Bennett J, et al. Childhood myelodysplastic syndrome. In: Swerdlow S, Campo E, Harris NL, et al, editors. WHO classification of tumors of haematopoietic and lymphoid tissue, vol. 2. Lyon (France): International Agency for Research on Cancer; 2008. p. 104–7; and Baumann I, Fuhrer M, Behrendt S, et al. Morphological differentiation of severe aplastic anaemia from hypocellular refractory cytopenia of childhood: reproducibility of histopathological diagnostic criteria. Histopathology 2012;61:10–7.

manifest as pallor, fatigue, or exercise intolerance. Neutropenia may predispose to infections and, thus, fever or focal signs of infection can occur as initial complaints. Hepatosplenomegaly and lymphadenopathy are typically absent. A history of jaundice often occurring 2 to 3 months before discovery of pancytopenia is consistent with hepatitis-associated AA.

ESTABLISHING THE DIAGNOSIS

A comprehensive history should include exposure to medications, recreational drugs, and chemicals as well as preceding infectious symptoms. The family history needs to be detailed, and assessed for diseases and signs suggestive of IBMFS (**Table 2**). A comprehensive laboratory panel is requested to establish the diagnosis of AA, classify

Table 1
Etiology associated with acquired AA

Infectious		Hepatitis-associated, typically seronegative
		Epstein-Barr virus
		Cytomegalovirus
		Parvovirus
		Mycobacterial infections
		Human immunodeficiency virus
		Human herpesvirus 6
		Varicella zoster virus
		Measles
		Adenovirus
		And others
Nutritional		Copper deficiency
		Vitamin B_{12}
		Folic acid
Drugs	Toxic	Nonsteroidal anti-inflammatory drugs
		Antibiotics
		Anticonvulsants
		Sulfonamides
		Gold salts
	Idiosyncratic	Many additional agents rarely associated with aplastic anemia
		Chloramphenicol
Chemicals		Benzene
		Insecticides
		Pesticides
		Solvents
Radiation		
Other associations		Pregnancy
		Inflammatory and autoimmune (eg, systemic lupus erythematosus)
		Graft-versus-host disease
Idiopathic		Of unknown etiology, this term is increasingly replaced by "immune-mediated AA"

its severity, and screen for potential causative factors (**Table 3**). A bone marrow aspirate and biopsy are needed to establish the diagnosis (see **Fig. 1**). A complete blood count, reticulocyte count, and review of the peripheral blood smear confirm existing cytopenias and exclude signs of dysplasia. Review of the biopsy is required to grade the severity of disease (see **Box 1**). AA can present with a hematopoietic cell clone that already lacks glycosyl phosphatidylinositol (GPI)-anchored proteins characteristic of paroxysmal nocturnal hemoglobinuria (PNH) at the time of diagnosis. Flow cytometry for the absence of GPI-anchored proteins is used to detect an early PNH cell clone.[11,12] However, because of leukopenia, testing for PNH at diagnosis has poor sensitivity and needs to be repeated when neutrophil counts are recovering. Patients with acquired AA have deceased numbers of regulatory T cells (Treg, CD4$^+$CD25$^+$ T cells). The number of Treg negatively correlates with the severity of disease, and low Treg numbers have been found to be associated with treatment failure.[13] At the Comprehensive Bone Marrow Failure Center of the Children's Hospital of Philadelphia (CHOP), the authors routinely assess peripheral lymphocytes with chromosome breakage studies to rule out Fanconi anemia (FA), and telomere-length analysis is performed to rule out dyskeratosis congenita (DC). Because these tests may take several days to complete, and because results have a great impact on treatment decisions, it

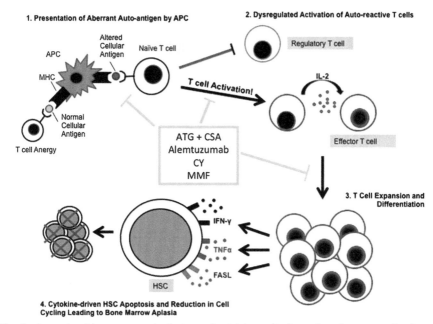

Fig. 3. Current evidence suggests that acquired AA results from the aberrant activation of one or more autoreactive T-cell clones caused by alteration of antigens presented by the major histocompatibility complex (MHC) on the surface of antigen-presenting cells (APC). This antigen alteration is triggered by viral infection, chemical exposure, or genetic mutation, and leads to the inappropriate activation of antigen-specific effector T cells and decreased activity of regulatory T cells, which normally serve to prevent autoimmunity. T-cell activation leads to interleukin (IL)-2–driven expansion and differentiation of T cells into effector and memory T cells. These proinflammatory T cells produce a variety of cytokines, including FAS ligand (FASL), interferon-γ (IFN-γ), and tumor necrosis factor α (TNFα), which (1) induce hematopoietic stem cell (HSC) apoptosis and (2) alter gene regulation and decrease protein synthesis to prevent HSC cycling, ultimately leading to bone marrow failure. Immunosuppressive therapy disrupts T-cell–driven HSC destruction by inhibiting T-cell responses at several points along this pathway. (*Data from* Young NS, Calado RT, Scheinberg P. Current concepts in the pathophysiology and treatment of aplastic anemia. Blood 2006;108:2509–19; and Shin SH, Lee JW. The optimal immunosuppressive therapy for aplastic anemia. Int J Hematol 2013;97:564–72.)

is recommended that these tests be performed early in the evaluation. The initial clinical presentation of patients with either FA or DC may be indistinguishable from that seen in patients with acquired AA. Genetic testing to confirm the diagnosis of DC is ordered when a patient with an aplastic marrow has a telomere length in peripheral blood lymphocytes that is far below the first percentile of that in healthy controls (of note, different criteria are used for dyskeratosis in a nonaplastic patient).[14]

Bone marrow examination usually includes cytogenetic studies, including a karyotype and fluorescence in situ hybridization (FISH) analysis for monosomy 7, trisomy 8, and others as indicated by the karyotype results. The utility of genome-wide single-nucleotide polymorphism (SNP) arrays performed in addition to conventional cytogenetics currently remains investigational, but may be helpful for the early detection of clonal hematopoiesis.[15,16]

The authors routinely obtain high-resolution HLA typing, including a preliminary donor search at diagnosis in all patients who present with severe AA (SAA) and very

Table 2
Features suggestive of inherited bone marrow failure syndromes (IBMFS) in a patient with pancytopenia

Clinical history	Failure to thrive
	History of cytopenia, easy bruising, frequent infections
	Malabsorption/maldigestion
	Developmental delay
Family history	Family members with cytopenias, myelodysplastic syndrome, or leukemia
	Cancer of the breast, lung, esophagus, head and neck in multiple family members
	Pulmonary fibrosis, liver fibrosis, early osteoporosis
	Family members with congenital anomalies associated with IBMFS
Physical examination	Short stature, congenital anomalies, dysmorphologies
	Abnormal skin pigmentation, birth marks
	Nail abnormalities
	Limb (especially forearm) abnormalities
	Other skeletal abnormalities
	Renal and genitourinary abnormalities
	Cardiac abnormalities
	Eye abnormalities
	Cleft lip/palate
	Hair or teeth abnormalities
	Developmental delay
Laboratory workup	Increased chromosomal breakage after exposure to cross-linking agents
	Very short telomere lengths in lymphocytes
	Macrocytosis
	Increased fetal hemoglobin

severe AA (vSAA) (see **Box 1**), even in the absence of a potential sibling donor. Early HLA typing will expedite an unrelated donor search for patients who are refractory to IST, and will be beneficial for patients in whom the initial investigations reveal an underlying IBMFS diagnosis.

Early therapeutic interventions (IST <4 weeks and bone marrow transplantation [BMT] <12 weeks from presentation) are associated with significantly improved outcomes in acquired AA.[17] Thus, every effort should be made to complete diagnostic evaluations and initiate therapy within 3 to 4 weeks of the initial diagnosis.

SUPPORTIVE CARE

Gains in survival for patients with acquired AA are due in part to the improvement in supportive therapy.[18] However, infections and bleeding still remain a major cause of morbidity and mortality in this patient population.[19,20] In an afebrile patient with a good performance status (Eastern Cooperative Oncology Group/WHO/Zubrod 0–2), the evaluation of AA may be performed in the outpatient setting in a center and by a care team experienced in treating AA patients.

Although there is a lack of strong evidence for most strategies in preventing neutropenic infections, the authors prescribe basic neutropenic precautions for patients with neutrophil counts lower than 500/μL (**Table 4**). Prophylactic antifungals are routinely used for AA patients with prolonged (>7 days) neutrophil counts of less than 500/μL[21] or for AA patients on IST (**Fig. 4**). In AA patients with lymphopenia

Table 3
Clinical evaluation of aplastic anemia

1. Establishing diagnosis and severity of AA	**Clinical history and physical examination**
	Complete blood count and differential
	Reticulocyte count
	Peripheral blood smear
	Bone marrow aspirate and biopsy
	Bone marrow cytogenetics
	Liver function tests, serum bilirubin, lactate dehydrogenase
2. Exclusion of inherited bone marrow failure syndromes (IBMFS)	**Clinical history**
	Family history
	Physical examination
	Chromosomal breakage studies in peripheral blood
	Telomere length measurement in peripheral blood
	Increased fetal hemoglobin (several IBMFS)
	Consider *c-mpl* testing
	Consider additional diagnostic and genetic testing for IBMFS if suspected
3. Assess for specific causes and association	**Viral serology** (hepatitis virus panel, CMV, EBV, parvovirus, VZV, HSV, HHV6, HIV, adenovirus)
	Flow cytometry of peripheral blood for paroxysmal nocturnal hemoglobinuria (PNH)
	Vitamin B$_{12}$ and folate
	Copper, ceruloplasmin, zinc
	Immunology: lymphocyte subsets (including CD4+, CD25+ regulatory T cells), quantitative immunoglobulins
	Autoimmune or inflammatory disease evaluation
	HLA typing
	Pregnancy test
	T-cell receptor rearrangement

In bold: tests routinely performed in all patients investigated for AA.
Abbreviations: CMV, cytomegalovirus; EBV, Epstein-Barr virus; HHV6, human herpesvirus 6; HIV, human immunodeficiency virus; HSV, herpes simplex virus; VZV, varicella zoster virus.

Table 4
Basic principles of neutropenic precaution for pediatric AA patients

Avoid	Recommend	Consider
Construction areas	Frequent hand washing	Air quality control
Garbage, compost, potted plants	Hospital guidelines for hygienic routine	Barrier isolation
Unpasteurized dairy products and fruit juices	Prophylactic antifungals	Prophylactic antibiotics
Uncooked meats, seafood, eggs		
Unwashed fruits and vegetables	G-CSF with IST	
Raw nuts and dried fruits		
Crowded rooms with no air-quality control		
Vaccinations with live vaccines		
Tampon use for women		
Situation whereby may get injured, ie, manicures or pedicures		

Abbreviations: G-CSF, granulocyte-colony stimulating factor; IST, immunosuppressive therapy.

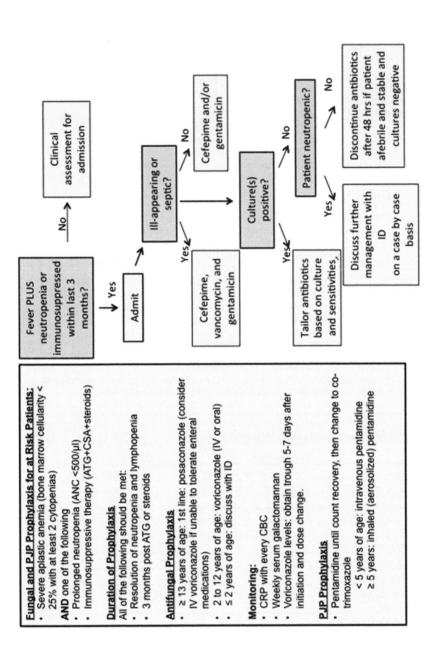

Fig. 4. Flow diagram for antimicrobial prophylaxis and empiric management of fever for patients with severe aplastic anemia, currently used at the Comprehensive Bone Marrow Failure Center, CHOP/University of Pennsylvania. ANC, absolute neutrophil count; ATG, antithymocyte globulin; CBC, complete blood count; CRP, C-reactive protein; CSA, cyclosporine; ID, infectious disease specialist; IV, intravenous; PJP, *Pneumocystis jirovecii* pneumonia. (*Courtesy of* Drs Talene Metjian, PharmD, Brian T. Fisher, DO MSCE, Infectious Diseases, and Shefali Parikh, MD, Hematology, The Children's Hospital of Philadelphia.)

(<500/µL) or those receiving IST, *Pneumocystis jirovecii* pneumonia (PJP) prophylaxis is provided. Trimethoprim/sulfamethoxazole (cotrimoxazole, TMP/SMX) three times weekly has been shown to be superior to oral dapsone, aerosolized pentamidine, or oral atovaquone in individuals with lymphopenia from human immunodeficiency virus or chemotherapy,[21] although owing to its potential bone marrow toxicity TMP/SMX is frequently abandoned when recovery of AA is delayed. The authors therefore use aerosolized pentamidine as a first-line PJP prophylaxis in children with AA, because it has good PJP protection in this patient population and has very good therapy-patient compliance rates attributable to its monthly dosing.[22]

Granulocyte-colony stimulating factor (G-CSF) alone is not a treatment of AA, and its routine use for patients with AA is controversial. At the authors' center, G-CSF is given to pediatric AA patients with neutrophil counts lower than 500/µL in combination with IST. Prolonged use of high doses of G-CSF may increase the risk of clonal hematopoiesis and malignant transformation to MDS/acute myelogenous leukemia.[23]

Neutropenic fever requires immediate attention and hospitalization with the initiation of antibiotic therapy according to preestablished hospital guidelines (see **Fig. 4**). For persistent fever or suspected fungal infection, galactomannan testing and a computed tomography scan of the chest are performed, and empiric antifungal agents are started. In life-threatening situations, the use of granulocyte infusions may be considered to provide a bridge between treatment response and neutrophil recovery.[24]

Platelet transfusions should be considered to prevent bleeding in asymptomatic patients with platelet counts lower than 10,000/µL. Higher thresholds for platelet transfusions are reserved for patients with either active bleeding or a history of significant bleeding complications. Higher thresholds (<20,000/µL) are also recommended in patients at risk for worsening thrombocytopenia (eg, febrile patients or those receiving IST).

Transfusion policies in patients with AA are, in general, restrictive. Institutional policies vary; in their practice the authors transfuse red blood cell concentrates for hemoglobin less than 8 g/dL or if symptomatic. Leukodepleted and irradiated blood products should be given to reduce the risk of transfusion-associated graft-versus-host disease (GVHD) and HLA sensitization.[25] Iron chelation is initiated for patients who remain transfusion dependent over a prolonged period. Iron chelation is performed with desferrioxamine or deferasirox. Deferiprone is not recommended for AA patients with iron overload because of the associated risk of agranulocytosis.[26]

Institutional policies and recommendations for vaccinations vary. The authors do not recommend vaccination until 1 year after the cessation of IST, at which time age-appropriate vaccines may be resumed. The use of inactivated vaccines is recommended. Because of potential infectious complications from live attenuated vaccines and the potential risk of AA relapse, live attenuated vaccines are not recommended in this population, although in each case the immunologic benefit of using attenuated live viruses has to be weighed against the potential risk of AA relapse.

Psychosocial support of patients and families and an age-appropriate explanation of disease, treatment, and prognosis are important at diagnosis and during the course of disease, and improve therapy adherence and disease outcomes. Psychosocial support is particularly important at the time of transition from pediatric to adult health care. Often there is a lack of ancillary support services to assist in care transition in the adult-care settings, which may result in a lack of continuity of care and poor therapy compliance.

DEFINITIVE TREATMENT

Once a diagnosis is firmly established, BMT and IST are currently the primary treatment options for AA patients, both children and adults. Numerous studies have established that BMT is highly successful when an HLA-matched sibling is available (matched related donor [MRD]), with 5-year survival rates of 90% and higher, making BMT the recommended first-line therapy in this setting (**Fig. 5**). In North America, the current practice is to reserve matched unrelated donor (URD) BMT for patients with SAA or vSAA who have failed IST.[27] However, with improved outcomes for patients who undergo matched URD transplant and with better donor availability, URD transplant may become a first-line therapy for patients with SAA or vSAA for whom a matched sibling is not available and for whom an excellent unrelated donor has been identified. Upfront URD transplant for children and young adults with SAA or vSAA is increasingly used in countries where horse antithymocyte globulin (ATG) is no longer available because IST using an alternative agent, rabbit ATG, is associated with a lower response rate (see later discussion).[28,29]

BONE MARROW TRANSPLANT

The current standard approach to BMT for pediatric patients with acquired AA is summarized in **Table 5**.

Matched Related Donor Bone Marrow Transplantation for Aplastic Anemia

Conditioning
Since the early 1990s, the standard conditioning regimen for MRD-BMT has been high-dose cyclophosphamide (CY; 200 mg/kg divided into 4 daily 50 mg/kg doses)

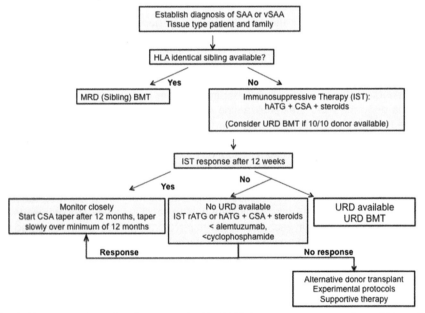

Fig. 5. Treatment algorithm for AA and sAA. BMT, bone marrow transplant; CSA, cyclosporine; hATG, horse antithymocyte globulin; IST, immunosuppressive therapy; MRD, matched related donor; rATG, rabbit antithymocyte globulin; URD, unrelated donor.

Table 5
Current approaches to BMT for pediatric patients with acquired AA

Conditioning	
Matched related donor	ATG + cyclophosphamide
Matched unrelated donor	ATG + fludarabine + cyclophosphamide[a] ± TBI[b]
Mismatched unrelated, haploidentical, or cord blood	Clinical trials ongoing
GVHD/Rejection Prophylaxis	
Agents	CSA/tacrolimus ± MTX/MMF
Duration of CSA/tacrolimus	≥6 mo followed by slow taper
Antimicrobial Prophylaxis	
Pneumocystis jirovecii	TMP/SMX (first-line) or alternative × 1 y
HSV/VZV	Acyclovir × 1 y if history of infection or positive HSV serology
CMV	Prophylaxis based on donor/recipient serology
Antifungal	Prophylaxis before neutrophil engraftment or during immunosuppression treatment for GVHD
Antibacterial	Penicillin if asplenic or for prolonged chronic GVHD

Abbreviations: ATG, antithymocyte globulin; CSA, cyclosporine; GVHD, graft-versus-host disease; MMF, mycophenolate mofetil; MTX, methotrexate; TBI, total body irradiation; TMP/SMX, trimethoprim-sulfamethoxazole.
[a] Optimal dose unknown, subject of ongoing clinical trials.
[b] Included in the United States, omitted in European regimens for younger pediatric patients.

plus ATG (CY-ATG).[30,31] Long-term analyses have shown that the Cy-ATG regimen in MRD-BMT for acquired AA results in decreased rates of GVHD and improved long-term overall survival in comparison with regimens that include total body irradiation (TBI).[32,33] At present, engraftment rates using CY-ATG are as high as 96%,[32] with overall survival (OS) in children estimated at 91% compared with 74% in adults.[17] Of interest, a recent randomized trial comparing outcomes for acquired AA patients receiving MRD-BMT with either CY alone or CY-ATG demonstrated no difference in graft failure, GVHD, or OS between the two regimens,[34] calling into question whether ATG is still needed in the MRD-BMT regimen for acquired AA, given the decreased risk of alloimmunization in the current era of first-line MRD-BMT therapy and leukoreduced blood products.

In older adults, fludarabine-containing regimens that enable dose reduction of CY (FLU-CY) are replacing CY 200 mg/kg regimens to reduce organ cytotoxicity and intensify immunosuppression, resulting in improved OS.[35] Small pediatric case series have shown excellent survival and engraftment with regimens containing fludarabine (180 mg/m^2) and dose-reduced CY (120 mg/kg).[36,37] Although such a regimen may decrease rates of alkylating agent–induced gonadal dysfunction,[38–40] prospective randomized trials are needed to compare its efficacy with that of standard CY-ATG regimens.

Graft source
Peripheral blood stem cells (PBSC) are increasingly used in matched sibling allogeneic transplantation for malignant conditions. However, retrospective analysis in patients undergoing MRD transplantation for acquired AA demonstrated a significant decrease in 5-year OS in pediatric acquired AA patients receiving PBSC (73%) versus bone

marrow (BM) (85%) grafts, likely because of a markedly increased incidence in chronic GVHD occurring in recipients of PBSCs in comparison with BM (27% vs 12%).[41] Therefore, unlike in transplantation for pediatric malignancies, whereby PBSC may elicit beneficial graft-versus-leukemia effects, BM is clearly the preferred stem-cell source for acquired AA patients.

Graft failure, GVHD, and donor chimerism

Rates of primary graft failure following MRD-BMT for acquired AA patients have declined from greater than 30% in early studies to current rates of less than 10%,[30,32] in large part due to decreased time to initial BMT, decreased transfusion exposure, and increased use of leukoreduced blood products.[42] Both acute and chronic GVHD remain a significant source of short-term and long-term morbidity for patients receiving MRD-BMT for acquired AA.[40] Prior studies demonstrated superiority of short-course methotrexate plus cyclosporine (MTX+CSA) versus cyclosporine (CSA) alone in prevention of GVHD and improvement in OS[43]; thus MTX-CSA remains the standard-of-care GVHD prophylaxis regimen. However, recent series have not identified differences in survival in comparisons of CSA with MTX+CSA prophylaxis regimens[17] while another prospective study has demonstrated equivalence of mycophenolate (MMF) plus CSA with MTX-CSA regimens in terms of GVHD incidence, with improvement in time to neutrophil engraftment in the MMF arm.[44] Tacrolimus appears to have efficacy equivalent to that of CSA in preventing GVHD.[45] CSA/tacrolimus should be continued for at least 6 months after transplantation in AA patients, followed by a slow taper, as this prolonged course serves not only to prevent GVHD but also to prevent secondary graft failure and relapse of BM aplasia.[46]

Mixed donor/recipient chimerism occurs in 44% to 55% of acquired AA patients following MRD-BMT.[40,46] A study of serial chimerism analysis in acquired AA patients indicates that while many develop transient or stable mixed chimerism, patients who exhibit progressive decline in donor chimerism, particularly during withdrawal of immunosuppression, are at highest risk for late graft rejection and poor OS.[46] In contrast to the standard approach following BMT for leukemia, whereby immunosuppression is withdrawn in response to falling donor chimerism, current recommendations include serial chimerism analysis and reinstitution of immunosuppression for acquired AA patients with falling donor chimerism after BMT.

Alternative Donor Bone Marrow Transplantation for Aplastic Anemia

Donor selection

Outcomes following URD-BMT for acquired AA have improved dramatically since the early 1990s, when OS was typically less than 40%.[43] This improvement is in large part due to improved sensitivity in methods of HLA typing and donor matching. In recent pediatric series using fully or closely matched donors, long-term OS following URD-BMT for acquired AA ranges from 78% to 94%[47,48] of patients, approaching the survival reported for MRD-BMT. Unfortunately, patients lacking a closely HLA-matched unrelated or related donor who undergo mismatched URD-BMT continue to exhibit poor outcomes, with several studies suggesting survival of less than 40%.[42] At present, therefore, transplant approaches for acquired AA patients without a closely matched URD should only be undertaken in the setting of ongoing clinical trials.

Unrelated cord blood transplantation (CBT) has had limited success in acquired AA patients. A large retrospective series including both pediatric and adult patients demonstrated a disappointing 3-year OS of 38%,[49] with graft failure the major cause of mortality. However, smaller case series restricted to pediatric patients have shown better rates of engraftment and OS, confirming the need for further pediatric studies.[42] Of note, the successful use of autologous cord blood units in restoring hematopoiesis in pediatric acquired AA patients has now been reported,[50] sparking new debate regarding the utility of private cord banking programs. Haploidentical stem cell transplantation (HaploSCT) from related donors using unmanipulated grafts has previously been associated with very poor outcomes; however, recent successes have been achieved with HaploSCT in pediatric acquired AA patients using partial T-cell depletion strategies to promote engraftment and OS.[51] Coinfusion of donor mesenchymal stem cells may promote immunologic tolerance, further enabling enhanced donor engraftment following haploSCT.[52]

Conditioning regimens

Optimal conditioning regimens for URD-BMT in acquired AA remain controversial.[53] Regimens using high-dose (HD) TBI can overcome the increased risk of graft failure in URD-BMT for pediatric acquired AA and, combined with partial T-cell depletion, can improve OS in comparison with regimens containing CY alone.[54] However, HD TBI regimens cause high rates of both early toxicity and late effects.[39] Subsequent studies have suggested that a lower dose of TBI (200 cGy) combined with full-dose CY enables high OS with lower regimen-related toxicity.[53] European data suggest that addition of fludarabine to regimens containing CY and ATG enables the elimination of TBI altogether for acquired AA patients younger than 14 years receiving URD-BMT, with an OS of 84% and a graft failure rate of 5%.[55] In the United States, ongoing studies including pediatric patients are using fludarabine with 200 cGy of TBI while investigating dose reduction of CY.[35] At CHOP the authors are conducting a prospective study of alemtuzumab, fludarabine, and melphalan reduced intensity conditioning for matched URD transplantation in patients with nonmalignant disorders including acquired AA. To date, 3 of 3 acquired AA patients have been treated successfully with this regimen with a follow-up of longer than 2 years posttransplantation (Nancy Bunin, personal communication, 2013).

Follow-Up and Late Effects After Stem Cell Transplantation for Acquired AA

For acquired AA patients receiving BMT, the authors require follow-up in a specialized blood and marrow transplant clinic for at least 1 year after transplantation. Because of limited adaptive immune reconstitution during this time, fevers are treated aggressively with blood cultures and parenteral antibiotics until systemic infection is ruled out. *Pneumocystis* prophylaxis is continued through the first year post-BMT, as is antiviral prophylaxis based on donor and recipient serologies. Following the first year posttransplant and in the absence of complications such as organ toxicity, GVHD, or graft failure, care is gradually transitioned back to the primary pediatrician. Full reimmunization is recommended beginning at 1 year after transplantation, or when adequate immune reconstitution is documented.

While follow-up continues in specialized transplant clinics beyond the first year post-BMT, general pediatricians often play a critical role in early recognition of the late complications of BMT (**Table 6**). Routine screening should include assessments of growth, endocrine function, pulmonary function, bone health, and cancer screening to ensure prompt detection and therapy for potential late effects. Long-term follow-up for late effects of therapy in pediatric AA patients is now available out to nearly 4 decades after treatment.[32,33,38,39] In general, pediatric acquired AA patients who receive MRD-BMT with CY-based regimens that do not contain TBI have excellent long-term outcomes, with normal growth rates and normal thyroid function. Although transient ovarian dysfunction is common, most prepubertal girls receiving MRD-BMT without

Table 6
Late effects of BMT for pediatric patients with acquired AA

	Conditioning Regimen	
	Chemotherapy Alone	**HD TBI + Chemotherapy**
Endocrine		
Growth abnormalities	Rare	Uncommon
Infertility	Rare in females, may occur in males	Common
Impaired pubertal development	Rare in females, may occur in males	Common
Thyroid dysfunction	Rare	Common
Second malignancy	Uncommon: skin/oral cancer[a]	Common: skin/oral[a], meningiomas, breast, thyroid, head/neck
Vision	Rare[a]	Cataracts
Cardiovascular	Hypertension[a]	Hypertension[a], metabolic syndrome
Pulmonary, hepatic, gastrointestinal	Uncommon[a]	Restrictive lung disease
Renal	Uncommon[b]	Uncommon[b]
Bone		
Avascular necrosis	Uncommon[a]	Uncommon[a]
Decreased bone density	Common[a]	Common[a]
Dental	Common[c]	Common[c]
Neurocognitive	Uncommon[d]	Uncommon[d]

Abbreviation: HD TBI, high-dose total body irradiation.
[a] Strongly associated with chronic GVHD and long-term steroid treatment.
[b] Usually associated with calcineurin inhibitors or nephrotoxic antimicrobials.
[c] Increased risk of abnormal development of permanent teeth, retention of primary teeth, poor mineralization, and caries: requires regular dental screening (every 6 months).
[d] True incidence of neurocognitive abnormalities following BMT is the subject of ongoing prospective studies.

TBI progress normally through puberty with preserved gonadal function and fertility, whereas males receiving high-dose CY regimens without TBI may develop prolonged azoospermia or exhibit abnormalities in pubertal development.[39] Recipients of TBI-containing regimens have much higher incidences of cataracts, thyroid abnormalities, gonadal dysfunction, and infertility than patients not receiving TBI,[50] although incidences of late effects caused specifically by low-dose TBI (200 cGy) regimens now used in URD-BMT are less well defined.

In contrast to acquired AA treated with IST, patients treated with BMT rarely develop leukemia or MDS. However, incidence of solid malignancy exceeds 10% when patient follow-up is extended beyond 15 years,[32,33,39] with major risk factors including TBI-based conditioning and chronic GVHD. A recent large series demonstrated a 5-year cumulative incidence of chronic GVHD of 22% and 37% for MRD-BMT and URD-BMT, respectively.[38] In addition to increased risk of malignancy, pediatric acquired AA patients who develop chronic GVHD after BMT have a much higher incidence of gonadal dysfunction, pulmonary function deficits, avascular necrosis, and abnormal bone density than patients without chronic GVHD.[38]

IMMUNOSUPPRESSIVE THERAPY

IST is currently the first-line therapy for patients with SAA or vSAA who lack an MRD (see **Fig. 5**). Most centers treating patients with AA use ATG and CSA as their first-line IST. In the United States, horse ATG (hATG, ATGAM; Upjohn, Kalamazoo, MI) is most commonly used. **Table 7** summarizes the IST treatment algorithm using hATG/ATGAM. A short course of corticosteroids is used to reduce the risk of serum sickness. There is no other role for corticosteroids in AA, thus dosing should be adjusted accordingly. The addition of CSA to hATG has significantly increased the response to treatment (65% hATG+CSA vs 31% ATG alone at 6 months),[56] and in multiple studies has shown an excellent overall 10-year survival of 82% to 93%.[57] CSA is usually started with ATG, but may also be given after the completion of ATG infusion, in patients with liver or kidney dysfunction or in those with preexisting hypertension, which often results in a better tolerance of the ATG+CSA regimen. In children, an increased rate of relapse was associated with a rapid CSA discontinuation (60% vs 7.6%),[58] and 15% to 25% of children remained CSA dependent.[58] Thus, it is recommended that CSA should generally be continued for at least 12 months in children after stable remission has been obtained, followed by a slow taper over a minimum of 12 months.[57,59]

In Europe, hATG (Lymphoglobuline; Genzyme Corp, Cambridge, MA) has most commonly been used until recently.[60] However, hATG is no longer available in Europe and Japan, so rabbit ATG (rATG, Thymoglobuline; Genzyme) currently is used (3.75 mg/kg for 5 days). Several important retrospective studies have demonstrated that rATG is inferior to hATG, with a lower response rate at 6 months and an increased rate of infections leading to a decreased OS at 2 years.[19,20] Although these findings

Table 7
Immunosuppressive therapy for severe aplastic anemia

Drug	Dose	Route	Schedule
ATGAM (equine antithymocyte globulin, hATG)[a]	40 mg/kg/d	IV	Days 1–4 Initial dose over 8–10 h, subsequent doses over 6–8 h
Cyclosporine[b] (CSA)	5–15 mg/kg/d Divided in 2 doses	PO	Starting on day 1 (or 5) Target trough blood level 200–400 ng/mL For 12 mo after stable CR or PR Then taper over 12 mo
Methylprednisolone[c]	1 or 2 mg/kg/d	IV/PO	Days 1–5, before ATG infusion Change to 1 mg/kg/d prednisone by mouth days 6–10, then individualize taper over 14 d
G-CSF	Starting dose 3–5 μg/kg daily	SQ	If ANC <500/μL Wean if consistently ANC >500/μL

Abbreviations: ANC, absolute neutrophil count; CR, complete response; IV, intravenous; PO, by mouth; PR, partial response; SQ, subcutaneous.

[a] Antihistamine and oral antipyretics are given before each ATG infusion (ie, acetaminophen and diphenhydramine).

[b] Reduce cyclosporine dose to 5mg/kg/day divided in 2 doses, maximum 200mg/kg/dose, when given concomitantly with voriconazole.

[c] H2-receptor antagonists (ranitidine) or a proton-pump inhibitor (latter might worsen CSA-associated hypomagnesemia) should be considered for peptic ulcer prophylaxis with high-dose steroids.

have not been observed in all primarily retrospectives studies, none of the studies have shown that rATG is superior to hATG. A recent retrospective study focusing on children confirmed a lower response rate at 6 months (36% for rATG and 65% for hATG) although, because of second-line URD-BMT, 3-year OS was similar, at 92% in both groups.[29] Thus, current IST recommendations for the treatment of children with AA should include hATG, and URD-BMT should be offered to all nonresponders early in the course of disease (3–6 months).[27]

G-CSF

Although G-CSF alone is not recommended for the treatment of AA, the addition of G-CSF to ATG and CSA in patients with SAA and vSAA increases neutrophil counts and reduces infections and days of hospitalization in the first 3 months of treatment, but has no impact on survival, response to treatment, or relapse.[61]

Alternative First-Line Therapies

Over the years several newer immunosuppressive agents have been investigated in hopes of improving the outcome of front-line IST in AA. These agents include mycophenolate mofetil, sirolimus, and alemtuzumab, none of which improved responses, or decreased relapse or clonal evolution. Tacrolimus as an alternative to CSA showed a comparable response rate in children, with a more favorable toxicity profile; however, this study was not powered to definitively assess the statistical analysis of relapse.[62] The addition of danazol to IST in children with AA was associated with a significant increase in relapse.[63] High-dose CY without stem cell support is used by the Johns Hopkins Group[64] as first-line therapy for pediatric and adult AA, with response rates comparable to those of IST with hATG and CSA. However, because of prolonged neutropenia associated with this protocol, high-dose CY is usually only considered as a second-line or third-line therapy by most centers.

Recently eltrombopag, a small, nonpeptide thrombopoietin receptor (c-MPL) agonist, has been shown to improve hematopoiesis in 11 of 25 adult AA patients who were refractory to IST; including 6 patients who showed improvement in all 3 blood cell lineages.[65] Although these results suggest that eltrombopag, and possibly other c-MPL agonists, may represent a new approach for the treatment of acquired AA, a major concern is the possible increased risk of clonal evolution and leukemia.[65] Thus, pending additional studies, eltrombopag or other c-MPL agonists should be restricted to clinical trial settings.

MODERATE OR NONSEVERE AA

The approach to patients with moderate AA is less defined. Studies on the natural history of nonsevere AA (NSAA) are inconsistent, most likely because of the heterogeneity of this patient population, differences in the study populations (pediatric vs adult NSAA), and the difficulty in excluding IBMFS and low-grade MDS. Often patients with NSAA require only supportive therapy and no specific treatment for their cytopenia. NSAA may resolve spontaneously or progress to SAA. In children, transformation to MDS or leukemia in patients who were cytogenetically normal at diagnosis is rare.[66–68] For NSAA patients who show signs of progression or who are transfusion dependent, IST is suggested as the first choice of treatment. In adult patients with NSAA, hATG+CSA was found to be superior to CSA alone (30% at 6 months for CSA alone and 65% for hATG+CSA); both groups had excellent long-term OS (>90%), although relapse was more frequent with CSA alone.[69]

RESPONSE, RELAPSE, AND LATE EFFECTS AFTER IST FOR ACQUIRED AA
Response

A complete response (CR) is defined as a normalization of peripheral blood values in at least 2 separate blood cell counts at least 4 weeks apart (**Box 3**). Response is usually assessed 3, 6, and 12 months after ATG initiation. Response to treatment usually occurs within 3 to 6 months of treatment initiation, but in some patients the response may be delayed. The 6-month response rate for hATG+CSA varies among studies from 60% to 77%, with these recent studies estimating a current 10-year OS of about 80% (in children about 90%–93%) and a relapse rate of 10% to 33%.[27] In adult AA patients there is an increased frequency for HLA-DR2, particularly HLA-DRB1*15, and this was associated with an improved response to IST with CSA.[70,71] Neither association was confirmed in children.[72,73] By contrast, in children an increased frequency of HLA-B14 was associated with SAA.[72]

Relapse

Relapse is highest during the first 3 years of IST therapy.[63,74]

Second-Line Therapy

For children without an MRD, who relapse or are refractory to first-line IST, URD transplant should be considered if a suitable matched donor is available (see **Fig. 5**).[28,75] In children with IST-refractory SAA or vSAA, an early URD-BMT is suggested (3–6 months after initial IST). If a matched URD is not available, relapse or initial IST-refractory patients are usually treated with a second course of hATG+CSA or with rATG+CSA. In contrast to its use in first-line therapy (response rate of 30%–40%, see above), rATG used at relapse has a response rate of 65%, though only 30% for patients who have failed first-line hATG+CSA.[76]

Late Complications

Clonal evolution of hematopoiesis and PNH is thought to occur in about 10% to 20% of AA patients, with the clonal abnormality frequently detected at diagnosis. Clonal hematopoiesis and PNH may also develop several years after IST treatment, when it is usually associated with either hemolysis (PNH) or a worsening of peripheral blood counts (clonal cytogenetic abnormality).[16]

Box 3	
Response after immunosuppressive therapy for acquired AA	
Complete response (CR)	• Red blood cell and platelet transfusion independence
	• Absolute neutrophil count >1500 × 10^6/L
	• Platelet count >150,000 × 10^6/L
Partial response (PR)	• Improvement of cytopenia with absolute neutrophil count ≥500 × 10^6/L and platelets ≥20,000 × 10^6/L
	• ± Transfusion dependent
No response	• Continues to meet SAA criteria
	• Ongoing transfusion dependence
Relapse	• Meets criteria of SAA or vSAA after initial response

> **Box 4**
> **Long-term follow-up after immunosuppressive therapy**
>
> - Complete blood count, reticulocyte counts, C-reactive protein, initially at least weekly
> - Cyclosporine level, creatinine, liver enzymes, serum bilirubin, magnesium monitoring
> - Transfusion support if hemoglobin <8 g/dL, platelets <10,000/μL
> - Close monitoring for infections
> - Repeat bone marrow aspirate, biopsy, and cytogenetics at 3 months and 12 months or at sustained worsening of cytopenias
> - Paroxysmal nocturnal hemoglobinuria testing annually
> - Autoimmune disease screening at regular intervals (every 2–3 years)
> - Transition to a specialty care center in the adult health care system which is familiar with the treatment and follow-up of patients with AA

The long-term follow-up of patients after IST is summarized in **Box 4**. The authors generally perform a repeat BM aspirate and biopsy at 3 and 12 months after IST initiation to assess for treatment response and monitor for clonal evolution. Monitoring for the development of PNH after IST is performed yearly using flow cytometry (see earlier discussion). In adult AA patients chromosomal abnormalities are seen in about 10% to 15% of patients, with many abnormalities being transient and not necessarily associated with a poor prognosis.[77,78] Persistent abnormalities of chromosome 7, however, are frequently associated with progression to MDS.[56,79] In children with AA, persistent chromosomal abnormalities of chromosome 7 and 8, or complex cytogenetic abnormalities, are generally considered as MDS and are associated with an increased risk of transformation, and are treated accordingly,[80] whereas the clinical significance of other chromosomal abnormalities (ie, copy-neutral 6pLOH) remains to be determined.

Patients after IST also have an increased risk for the development of autoimmune disease (10%)[81] and solid tumors (11%).[82] Thus children with a history of AA should be followed indefinitely, and age-appropriately, in a specialized bone marrow failure center, irrespective of whether they have undergone BMT or IST.

SUMMARY

Acquired AA is a rare, life-threatening disorder, which is thought to be due to immune-mediated destruction of hematopoietic cells in the BM. Great advances have been made in the last decade in the understanding of its pathogenesis, as well as in the care and treatment of children with AA, which is now associated with excellent OS surpassing 90%. Allogeneic BMT offers the opportunity for cure in children if a suitable histocompatible donor is available. Comparable long-term survival in SAA is achieved with IST. However, one-quarter of children with AA will not respond to primary IST and will require second-line therapy, 10% to 30% of responders will relapse, and there is an increased risk of clonal hematopoiesis, leukemia, autoimmunity, and cancer that requires long-term follow-up by a specialized care center knowledgable in late manifestations of disease. With an increased understanding of the pathogenesis of AA and its specific late manifestations, targeted preventive strategies and more personalized treatment options are likely to further improve outcomes and decrease late complications in children (and adults) with acquired AA.

ACKNOWLEDGMENTS

The authors thank all patients with AA for participating in their BMF studies at CHOP/UPENN; Beverly J. Paul, RN, for her contributions in the care of BMF patients; Michele E. Paessler, DO, Pathology, CHOP, for providing the images used in **Fig. 1**; Talene Metjian, PharmD, Brian T. Fisher, DO, MSCE, Infectious Diseases, and Shefali Parikh, MD, Hematology, The Children's Hospital of Philadelphia, for sharing the algorithm for anti-infective prophylaxis in patients with SAA shown in **Fig. 5**; Neil Patel, PharmD, BCOP, Clinical Pharmacists, CHOP, for input and discussions on the IST therapy protocol; and Daria Babushok, MD, PhD, and Philip Mason, PhD for reading the article.

REFERENCES

1. Camitta BM, Rappeport JM, Parkman R, et al. Selection of patients for bone marrow transplantation in severe aplastic anemia. Blood 1975;45:355–63.
2. Bacigalupo A, Hows J, Gluckman E, et al. Bone marrow transplantation (BMT) versus immunosuppression for the treatment of severe aplastic anaemia (SAA): a report of the EBMT SAA working party. Br J Haematol 1988;70: 177–82.
3. Bessler M, Mason P, Link D, et al. Inherited bone marrow failure syndromes. In: Orkin SE, Nathan DG, Ginsberg D, et al, editors. Nathans and Oski's hematology of infancy and childhood. 8th edition. Philadelphia: W.B. Saunders Co; 2013, in press.
4. Baumann I, Niemeyer C, Bennett J, et al. Childhood myelodysplastic syndrome. In: Swerdlow S, Campo E, Harris NL, et al, editors. WHO classification of tumors of haematopoietic and lymphoid tissue, vol. 2. Lyon (France): International Agency for Research on Cancer; 2008. p. 104–7.
5. Baumann I, Fuhrer M, Behrendt S, et al. Morphological differentiation of severe aplastic anaemia from hypocellular refractory cytopenia of childhood: reproducibility of histopathological diagnostic criteria. Histopathology 2012;61:10–7.
6. Montane E, Ibanez L, Vidal X, et al. Epidemiology of aplastic anemia: a prospective multicenter study. Haematologica 2008;93:518–23.
7. Kagan WA, Ascensao JA, Pahwa RN, et al. Aplastic anemia: presence in human bone marrow of cells that suppress myelopoiesis. Proc Natl Acad Sci U S A 1976;73:2890–4.
8. Risitano AM, Maciejewski JP, Green S, et al. In-vivo dominant immune responses in aplastic anaemia: molecular tracking of putatively pathogenetic T-cell clones by TCR beta-CDR3 sequencing. Lancet 2004;364:355–64.
9. Kordasti S, Marsh J, Al-Khan S, et al. Functional characterization of CD4+ T cells in aplastic anemia. Blood 2012;119:2033–43.
10. Katagiri T, Sato-Otsubo A, Kashiwase K, et al. Frequent loss of HLA alleles associated with copy number-neutral 6pLOH in acquired aplastic anemia. Blood 2011;118:6601–9.
11. Sutherland DR, Kuek N, Davidson J, et al. Diagnosing PNH with FLAER and multiparameter flow cytometry. Cytometry B Clin Cytom 2007;72:167–77.
12. Bessler M, Fehr J. Fc III receptors (FcRIII) on granulocytes: a specific and sensitive diagnostic test for paroxysmal nocturnal hemoglobinuria (PNH). Eur J Haematol 1991;47:179–84.
13. Sutton KS, Shereck EB, Nemecek ER, et al. Immune markers of disease severity and treatment response in pediatric acquired aplastic anemia. Pediatr Blood Cancer 2013;60:455–60.

14. Du HY, Pumbo E, Ivanovich J, et al. TERC and TERT gene mutations in patients with bone marrow failure and the significance of telomere length measurements. Blood 2009;113:309–16.

15. Kojima S, Nakao S, Young N, et al. The Third Consensus Conference on the treatment of aplastic anemia. Int J Hematol 2011;93:832–7.

16. Babushok DV, Xie HM, Roth JJ, et al. Single Nucleotide Polymorphism Array Analysis of Bone Marrow Failure Patients Reveals Characteristic Patterns of Genetic Changes. Brit J Haematol 2013, in press.

17. Locasciulli A, Oneto R, Bacigalupo A, et al. Outcome of patients with acquired aplastic anemia given first line bone marrow transplantation or immunosuppressive treatment in the last decade: a report from the European Group for Blood and Marrow Transplantation (EBMT). Haematologica 2007; 92:11–8.

18. Valdez JM, Scheinberg P, Nunez O, et al. Decreased infection-related mortality and improved survival in severe aplastic anemia in the past two decades. Clin Infect Dis 2011;52:726–35.

19. Marsh JC, Bacigalupo A, Schrezenmeier H, et al. Prospective study of rabbit antithymocyte globulin and cyclosporine for aplastic anemia from the EBMT Severe Aplastic Anaemia Working Party. Blood 2012;119:5391–6.

20. Scheinberg P, Nunez O, Weinstein B, et al. Horse versus rabbit antithymocyte globulin in acquired aplastic anemia. N Engl J Med 2011;365:430–8.

21. Neumann S, Krause SW, Maschmeyer G, et al. Primary prophylaxis of bacterial infections and *Pneumocystis jirovecii* pneumonia in patients with hematological malignancies and solid tumors: guidelines of the Infectious Diseases Working Party (AGIHO) of the German Society of Hematology and Oncology (DGHO). Ann Hematol 2013;92:433–42.

22. Quarello P, Saracco P, Giacchino M, et al. Epidemiology of infections in children with acquired aplastic anaemia: a retrospective multicenter study in Italy. Eur J Haematol 2012;88:526–34.

23. Ohara A, Kojima S, Hamajima N, et al. Myelodysplastic syndrome and acute my-elogenous leukemia as a late clonal complication in children with acquired aplastic anemia. Blood 1997;90:1009–13.

24. Quillen K, Wong E, Scheinberg P, et al. Granulocyte transfusions in severe aplastic anemia: an eleven-year experience. Haematologica 2009;94:1661–8.

25. Marsh J, Socie G, Tichelli A, et al. Should irradiated blood products be given routinely to all patients with aplastic anaemia undergoing immunosuppressive therapy with antithymocyte globulin (ATG)? A survey from the European Group for Blood and Marrow Transplantation Severe Aplastic Anaemia Working Party. Br J Haematol 2010;150:377–9.

26. Jamuar SS, Lai AH. Safety and efficacy of iron chelation therapy with deferi-prone in patients with transfusion-dependent thalassemia. Ther Adv Hematol 2012;3:299–307.

27. Samarasinghe S, Steward C, Hiwarkar P, et al. Excellent outcome of matched unrelated donor transplantation in paediatric aplastic anaemia following failure with immunosuppressive therapy: a United Kingdom multicentre retrospective experience. Br J Haematol 2012;157:339–46.

28. Bacigalupo A, Marsh JC. Unrelated donor search and unrelated donor trans-plantation in the adult aplastic anaemia patient aged 18-40 years without an HLA-identical sibling and failing immunosuppression. Bone Marrow Transplant 2013;48:198–200.

29. Yoshimi A, Niemeyer CM, Fuhrer MM, et al. Comparison of the efficacy of rabbit and horse antithymocyte globulin for the treatment of severe aplastic anemia in children. Blood 2013;121:860–1.
30. Armand P, Antin JH. Allogeneic stem cell transplantation for aplastic anemia. Biol Blood Marrow Transplant 2007;13:505–16.
31. Bunin N, Leahey A, Kamani N, et al. Bone marrow transplantation in pediatric patients with severe aplastic anemia: cyclophosphamide and anti-thymocyte globulin conditioning followed by recombinant human granulocyte-macrophage colony stimulating factor. J Pediatr Hematol Oncol 1996;18:68–71.
32. Kahl C, Leisenring W, Deeg HJ, et al. Cyclophosphamide and antithymocyte globulin as a conditioning regimen for allogeneic marrow transplantation in patients with aplastic anaemia: a long-term follow-up. Br J Haematol 2005;130: 747–51.
33. Ades L, Mary JY, Robin M, et al. Long-term outcome after bone marrow transplantation for severe aplastic anemia. Blood 2004;103:2490–7.
34. Champlin RE, Perez WS, Passweg JR, et al. Bone marrow transplantation for severe aplastic anemia: a randomized controlled study of conditioning regimens. Blood 2007;109:4582–5.
35. Pulsipher MA, Young NS, Tolar J, et al. Optimization of therapy for severe aplastic anemia based on clinical, biologic, and treatment response parameters: conclusions of an international working group on severe aplastic anemia convened by the Blood and Marrow Transplant Clinical Trials Network, March 2010. Biol Blood Marrow Transplant 2011;17:291–9.
36. George B, Mathews V, Viswabandya A, et al. Fludarabine based reduced intensity conditioning regimens in children undergoing allogeneic stem cell transplantation for severe aplastic anemia. Pediatr Transplant 2008;12:14–9.
37. Resnick IB, Aker M, Shapira MY, et al. Allogeneic stem cell transplantation for severe acquired aplastic anaemia using a fludarabine-based preparative regimen. Br J Haematol 2006;133:649–54.
38. Buchbinder D, Nugent DJ, Brazauskas R, et al. Late effects in hematopoietic cell transplant recipients with acquired severe aplastic anemia: a report from the late effects working committee of the center for international blood and marrow transplant research. Biol Blood Marrow Transplant 2012;18: 1776–84.
39. Sanders JE, Woolfrey AE, Carpenter PA, et al. Late effects among pediatric patients followed for nearly 4 decades after transplantation for severe aplastic anemia. Blood 2011;118:1421–8.
40. Konopacki J, Porcher R, Robin M, et al. Long-term follow up after allogeneic stem cell transplantation in patients with severe aplastic anemia after cyclophosphamide plus antithymocyte globulin conditioning. Haematologica 2012; 97:710–6.
41. Schrezenmeier H, Passweg JR, Marsh JC, et al. Worse outcome and more chronic GVHD with peripheral blood progenitor cells than bone marrow in HLA-matched sibling donor transplants for young patients with severe acquired aplastic anemia. Blood 2007;110:1397–400.
42. Myers KC, Davies SM. Hematopoietic stem cell transplantation for bone marrow failure syndromes in children. Biol Blood Marrow Transplant 2009;15: 279–92.
43. Young NS, Bacigalupo A, Marsh JC. Aplastic anemia: pathophysiology and treatment. Biol Blood Marrow Transplant 2010;16:S119–25.

44. Ostronoff F, Ostronoff M, Souto-Maior AP, et al. Prospective trial of mycopheno-late mofetil-cyclosporine A prophylaxis for acute GVHD after G-CSF stimulated allogeneic bone marrow transplantation with HLA-identical sibling donors in pa-tients with severe aplastic anemia and hematological malignancies. Clin Trans-plant 2009;23:33–8.

45. Yagasaki H, Kojima S, Yabe H, et al. Tacrolimus/methotrexate versus cyclo-sporine/methotrexate as graft-versus-host disease prophylaxis in patients with severe aplastic anemia who received bone marrow transplantation from unre-lated donors: results of matched pair analysis. Biol Blood Marrow Transplant 2009;15:1603–8.

46. Lawler M, McCann SR, Marsh JC, et al. Serial chimerism analyses indicate that mixed haemopoietic chimerism influences the probability of graft rejection and disease recurrence following allogeneic stem cell transplantation (SCT) for se-vere aplastic anaemia (SAA): indication for routine assessment of chimerism post SCT for SAA. Br J Haematol 2009;144:933–45.

47. Maury S, Bacigalupo A, Anderlini P, et al. Improved outcome of patients older than 30 years receiving HLA-identical sibling hematopoietic stem cell transplan-tation for severe acquired aplastic anemia using fludarabine-based condition-ing: a comparison with conventional conditioning regimen. Haematologica 2009;94:1312–5.

48. Yagasaki H, Takahashi Y, Hama A, et al. Comparison of matched-sibling donor BMT and unrelated donor BMT in children and adolescent with acquired severe aplastic anemia. Bone Marrow Transplant 2010;45:1508–13.

49. Peffault de Latour R, Purtill D, Ruggeri A, et al. Influence of nucleated cell dose on overall survival of unrelated cord blood transplantation for patients with se-vere acquired aplastic anemia: a study by Eurocord and the Aplastic Anemia Working Party of the European Group for Blood and Marrow Transplantation. Biol Blood Marrow Transplant 2011;17:78–85.

50. Buchbinder D, Hsieh L, Puthenveetil G, et al. Successful autologous cord blood transplantation in a child with acquired severe aplastic anemia. Pediatr Trans-plant 2013;17:E104–7.

51. Im HJ, Koh KN, Choi ES, et al. Excellent outcome of haploidentical hematopoi-etic stem cell transplantation in children and adolescents with acquired severe aplastic anemia. Biol Blood Marrow Transplant 2013;19:754–9.

52. Wang H, Yan H, Wang Z, et al. Cotransplantation of allogeneic mesenchymal and hematopoietic stem cells in children with aplastic anemia. Pediatrics 2012;129:e1612–5.

53. Eapen M, Horowitz MM. Alternative donor transplantation for aplastic anemia. Hematology Am Soc Hematol Educ Program 2010;2010:43–6.

54. Bunin N, Aplenc R, Iannone R, et al. Unrelated donor bone marrow transplantation for children with severe aplastic anemia: minimal GVHD and durable engraftment with partial T cell depletion. Bone Marrow Transplant 2005;35:369–73.

55. Bacigalupo A, Locatelli F, Lanino E, et al. Fludarabine, cyclophosphamide and anti-thymocyte globulin for alternative donor transplants in acquired severe aplastic anemia: a report from the EBMT-SAA Working Party. Bone Marrow Transplant 2005;36:947–50.

56. Frickhofen N, Heimpel H, Kaltwasser JP, et al. Antithymocyte globulin with or without cyclosporin A: 11-year follow-up of a randomized trial comparing treat-ments of aplastic anemia. Blood 2003;101:1236–42.

57. Samarasinghe S, Webb DK. How I manage aplastic anaemia in children. Br J Haematol 2012;157:26–40.

58. Saracco P, Quarello P, Iori AP, et al. Cyclosporin A response and dependence in children with acquired aplastic anaemia: a multicentre retrospective study with long-term observation follow-up. Br J Haematol 2008;140:197–205.
59. Dufour C, Svahn J, Bacigalupo A. Front-line immunosuppressive treatment of acquired aplastic anemia. Bone Marrow Transplant 2013;48:174–7.
60. Fuhrer M, Rampf U, Baumann I, et al. Immunosuppressive therapy for aplastic anemia in children: a more severe disease predicts better survival. Blood 2005; 106:2102–4.
61. Tichelli A, Schrezenmeier H, Socie G, et al. A randomized controlled study in patients with newly diagnosed severe aplastic anemia receiving antithymocyte globulin (ATG), cyclosporine, with or without G-CSF: a study of the SAA Working Party of the European Group for Blood and Marrow Transplantation. Blood 2011; 117:4434–41.
62. Alsultan A, Goldenberg NA, Kaiser N, et al. Tacrolimus as an alternative to cyclosporine in the maintenance phase of immunosuppressive therapy for severe aplastic anemia in children. Pediatr Blood Cancer 2009;52:626–30.
63. Kamio T, Ito E, Ohara A, et al. Relapse of aplastic anemia in children after immunosuppressive therapy: a report from the Japan Childhood Aplastic Anemia Study Group. Haematologica 2011;96:814–9.
64. Brodsky RA, Chen AR, Dorr D, et al. High-dose cyclophosphamide for severe aplastic anemia: long-term follow-up. Blood 2010;115:2136–41.
65. Olnes MJ, Scheinberg P, Calvo KR, et al. Eltrombopag and improved hematopoiesis in refractory aplastic anemia. N Engl J Med 2012;367:11–9.
66. Nishio N, Yagasaki H, Takahashi Y, et al. Natural history of transfusion-independent non-severe aplastic anemia in children. Int J Hematol 2009;89:409–13.
67. Howard SC, Naidu PE, Hu XJ, et al. Natural history of moderate aplastic anemia in children. Pediatr Blood Cancer 2004;43:545–51.
68. Brock K, Goldenberg N, Graham DK, et al. Moderate aplastic anemia in children: preliminary outcomes for treatment versus observation from a single-institutional experience. J Pediatr Hematol Oncol 2013;35:148–52.
69. Marsh J, Schrezenmeier H, Marin P, et al. Prospective randomized multicenter study comparing cyclosporin alone versus the combination of antithymocyte globulin and cyclosporin for treatment of patients with nonsevere aplastic anemia: a report from the European Blood and Marrow Transplant (EBMT) Severe Aplastic Anaemia Working Party. Blood 1999;93:2191–5.
70. Nimer SD, Ireland P, Meshkinpour A, et al. An increased HLA DR2 frequency is seen in aplastic anemia patients. Blood 1994;84:923–7.
71. Sugimori C, Yamazaki H, Feng X, et al. Roles of DRB1 *1501 and DRB1 *1502 in the pathogenesis of aplastic anemia. Exp Hematol 2007;35:13–20.
72. Fuhrer M, Durner J, Brunnler G, et al. HLA association is different in children and adults with severe acquired aplastic anemia. Pediatr Blood Cancer 2007;48: 186–91.
73. Yoshida N, Yagasaki H, Takahashi Y, et al. Clinical impact of HLA-DR15, a minor population of paroxysmal nocturnal haemoglobinuria-type cells, and an aplastic anaemia-associated autoantibody in children with acquired aplastic anaemia. Br J Haematol 2008;142:427–35.
74. Scheinberg P, Wu CO, Nunez O, et al. Long-term outcome of pediatric patients with severe aplastic anemia treated with antithymocyte globulin and cyclosporine. J Pediatr 2008;153:814–9.
75. Kosaka Y, Yagasaki H, Sano K, et al. Prospective multicenter trial comparing repeated immunosuppressive therapy with stem-cell transplantation from an

alternative donor as second-line treatment for children with severe and very severe aplastic anemia. Blood 2008;111:1054–9.

76. Scheinberg P, Nunez O, Young NS. Retreatment with rabbit anti-thymocyte globulin and ciclosporin for patients with relapsed or refractory severe aplastic anaemia. Br J Haematol 2006;133:622–7.

77. Gupta V, Brooker C, Tooze JA, et al. Clinical relevance of cytogenetic abnormalities at diagnosis of acquired aplastic anaemia in adults. Br J Haematol 2006; 134:95–9.

78. Afable MG 2nd, Wlodarski M, Makishima H, et al. SNP array-based karyotyping: differences and similarities between aplastic anemia and hypocellular myelodysplastic syndromes. Blood 2011;117:6876–84.

79. Socie G, Mary JY, Schrezenmeier H, et al. Granulocyte-stimulating factor and severe aplastic anemia: a survey by the European Group for Blood and Marrow Transplantation (EBMT). Blood 2007;109:2794–6.

80. Niemeyer CM, Baumann I. Myelodysplastic syndrome in children and adolescents. Semin Hematol 2008;45:60–70.

81. Stalder MP, Rovo A, Halter J, et al. Aplastic anemia and concomitant autoimmune diseases. Ann Hematol 2009;88:659–65.

82. Socie G, Henry-Amar M, Bacigalupo A, et al. Malignant tumors occurring after treatment of aplastic anemia. European Bone Marrow Transplantation-Severe Aplastic Anaemia Working Party. N Engl J Med 1993;329:1152–7.

83. Chapuis B, Von Fliedner VE, Jeannet M, et al. Increased frequency of DR2 in patients with aplastic anaemia and increased DR sharing in their parents. Br J Haematol 1986;63:51–7.

84. Babushok DV, Li Y, Roth JJ, et al. Common polymorphic deletion of glutathione S-transferase theta predisposes to acquired aplastic anemia: independent cohort and meta-analysis of 609 patients. Am J Hematol 2013;88(10):862–7.

Hematologic Manifestations of Systemic Disease (Including Iron Deficiency, Anemia of Inflammation and DIC)

Char M. Witmer, MD, MSCE

KEYWORDS

- Function of hemoglobin • Anemia of inflammation • Iron deficiency anemia
- Disseminated intravascular coagulation

KEY POINTS

- A complete blood cell count (CBC) is a frequent test sent to aid in the diagnostic evaluation of ill patients.
- Not uncommonly hematologic abnormalities may be the first sign of an underlying systemic disorder.
- The astute clinician needs to understand how systemic disease can affect the CBC to direct further diagnostic investigations.

INTRODUCTION

A complete blood cell count (CBC) is a frequent test sent to aid in the diagnostic evaluation of ill patients. Not uncommonly hematologic abnormalities may be the first sign of an underlying systemic disorder. The astute clinician needs to understand how systemic disease can affect the CBC to direct further diagnostic investigations. This article focuses on the 2 most common acquired anemias including iron deficiency and anemia of inflammation (AI) as well as disseminated intravascular coagulation (DIC).

STRUCTURE AND FUNCTION OF HEMOGLOBIN

A red blood cell (RBC) is nonnucleated and survives for 120 days. The key functional component of an RBC is hemoglobin, a nearly spherical protein composed of

Conflict of Interest: The author has no relevant financial disclosures or conflict of interests to report.
Division of Hematology, Department of Pediatrics, Children's Hospital of Philadelphia, Perelman School of Medicine, University of Pennsylvania, 3501 Civic Center Boulevard, CTRB 11th Floor, Room 11-026, Philadelphia, PA 19104, USA
E-mail address: witmer@email.chop.edu

tetramers of 2 alphalike globin chains and 2 betalike globin chains. The primary physiologic function of hemoglobin is to transport oxygen to the tissues from the lungs. Each of the subunits in the hemoglobin tetramer contains a heme prosthetic group. Heme is an iron-containing protoporphyrin IX with an iron atom at the center, typically in the ferrous form (+2). In the ferrous form the heme group can bind gaseous ligands specifically O_2, CO, and NO. Hemoglobin also binds and transports CO_2 (on a different binding site than O_2) to the lungs from the tissues.

Physiologically anemia compromises oxygen delivery to tissues. Symptoms depend on how severely anemic a patient is, how slowly they became anemic, and underlying comordibities. Many patients may be asymptomatic or have vague generalized symptoms like fatigue. On physical exam, pallor is manifest as pale skin, mucosa, and palmar creases. More severe anemia will have evidence of a hyperdynamic circulation with tachycardia, a systolic flow murmur (more common once the hemoglobin is less than 8 g/dL), and potentially signs of heart failure.

IRON DEFICIENCY ANEMIA
Epidemiology

Iron deficiency is the most common nutrient deficiency worldwide and accounts for 50% of the world's anemia burden.[1] It is the only nutrient deficiency that is found in both industrialized and nonindustrialized countries.[1] There is a bimodal peak of occurrence in pediatrics with increased rates seen in infancy and menstruating adolescent women. It is estimated in the United States that up to 7% of toddlers, 9% of adolescents, and 16% of women of childbearing age is iron deficient.[2]

Pathophysiology

Iron is a ubiquitous metal that is found in most cells within the human body. It is a critical ingredient for effective red cell production but also plays a role in other biochemical pathways including myoglobin formation, energy metabolism, neurotransmitter production, collagen formation, and immune system function.[3] Approximately 1 to 2 mg of iron enters and leaves the body daily. Gastrointestinal (GI) absorption of iron occurs primarily in the proximal duodenum and is a tightly controlled process that is responsive to iron status, erythropoietin demand, hypoxia, and inflammation. The main regulator of iron absorption is hepcidin, which serves as a negative regulator of iron absorption and macrophage iron release.[4]

Within the body, iron is distributed in 3 pools including transport, functional, and storage iron.[3] Absorbed iron is bound to transferrin for transport in the plasma and accounts for only 0.1% of total body iron. Functional iron accounts for 75% of the total body iron and is predominantly used for hemoglobin production (70%) with the remaining in muscle and other tissues. Excess iron is stored in tissues (primarily liver, bone marrow, and spleen) as ferritin. The amount of daily iron absorption is low relative to ongoing demands necessitating iron recycling of senescent red cells by macrophages. Although iron absorption is tightly regulated, there is no mechanism to regulate iron loss.

At birth, infants have high total body iron stores (75 mg/kg of iron).[5,6] These iron stores support rapid neonatal growth but are only adequate until about 6 months of age. At this point, iron-enriched cereals should be included in the first foods introduced into an infant's diet. In preterm infants, the total body iron stores are decreased compared with full-term infants although the proportion to body weight is similar.[7] Preterm infants should receive iron supplementation because they undergo more rapid postnatal growth than full-term infants and exhaust their iron stores by 2 to 3 months of age. This high iron requirement will decrease toward the end of the second year of life as the rate of growth decreases. Iron requirements again rise with the rapid growth seen in adolescents, and this is further compounded by adolescent women who have ongoing iron losses through menstruation.

Iron deficiency is always secondary to an underlying source and results from an interplay between increasing iron requirements with growth, inadequate iron intake, excessive iron losses, or poor absorption. **Table 1** provides a list of potential causes of iron deficiency. Further discussion is warranted on the most common causes of iron deficiency in pediatric patients, including cow's milk ingestion in toddlers, menstruating adolescents, and celiac disease (CD).

For many toddlers, the transition from drinking breast milk or formula to solid food can be a challenge. This is further compounded by the continued use of a bottle after the age of 12 months. With the transition to cow's milk many toddlers drink excessive amounts (>24 ounces per day) preferentially over solid food. Cow's milk contributes to the development of iron deficiency through multiple mechanisms. It is a poor source of iron and its excessive use displaces iron-rich foods. Components in cow's milk, casein and calcium, in high amounts directly interfere with iron absorption.[8] Excess cow's milk can also lead to GI inflammation, which can result in occult GI blood loss.[8]

For menstruating women, dysfunctional uterine bleeding or menorrhagia can result in significant iron loss over time. The definition of menorrhagia is a blood loss of

Table 1
Causes of iron deficiency

Category	Conditions
Inadequate oral iron intake	Excessive/exclusive cow's milk intake in toddlers Restrictive diet

Inadequate iron absorption	Loss or dysfunction of absorptive enterocytes
	    Celiac disease
	    Inflammatory bowel disease
	    Bowel resection (proximal duodenum)
	Antacid therapy/high gastric pH
	Genetic defects in intestinal iron uptake
	    Iron refractory iron deficiency anemia-TMPRSS6 mutations

Excessive blood loss	Gastrointestinal blood loss
	    Anatomic defects (Meckel diverticulum)
	    Gastritis
	    Ulcer
	    Inflammatory bowel disease
	    Vascular malformations
	    Varices
	    Parasitic infection
	    Cow's milk–induced enteropathy
	    Tumor (rare in children)
	Hematuria
	Menstrual blood loss
	Other excessive bleeding (ie, epistaxis)
	Pulmonary hemosiderosis

Increased iron demand	Neonatal growth Adolescent growth Pregnancy

greater than 80 mL in one menstrual cycle. Unfortunately this is not a practical definition and leaves clinicians with little guidance as to how to make this diagnosis. Just asking an adolescent if her period is "heavy" is fraught with pitfalls. A more thorough clinical history is needed. **Table 2** provides clinical pearls for diagnosing menorrhagia.

CD is a chronic immune-mediated enteropathy secondary to a sensitivity to gluten proteins. The prevalence of CD is estimated to be 1% in the United States and European countries.[9] The classic symptoms of pediatric CD include failure to thrive, malnutrition, and diarrhea. Recently new clinical patterns of CD presentation in pediatric patients are emerging, thus requiring a higher index of suspicion on the clinician's part. There has been a shift toward CD being diagnosed at a later age, most do not present with classic symptoms, there is little to mild GI symptoms, associated non-GI symptoms are common, and 10% are overweight.[10] High-risk groups for CD include patients with a first-degree family member with CD, specific genetic disorders (Turner, Williams, and Down syndromes), type 1 diabetes mellitus, other autoimmune disorders, iron deficiency anemia (especially recurrent), and persistently elevated aminotransferase levels. In pediatric patients with iron deficiency it has been reported that 4.4% to 15.5% will have CD.[11,12]

Clinical Manifestations

The consequences of iron deficiency are systemic and include neurocognitive effects, epithelial changes, and the systemic consequences of anemia.[13] Studies have repeatedly demonstrated that children with iron deficiency have an associated impaired motor and mental functioning.[14–20] Effects on epithelial cells include angular stomatitis and glossitis. Rarely patients can develop Plummer-Vinson syndrome with the formation of an esophageal web. Long-standing iron deficiency can lead to koilonychias, which is "spooning" of the nails. Some iron-deficient patients may develop pica, which is the compulsion to consume nonfood items like ice, dirt, or clay. The associated signs of anemia depend on the severity of the anemia as previously discussed.

Diagnostic Evaluation

Table 3 describes the common tests of iron. As a person becomes iron deficient, there are progressive changes that occur initially in iron stores and ultimately to the production of RBCs (**Table 4**). Depending on the time in which laboratory testing is obtained there will be variable laboratory findings. Using a CBC as a screen for iron deficiency only detects the more severe forms as it is a late clinical finding. Although iron deficiency anemia is classically described as a microcytic anemia, there is a brief time when it is a normocytic anemia. The reticulocyte count is low relative to the degree of anemia. Mild to moderate thrombocytosis (range of 500–700,000/mcL) occurs frequently. **Table 5** lists common laboratory findings in iron deficiency anemia and how to differentiate from AI and thalassemia trait.

Table 2 Clinical symptoms of menorrhagia	
Definition	Blood loss of >80 mL per menstrual cycle
Clinical symptoms suggestive of menorrhagia	Duration of menses longer than 7 d Changing of a "soaked" product every 1–2 h Flooding Passage of blood clots >1 inch in size

Table 3
Common tests of iron

Test	Description	Pitfalls with Testing
Serum iron	Measures the amount of iron in circulation.	The serum iron fluctuates with recent oral iron intake, infection, and inflammation. Diurnal variation is also seen.
TIBC	Indirect measure of serum transferrin, which is the iron transport protein. Measures the availability of iron-binding sites on transferrin.	It is decreased in malnutrition, inflammation, chronic infection, and cancer.
Transferrin saturation	The percentage of iron-binding sites on transferrin that are occupied by iron. Calculated = (serum iron/TIBC) × 100	Influenced by the same factors that affect serum iron and TIBC.
Ferritin	Storage compound for iron. In general serum levels correlate with total iron stores.	Ferritin is an acute phase reactant so will be elevated during inflammation.

Abbreviation: TIBC, total iron binding capacity.

Treatment

Imperative to treatment is identifying the underlying cause of iron deficiency. Oral iron replacement is preferentially used to replete iron stores. Ferrous sulfate is the most common oral supplement used. Dosing is based on elemental iron:

- Children:
  - severe iron deficiency anemia 4–6 mg/kg of elemental iron divided tid
  - Mild to moderate iron deficiency anemia: 3 mg/kg of elemental iron in 1–2 divided doses
  - Prophylaxis: 1–2 mg/kg up to a maximum of 15 mg/d
- Adolescents:
  - Iron deficiency anemia: 60–65 mg of elemental iron 2–4 times/d
  - Prophylaxis: 60–65 mg of elemental iron daily

To fully replete the iron stores, iron replacement should be continued for 2 to 3 months. Side effects of iron therapy include staining of teeth from liquid preparations, epigastric pain, nausea, dark stools, and constipation. Parenteral iron is used if oral

Table 4
Laboratory findings during the stages of iron depletion

Clinical Test	Deplete Iron Stores	Iron Deficiency Without Anemia	Iron Deficiency Anemia
Decreased serum ferritin	████████████████████████████████▶		
Decreased transferrin saturation		████████████████████▶	
Decreased hemoglobin			███████████▶
Elevated RDW			███████████▶
Decreased MCV			███████████▶

Abbreviations: MCV, mean corpuscular volume; RDW, red cell distribution width.

Table 5
Laboratory differences between iron deficiency anemia, AI, and thalassemia trait

Clinical Test	Iron Deficiency Anemia	Anemia of Inflammation	Thalassemia Trait
Serum ferritin	Low	Normal to high	Normal
Serum iron	Low	Low	Normal
TIBC	High	Low	Normal
Transferrin saturation	Low	Low	Normal
MCV	Low	Low to normal	Low
RDW	High	High	Normal

Abbreviations: MCV, mean corpuscular volume; RDW, red cell distribution width; TIBC, total iron binding capacity.

iron is not effective secondary to intolerance or poor GI absorption. A red cell transfusion should only be used in the setting of severe anemia.

To ensure your patient is responding appropriately to iron therapy, it is essential to be aware of the predictable hematological response to therapy. **Table 6** provides a timeline for hematologic response to therapy. If a patient does not have an adequate response to iron replacement or if the iron deficiency reoccurs, additional investigations should be considered.

ANEMIA OF INFLAMMATION
Epidemiology

AI, also called anemia of chronic disease, is the second most common cause of anemia after iron deficiency anemia.[21] It is an underrecognized cause of anemia in children and can occur in the setting of acute as well as chronic illness.

Pathophysiology

AI is an acquired immune-mediated disorder with a pathophysiology that is multifactorial including abnormal iron homeostasis, impaired erythropoiesis and a blunted erythropoietin response.[21] Impaired iron hemostasis is secondary to cytokine stimulation of hepcidin.[22] As mentioned previously, hepcidin is a negative regulator of iron. When hepcidin levels are increased, there is a resultant decrease in GI iron absorption as well as a sequestration of macrophage iron, which limits iron availability for erythropoiesis, thus inhibiting the most important source of iron for erythropoiesis and

Table 6
Hematologic response to iron replacement therapy

Hematologic Response	Timing
Increase in the reticulocyte count	Within 2–3 d of starting iron therapy
Increase in the hemoglobin	Within 1 wk of starting iron therapy
Normalization in the hemoglobin	After 4–6 wk of iron therapy
Normalization in the RDW	After 3 mo of iron therapy. The RDW will initially increase with starting iron therapy.

Abbreviation: RDW, red cell distribution width.

causing an iron restricted anemia. Cytokines also exert inhibitory effects against red cell progenitors limiting proliferation and differentiation, which is further complicated with decreased response to erythropoietin.[21,23,24] **Table 7** provides a list of common conditions associated with AI.

Clinical Manifestations

The clinical manifestations will vary with the underlying cause as well as the degree of anemia.

Diagnostic Evaluation

Common tests used to diagnosis AI include a CBC with reticulocyte count and iron studies. AI is a mild to moderate anemia that is typically normocytic but can be microcytic. There is also a relative reticulocytopenia for the degree of anemia and the red cell distribution width is elevated. **Table 5** provides laboratory findings to aid clinicians in differentiating between iron deficiency, AI, and thalassemia trait. Inflammatory markers (ie, C-reactive protein) may be elevated but this is nonspecific.

Currently, hepcidin levels are not clinically available although many different methods are in development.[25–27] Many of these methods have not been reliable or reproducible in actual human samples and the need for harmonization and universal reference ranges is ongoing.[28] Recently a large population-based study provided information regarding hepcidin levels in 2998 healthy adult patients and smaller studies have been completed in pediatric patients.[29,30] These studies demonstrate significant interindividual variation in hepcidin levels and the need for sex- and age-specific ranges.[29,30] It also appears that hepcidin levels need to be interpreted within the context of iron indices.[29,30]

Treatment

The primary treatment of AI is to treat the underlying disorder, although treating the underlying condition is not always a viable option. RBC transfusions are used in the setting of severe, symptomatic anemia or anemia with cardiovascular compromise. Animal models are currently being used to investigate the use of hepcidin inhibitors to increase the systemic availability of iron.[31]

Table 7
Conditions associated with anemia of inflammation

Category	Conditions
Infection (can be acute or chronic)	Bacterial Viral Parasitic Fungal
Autoimmune disorders	Systemic lupus erythematosus Rheumatoid arthritis Vasculitis Sarcoidosis Inflammatory bowel disease
Malignancy	Lymphoma Solid tumors
Chronic disease	Congestive heart failure Chronic renal disease

DISSEMINATED INTRAVASCULAR COAGULATION
Epidemiology

The epidemiology of DIC in pediatrics is not well described. A retrospective single institutional study estimated a prevalence of DIC as 1% of hospitalized pediatric patients.[32] The presence of DIC in term and preterm neonates is likely under recognized.[33]

Pathophysiology

DIC is an acquired syndrome characterized by the systemic activation of coagulation with resultant diffuse microvascular thrombosis with a concomitant consumption of coagulation factors and platelets. It is not a disease in itself and is always secondary to an underlying disorder. **Table 8** provides a list of conditions associated with DIC.

The disorders implicated in DIC all share the ability to induce systemic activation of coagulation, mediated primarily through either the release of activating cytokines or procoagulant substances.[34] These mediators activate coagulation exclusively through the tissue factor/factor VIIa pathway.[35] The source of tissue factor includes mononuclear cells in response to cytokines, injured vascular endothelial cells, or cancer cells. Concurrent with the systemic activation of coagulation, there is also an impairment of the major anticoagulant pathways including antithrombin, protein C, and protein S.[36]

Table 8
Conditions associated with disseminated intravascular coagulation

Category	Conditions
Fetal	Perinatal asphyxia Necrotizing enterocolitis Metabolic disorders Respiratory distress syndrome Amniotic fluid aspiration Respiratory distress syndrome Homozygous protein C/S deficiency
Immunologic	Transfusion reaction Transplant rejection
Infection	Bacterial *(gram positive and negative)* Viral *(hemorrhagic fevers, cytomegalovirus, influenza)* Parasites *(malaria)*
Malignancy	Solid tumors *(disseminated adenocarcinoma)* Leukemia *(acute promyelocytic leukemia)*
Obstetric	Amniotic fluid embolism Abruption placentae Preeclampsia/eclampsia Intrauterine fetal demise
Organ destruction	Pancreatitis Severe liver failure
Severe trauma	Poly trauma Neurotrauma Fat embolism
Toxic	Snake bites Drugs
Vascular abnormalities	Kaposiform hemangioendothelioma Tufted angioma Large vascular aneurysm

Additional derangement is also seen within the fibrinolytic system, resulting in hypofibrinolysis with decreased clot dissolution.[37]

The clinical complications of DIC are related to thrombosis and bleeding. Thrombotic complications are more common than bleeding.[34] The most common thrombotic complication is from microvascular thrombi that lead to organ dysfunction. Less common is *purpura fulminans*, a hemorrhagic necrosis of the skin due to dermal vascular thrombosis.

Diagnostic Evaluation

No single laboratory test will accurately diagnose the presence of DIC.[38,39] The diagnosis is made by evaluating a combination of tests and their change over time. **Table 9** lists the laboratory tests available for the diagnosis of DIC, the patterns seen in DIC, and the clinical utility of each test. In making the diagnosis of DIC, it is imperative to incorporate both clinical and laboratory information.

Treatment

The effective management of DIC hinges on the ability to diagnose and treat the underlying cause. Additional interventions are purely supportive and include respiratory, circulatory, replacement of organ function (ie, dialysis), and coagulation interventions. In this article, only treatment with anticoagulant and hemostatic therapies are discussed.

As mentioned previously, thrombosis is the most significant complication found in DIC. Experimental animal and human DIC models have demonstrated a benefit with heparin therapy.[40–43] Unfortunately, no randomized clinical trial has been able to demonstrate an improvement in mortality.[44] The current recommendation regarding anticoagulation in DIC is to consider deep vein thrombosis prophylaxis (no well-established pediatric recommendations) but to balance this with the patient's risk of

Table 9		
Laboratory testing in disseminated intravascular coagulation		
Test	**Laboratory Findings in DIC**	**Clinical Utility**
Platelet count	• Initially normal followed by a declining platelet count. <or> • Thrombocytopenia at presentation	Limited specificity, common finding in critically ill patients.
PT and PTT	• Normal <or> • Prolongation	Poorly reflects in vivo hemostasis. Prolongation is not specific for DIC and normal values do not exclude DIC.
D-dimer	Elevated	An elevated D-dimer is not specific for DIC. It is elevated in other conditions including venous thrombosis, inflammatory conditions, and recent surgery. *A normal D-dimer rules out DIC.*
Fibrinogen	• Elevated/normal in early DIC with decreased levels over time. • Can be decreased in severe DIC.	Overall poor sensitivity because it is an acute phase reactant. Sensitivity is only 28%.

Abbreviations: DIC, disseminated intravascular coagulation; PT, prothrombin time; PTT, partial thromboplastin time.

bleeding.[45,46] If there is a thrombotic event (arterial, venous, or *purpura fulminans*), proceed with anticoagulation.[45,46]

Hemostatic therapy in DIC should not be used to treat isolated laboratory abnormalities. Correction of the coagulopathy should only occur when there is bleeding or before an invasive procedure. Therapy should be directed toward the identified deficiencies using blood component therapy. Recommended hemostatic therapies include blood product components (fresh frozen plasma, cryoprecipitate, or platelets).[45,46] In general, procoagulant factor concentrates (prothrombin complex concentrate or recombinant factor VIIa) are not recommended for the treatment of coagulopathy associated with DIC because they are prothrombotic and could theoretically worsen the coagulopathy. For most causes of DIC, antifibrinolytic therapy is not recommended because there is significant hypofibrinolysis in DIC and further suppression could be prothrombotic.

The use of anticoagulant factors (antithrombin or activated protein C) to restore the anticoagulant pathways in DIC is not recommended for pediatric patients. Antithrombin has been available since the 1980s, but no clinical trial has been able to demonstrate improved mortality.[45,47] Unlike in adults, activated protein C is not recommended in children with DIC.[46] A randomized clinical trial of activated protein C in children with severe sepsis was stopped early secondary to an increased risk of bleeding and no evidence of efficacy.[48]

REFERENCES

1. World Health Organization. Iron deficiency anaemia: assessment, prevention, and control. A guide for programme managers. Geneva (Switzerland): World Health Organization; 2001.
2. Looker A. Iron Deficiency-United States, 1999-2000: Centers for Disease Control and Prevention. 2002.
3. Edison ES, Bajel A, Chandy M. Iron homeostasis: new players, newer insights. Eur J Haematol 2008;81(6):411–24.
4. Nemeth E, Tuttle MS, Powelson J, et al. Hepcidin regulates cellular iron efflux by binding to ferroportin and inducing its internalization. Science 2004;306(5704): 2090–3.
5. Widdowson EM, Spray CM. Chemical development in utero. Arch Dis Child 1951; 26(127):205–14.
6. Dallman PR, Siimes MA, Stekel A. Iron deficiency in infancy and childhood. Am J Clin Nutr 1980;33(1):86–118.
7. Worwood M. The clinical biochemistry of iron. Semin Hematol 1977;14(1):3–30.
8. Agostoni C, Turck D. Is cow's milk harmful to a child's health? J Pediatr Gastroenterol Nutr 2011;53(6):594–600.
9. Reilly NR, Green PH. Epidemiology and clinical presentations of celiac disease. Semin Immunopathol 2012;34(4):473–8.
10. Telega G, Bennet TR, Werlin S. Emerging new clinical patterns in the presentation of celiac disease. Arch Pediatr Adolesc Med 2008;162(2):164–8.
11. Ferrara M, Coppola L, Coppola A, et al. Iron deficiency in childhood and adolescence: retrospective review. Hematology 2006;11(3):183–6.
12. Kalayci AG, Kanber Y, Birinci A, et al. The prevalence of coeliac disease as detected by screening in children with iron deficiency anaemia. Acta Paediatr 2005; 94(6):678–81.
13. Orkin S, Nathan D, Ginsburg D, et al. Nathan and Oski's Hematology of Infancy and Childhood. 7th edition. Philadelphia: Saunders Elsevier; 2009.

14. Oski FA, Honig AS, Helu B, et al. Effect of iron therapy on behavior performance in nonanemic, iron-deficient infants. Pediatrics 1983;71(6):877–80.
15. Lozoff B, Brittenham GM, Viteri FE, et al. Developmental deficits in iron-deficient infants: effects of age and severity of iron lack. J Pediatr 1982;101(6):948–52.
16. Akman M, Cebeci D, Okur V, et al. The effects of iron deficiency on infants' developmental test performance. Acta Paediatr 2004;93(10):1391–6.
17. Halterman JS, Kaczorowski JM, Aligne CA, et al. Iron deficiency and cognitive achievement among school-aged children and adolescents in the United States. Pediatrics 2001;107(6):1381–6.
18. Congdon EL, Westerlund A, Algarin CR, et al. Iron deficiency in infancy is associated with altered neural correlates of recognition memory at 10 years. J Pediatr 2012;160(6):1027–33.
19. Chang S, Wang L, Wang Y, et al. Iron-deficiency anemia in infancy and social emotional development in preschool-aged Chinese children. Pediatrics 2011; 127(4):e927–33.
20. Corapci F, Calatroni A, Kaciroti N, et al. Longitudinal evaluation of externalizing and internalizing behavior problems following iron deficiency in infancy. J Pediatr Psychol 2010;35(3):296–305.
21. Weiss G, Goodnough LT. Anemia of chronic disease. N Engl J Med 2005;352(10): 1011–23.
22. Nemeth E, Rivera S, Gabayan V, et al. IL-6 mediates hypoferremia of inflammation by inducing the synthesis of the iron regulatory hormone hepcidin. J Clin Invest 2004;113(9):1271–6.
23. Wang CQ, Udupa KB, Lipschitz DA. Interferon-gamma exerts its negative regulatory effect primarily on the earliest stages of murine erythroid progenitor cell development. J Cell Physiol 1995;162(1):134–8.
24. Taniguchi S, Dai CH, Price JO, et al. Interferon gamma downregulates stem cell factor and erythropoietin receptors but not insulin-like growth factor-I receptors in human erythroid colony-forming cells. Blood 1997;90(6):2244–52.
25. Schwarz P, Strnad P, von Figura G, et al. A novel monoclonal antibody immunoassay for the detection of human serum hepcidin. J Gastroenterol 2011;46(5): 648–56.
26. Scarano S, Vestri A, Ermini ML, et al. SPR detection of human hepcidin-25: a critical approach by immuno-and biomimetic-based biosensing. Biosens Bioelectron 2013;40(1):135–40.
27. Grebenchtchikov N, Geurts-Moespot AJ, Kroot JJ, et al. High-sensitive radioimmunoassay for human serum hepcidin. Br J Haematol 2009;146(3):317–25.
28. Kroot JJ, Kemna EH, Bansal SS, et al. Results of the first international round robin for the quantification of urinary and plasma hepcidin assays: need for standardization. Haematologica 2009;94(12):1748–52.
29. Galesloot TE, Vermeulen SH, Geurts-Moespot AJ, et al. Serum hepcidin: reference ranges and biochemical correlates in the general population. Blood 2011; 117(25):e218–25.
30. Cangemi G, Pistorio A, Miano M, et al. Diagnostic potential of hepcidin testing in pediatrics. Eur J Haematol 2013;90(4):323–30.
31. Sun CC, Vaja V, Chen S, et al. A hepcidin lowering agent mobilizes iron for incorporation into red blood cells in an adenine-induced kidney disease model of anemia in rats. Nephrol Dial Transplant 2013;28(7):1733–43.
32. Oren H, Cingoz I, Duman M, et al. Disseminated intravascular coagulation in pediatric patients: clinical and laboratory features and prognostic factors influencing the survival. Pediatr Hematol Oncol 2005;22(8):679–88.

33. Veldman A, Fischer D, Nold MF, et al. Disseminated intravascular coagulation in term and preterm neonates. Semin Thromb Hemost 2010;36(4):419–28.
34. Levi M. Disseminated intravascular coagulation. Crit Care Med 2007;35(9):2191–5.
35. Levi M, van der Poll T, ten Cate H. Tissue factor in infection and severe inflammation. Semin Thromb Hemost 2006;32(1):33–9.
36. Levi M. The imbalance between tissue factor and tissue factor pathway inhibitor in sepsis. Crit Care Med 2002;30(8):1914–5.
37. Levi M, van der Poll T, ten Cate H, et al. The cytokine-mediated imbalance between coagulant and anticoagulant mechanisms in sepsis and endotoxaemia. Eur J Clin Invest 1997;27(1):3–9.
38. Favaloro EJ. Laboratory testing in disseminated intravascular coagulation. Semin Thromb Hemost 2010;36(4):458–67.
39. Levi M, Meijers JC. DIC: which laboratory tests are most useful. Blood Rev 2011; 25(1):33–7.
40. Pernerstorfer T, Hollenstein U, Hansen J, et al. Heparin blunts endotoxin-induced coagulation activation. Circulation 1999;100(25):2485–90.
41. Griffin MP, Gore DC, Zwischenberger JB, et al. Does heparin improve survival in experimental porcine gram-negative septic shock? Circ Shock 1990;31(3):343–9.
42. Meyer J, Cox CS, Herndon DN, et al. Heparin in experimental hyperdynamic sepsis. Crit Care Med 1993;21(1):84–9.
43. Boldt J, Papsdorf M, Piper SN, et al. Continuous heparinization and circulating adhesion molecules in the critically ill. Shock 1999;11(1):13–8.
44. Jaimes F, De La Rosa G, Morales C, et al. Unfractioned heparin for treatment of sepsis: a randomized clinical trial (The HETRASE Study). Crit Care Med 2009; 37(4):1185–96.
45. Levi M, Toh CH, Thachil J, et al. Guidelines for the diagnosis and management of disseminated intravascular coagulation. British Committee for Standards in Haematology. Br J Haematol 2009;145(1):24–33.
46. Dellinger RP, Levy MM, Carlet JM, et al. Surviving Sepsis Campaign: international guidelines for management of severe sepsis and septic shock: 2008. Crit Care Med 2008;36(1):296–327.
47. Warren BL, Eid A, Singer P, et al. Caring for the critically ill patient. High-dose antithrombin III in severe sepsis: a randomized controlled trial. JAMA 2001;286(15): 1869–78.
48. Nadel S, Goldstein B, Williams MD, et al. Drotrecogin alfa (activated) in children with severe sepsis: a multicentre phase III randomised controlled trial. Lancet 2007;369(9564):836–43.

Abnormalities of the Erythrocyte Membrane

Patrick G. Gallagher, MD

KEYWORDS

- Hereditary spherocytosis • Hereditary elliptocytosis • Hereditary pyropoikilocytosis
- Erythrocyte membrane • Anemia • Splenectomy

KEY POINTS

- Disorders of the erythrocyte membrane are an important group of inherited hemolytic anemias.
- Red cell membrane disorders are marked by clinical, laboratory, and genetic heterogeneity.
- Abnormalities of erythrocyte shape on peripheral blood smear provide clues to the underlying diagnosis.
- Hereditary spherocytosis is the most common membrane disorder associated with hemolytic anemia.
- Splenectomy is curative in most patients with membrane-associated hemolytic anemia.
- Growing recognition of long-term risks associated with splenectomy has led to re-evaluation of its use in subsets of patients.

INTRODUCTION

Primary abnormalities of the erythrocyte membrane lead to a variety of clinical syndromes, including hereditary spherocytosis (HS), hereditary elliptocytosis, and related disorders.[1] Clinical and laboratory manifestations, as well as associated molecular defects, of these disorders vary widely. Abnormalities of erythrocyte shape on peripheral blood smear often provide clues to the underlying pathobiology and clinical diagnosis of the underlying disorder.

HEREDITARY SPHEROCYTOSIS

HS syndromes are a group of disorders associated with a primary defect in erythrocyte membrane proteins.[2] HS was first described based on the finding of spherocytes, characteristic erythrocytes lacking central pallor, on peripheral blood smear. HS

Supported in part by grants from the NHLBI, NIH.
Department of Pediatrics, Yale University School of Medicine, 333 Cedar Street, PO Box 208064, New Haven, CT 06520-8064, USA
E-mail address: patrick.gallagher@yale.edu

Pediatr Clin N Am 60 (2013) 1349–1362
http://dx.doi.org/10.1016/j.pcl.2013.09.001 **pediatric.theclinics.com**

occurs worldwide in all racial and ethnic groups. It is the most common inherited anemia in individuals of northern European ancestry, affecting approximately 1 person per 2500 individuals in the United States. Clinical, laboratory, and molecular heterogeneity characterize the HS syndromes.[3]

The principal abnormality in HS erythrocytes is loss of membrane surface area relative to intracellular volume, which leads to spherically shaped erythrocytes with decreased deformability.[4] The loss of surface area results from increased membrane fragility due to primary and secondary abnormalities in erythrocyte membrane proteins, particularly ankyrin, α- and β-spectrin, band 3, and protein 4.2 (**Fig. 1**).[2] Increased erythrocyte fragility leads to vesiculation and membrane loss. Splenic destruction of poorly deformable HS erythrocytes is the primary cause of hemolysis experienced by HS patients.[5,6]

HS is inherited as in autosomal-dominant manner in approximately two-thirds of patients, associated with mutations in the ankyrin, β-spectrin, or band 3 genes.[2] In the remaining patients, inheritance is not dominant because of autosomal recessive inheritance or a de novo mutation.[3,7] Autosomal recessive inheritance is associated with mutations of either the α-spectrin or protein 4.2 genes. Several de novo mutations have been reported in the HS genes.[8,9]

CLINICAL MANIFESTATIONS AND CLASSIFICATION

Clinical manifestations of the spherocytosis syndromes vary widely. Typical HS is associated with pallor, jaundice, splenomegaly, anemia, reticulocytosis, spherocytes on peripheral blood smear, positive osmotic fragility or flow cytometric analysis of eosin-5-maleimide-labeled erythrocytes (EMA binding) (see below), and a positive family history. Mild, moderate, and severe forms of HS have been defined according

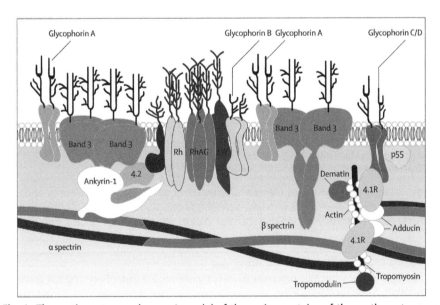

Fig. 1. The erythrocyte membrane. A model of the major proteins of the erythrocyte membrane is shown: α- and β-spectrin, ankyrin, band 3 (the anion exchanger), 4.1 (protein 4.1) and 4.2 (protein 4.2), actin and glycophorin. (*From* Perrotta S, Gallagher PG, Mohandas N. Hereditary spherocytosis. Lancet 2008;372:1412; with permission.)

to the severity of anemia and the degree of compensation for the hemolysis (**Table 1**).[10]

HS may present at any age, but typically it presents in childhood. Anemia is the most frequent finding at presentation (50%), followed by splenomegaly, jaundice, or a positive family history.[3] Most HS patients have incompletely compensated hemolysis with mild-to-moderate anemia that is asymptomatic except for fatigue and pallor. Jaundice is visible at some time in over half of HS patients, usually in association with viral infection or other stress. The jaundice is typically acholuric (ie, unconjugated hyperbilirubinemia without detectable bilirubinuria). By late childhood, palpable splenomegaly is found in most HS patients. Approximately 25% of HS patients have compensated hemolysis (ie, erythrocyte production and destruction are balanced).[11] These patients are not anemic and are usually asymptomatic. The remaining 5% to 10% of HS patients experience moderate-to-severe anemia. This category includes patients with both dominant and recessive HS. The most severely affected patients are transfusion-dependent and almost always have recessive HS.[12–14] Chronically transfused patients are at risk for developing complications of recurrent transfusion and iron overload.

HS may present in the neonatal period. Some patients present with significant neonatal jaundice requiring phototherapy or even exchange transfusion.[15,16] Others present with significant anemia presenting in the first few weeks of life and may require several transfusions in infancy. Most of these patients become transfusion-independent during the first year of life. A subset of patients presents with severe anemia in utero or immediately after birth and requires red blood cell transfusion.[17–19] These patients frequently remain transfusion-dependent and suffer from severe HS.

INITIAL ASSESSMENT/PHYSICAL EXAMINATION

Initial assessment of a patient with suspected HS includes a detailed family history and questions about a history of pallor, jaundice, anemia, gallstones, and splenectomy. Physical examination includes attention to pallor, scleral icterus, and splenomegaly.

After diagnosing a patient with HS, family members should be examined for the presence of HS.

Table 1
Classification of hereditary spherocytosis

	Carrier	Mild Spherocytosis	Moderate Spherocytosis	Severe Spherocytosis[a]
Hemoglobin (g/dL)	Normal	11–15	8–12	6–8
Reticulocytes (%)	≤3	3–6	≥6	≥10
Bilirubin (mg/dL)	0–1	1–2	≥2	≥2
Spectrin content (% of normal)	100	80–100	50–80	40–60
Peripheral smear	Normal	Mild spherocytosis	Spherocytosis	Spherocytosis
Osmotic fragility fresh blood	Normal	Normal or slightly increased	Distinctly increased	Distinctly increased
Incubated blood	Slightly increased	Distinctly increased	Distinctly increased	Distinctly increased

[a] Values in untransfused patients.

From Eber SW, Armbrust R, Schroter W. Variable clinical severity of hereditary spherocytosis: relation to erythrocytic spectrin concentration, osmotic fragility, and autohemolysis. J Pediatr 1990;117:409–16.

LABORATORY FINDINGS

Laboratory findings in HS are heterogeneous. Initial studies in a patient with suspected HS include:

- Complete blood count/erythrocyte indices
- Peripheral blood smear
- Reticulocyte count
- Bilirubin
- Flow cytometric analysis of eosin-5-maleimide-labeled erythrocytes (EMA binding) or incubated osmotic fragility

Erythrocyte Indices

Most HS patients have some degree of anemia with reticulocytosis.[11,20] The mean corpuscular volume (MCV) is normal or slightly decreased in most patients, except in severe cases, when it is decreased despite reticulocytosis, reflecting membrane loss and cellular dehydration.[21] The mean corpuscular hemoglobin concentration (MCHC) is increased ($\geq$34.5 g/dL) due to relative cellular dehydration in more than 50% of patients.[22] The red cell distribution width (RDW) is increased (>14) in most patients. Combining the MCHC and red cell distribution width (>35.4 g/dL and >14, respectively), or combining the MCHC with histograms of hyperdense erythrocytes (MCHC>40 g/dL) obtained from laser-based cell counters, has been utilized to rapidly identify HS patients.[21,23]

Peripheral Blood Smear

Typical HS patients have blood smears with easily detectable spherocytes (ie, erythrocytes lacking central pallor), which are distinctive but not diagnostic (**Fig. 2**A). Occasionally, only a few spherocytes are seen on peripheral smear, or, in contrast, numerous small, dense spherocytes and bizarre erythrocyte morphology with anisocytosis and poikilocytosis may be observed in severely affected patients (see **Fig. 2**B). Specific findings have been identified in some patients with specific membrane protein abnormalities such as pincered erythrocytes (band 3) or spherocytic acanthocytes (β spectrin).[24,25]

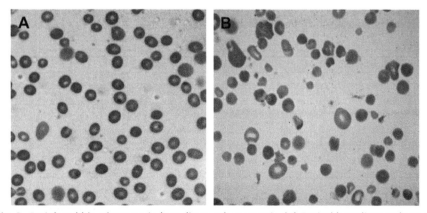

Fig. 2. Peripheral blood smears in hereditary spherocytosis. (*A*) Typical hereditary spherocytosis. Characteristic spherocytes lacking central pallor are seen. (*B*) Severe, recessively inherited spherocytosis. Numerous small, dense spherocytes and bizarre erythrocyte morphology with anisocytosis and poikilocytosis associated with severe hemolysis are seen.

EMA Binding and Osmotic Fragility

The EMA (eosin-5-maleimide) binding test is a flow cytometry-based analysis of the relative amounts of fluorescence, reflecting the amount EMA binding to band 3 and Rh-related proteins in the erythrocyte membrane.[26,27] The basis of the test is the reduction in band 3 and related membrane proteins, leading to a decrease in fluorescence intensity, typically to approximately 65% of normal (**Fig. 3**A).[28] Although defects of band 3 protein are only found in approximately 25% of typical HS patients, decreased fluorescence intensity is also observed in HS erythrocytes with defects in ankyrin and spectrin, thought to be due to transmission of long range effects of varying protein defects across the membrane, thereby influencing EMA binding to band 3. In laboratories with the ability to perform Fluorescence-activated cell sorting-based studies, EMA binding has high sensitivity and specificity and is simple and rapidly

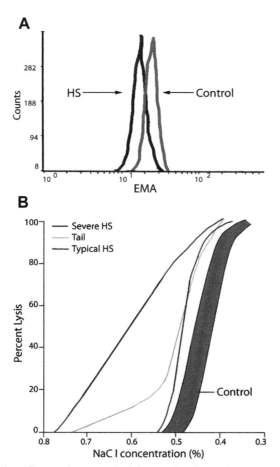

Fig. 3. Testing in hereditary spherocytosis. (*A*). EMA binding. Histogram of fluorescence of EMA-labeled erythrocytes from a normal control and a patient with typical hereditary spherocytosis. Decreased fluorescence in observed from HS erythrocytes. (*B*) Osmotic fragility curves in hereditary spherocytosis. The shaded region is the normal range. Results representative of typical and severe spherocytosis are shown. A tail, representing fragile erythrocytes conditioned by the spleen, is common in spherocytosis patients prior to splenectomy.

performed.[29] EMA binding results are not influenced by shipping or storage for several days, and may be suitable for study of patients who have been recently transfused.

The osmotic fragility (OF) test, which measures the in vitro lysis of erythrocytes suspended in solutions of decreasing osmolarity, is frequently utilized in the diagnosis of HS. Because of the loss of membrane surface area relative to intracellular volume, HS erythrocytes are unable to withstand the introduction of small amounts of free water that occur when they are placed in increasingly hypotonic saline solutions. As a consequence, HS erythrocytes hemolyze more readily than normal erythrocytes at any saline concentration. Hemolysis is determined by measuring the amount of hemoglobin released from red cells into the extracellular fluid. Approximately 25% of HS patients have a normal OF on freshly drawn blood, with the OF curve approximating the number of spherocytes on peripheral smear. After incubation at 37°C for 24 hours, HS erythrocytes lose membrane surface area more readily than normal, because their membranes are leaky and unstable, revealing the membrane defect in OF testing. When the spleen is present, a subpopulation of fragile erythrocytes that have been conditioned by the spleen form the tail of the OF curve that disappears after splenectomy (see **Fig. 3**B).

Neither EMA binding nor OF testing detects all HS patients. Both tests struggle in the identification of cases of mild HS, with OF suffering from poorer sensitivity.[30] Other conditions such as congenital dyserythropoietic anemia type 2, southeast Asian ovalocytosis, and hereditary pyropoikilocytosis may yield reduced fluorescence in EMA binding.[31] OF testing is unreliable in patients who have small numbers of spherocytes, including those who have been recently transfused, and it is abnormal in other conditions where spherocytes are present. Although some laboratories in Europe combine EMA-binding studies with the acidified glycerol lysis test to improve diagnostic sensitivity,[27] this test is not available in most clinical laboratories in North America.

Specialized Testing and Molecular Studies

Ektacytometry is a highly sensitive test of membrane deformability. It is available only in a few specialized centers. Similarly, quantitation of major erythrocyte membrane proteins via sodium dodecyl sulfate-polyacrylamide gel electrophoresis has limited availability. Mutation detection in the major erythrocyte membrane protein genes is now available commercially in the United States. It will be of use in diagnosing difficult cases and in cases in which a molecular diagnosis is desired.

Other Laboratory Findings

Nonspecific markers of ongoing hemolysis, increased bilirubin, increased lactate dehydrogenase, increased urinary and fecal urobilinogen, and decreased haptoglobin may be found, reflecting increased erythrocyte production and/or destruction.

DIAGNOSIS OF HS IN THE NEONATE

The diagnosis of HS in the neonate requires careful consideration of clinical and laboratory findings.[15] In the neonatal period, findings on peripheral smear are variable, with anemia and hyperbilirubinemia typically present. Elevated MCHC is often a clue to underlying HS, especially when greater than 36 g/dL.[16] If specific diagnostic testing is pursued, the diagnosis can be established in the neonatal period. However, EMA binding or osmotic fragility testing must utilize appropriate age-matched controls, and then, the results should be interpreted in concert with clinical course, family history, and detailed examination of the peripheral smear and complete blood cell indices.

IMAGING STUDIES

Splenomegaly is typically detected on abdominal ultrasound examination or radionuclide scanning. Cholelithiasis may be detected on abdominal ultrasound.

DIFFERENTIAL DIAGNOSIS

Hemolytic anemia with spherocytes on peripheral blood smear is found in a number of conditions including autoimmune hemolytic anemia, liver disease, thermal injury, micro- and macroangiopathic hemolytic anemias, clostridial sepsis, transfusion reaction with hemolysis, severe hypophosphatemia, ABO incompatibility, and poisoning with certain snake, spider, and hymenoptera venoms. It is usually not difficult to distinguish HS from other disorders by additional diagnostic testing, such as autoimmune hemolytic anemia via a Coombs test (the direct antiglobulin test or DAT), or by viewing the condition in the appropriate clinical context.

COMPLICATIONS

Complications include gallbladder disease, hemolytic crisis, aplastic crisis, megaloblastic crisis, and uncommon complications such as chronic leg ulceration, cardiomyopathy, neuromuscular abnormalities, and tumors caused by extramedullary erythropoiesis.[32,33]

Gallbladder Disease

Chronic hemolysis may lead to the formation of bilirubinate gallstones, the most common complication in HS patients. In most HS patients, gallstones become apparent in childhood and young adulthood. Interval ultrasonography to detect gallstones is recommended to allow timely diagnosis and treatment, thereby preventing complications of symptomatic biliary tract disease such as biliary obstruction, cholecystitis, and cholangitis.

Crises

Similar to other chronic hemolytic diseases, HS patients suffer from a variety of crises. Hemolytic crises present with jaundice, increased splenomegaly, decreased hematocrit, and reticulocytosis. They are generally mild and are associated with viral infection. Rarely, in severe cases, there is marked jaundice, lethargy, abdominal pain, tender splenomegaly, and significant anemia requiring hospitalization and erythrocyte transfusion. Aplastic crises are typically caused by viral bone marrow suppression by parvovirus B19 infection, which selectively infects erythropoietic progenitor cells and inhibits their growth.[34] During the aplastic phase, the hemoglobin and reticulocyte counts fall, paralleling a decrease in the production of new red blood cells. Aplastic crises usually last 7 to 10 days, about half the life span of typical HS erythrocytes, with the hemoglobin falling to about approximately 50% of its normal level before recovery. In severe HS cases, the anemia may be severe due to extremely short life span of erythrocytes, requiring hospitalization and transfusion. Parvovirus infection may be the first manifestation of HS, and multiple HS family members infected with parvovirus have developed aplastic crises at the same time, leading to descriptions of epidemics of HS.[35] Megaloblastic crises with exaggeration of anemia occur due to exhaustion of folate reserves by the sustained increase in net DNA synthesis associated with increased folate demands,[36] such as during pregnancy, during periods of rapid growth in childhood, and during the recovery phase of an aplastic crisis.

TREATMENT

Treatment of HS encompasses supportive care and when appropriate, splenectomy.[30] HS patients should be followed regularly to assess the degree of anemia, development of complications such as gallstones, and in children, to monitor growth and development. Folate supplementation should be provided to patients with moderate and severe HS. Counseling of the patient regarding HS and its complications as well as investigation of other family members should be provided when appropriate. There should be close observation for hematologic decompensation during acute illnesses or stress. Many care providers obtain serial parvovirus B19 antibody titers until positive to assess risk for parvovirus-associated aplastic crisis.

Splenectomy

Splenic sequestration and destruction are the primary determinants of erythrocyte survival in HS patients. Thus in most HS patients, splenectomy cures the anemia, and decreases the incidence of cholelithiasis.[37] Even severe HS cases experience marked improvement in anemia after splenectomy.[12] Early complications of splenectomy include local infection, bleeding, and pancreatitis caused injury to the tail of the pancreas during surgery. Overwhelming postsplenectomy infection (OPSI), typically from encapsulated organisms, is an uncommon but significant late complication of splenectomy, especially in the first few years of life.[38] Immunization with pneumococcal vaccine and promotion of early antibiotic therapy for asplenic febrile children have led to decreases in the incidence of OPSI. However, increasing rates of penicillin-resistant pneumococci have raised concerns about the potential increases in infection with this virulent organism. Another postsplenectomy complication is an increased risk of cardiovascular disease, particularly thrombosis and pulmonary hypertension.[39–41] Finally, as global travel increases, increasing consideration has been given to the contribution of the spleen in protection from parasitic diseases such as malaria and babesiosis.

For many years, splenectomy was considered a routine procedure in HS patients. However, the risk of OPSI with penicillin-resistant pneumococci, increased recognition of postsplenectomy cardiovascular disease, and increased international travel have contributed to a re-evaluation of the role of splenectomy in the treatment of HS.[42] Health care providers, patients, and family members should review the risks and benefits when considering splenectomy.[38,42] Most experts agree that is reasonable to splenectomize all patients with severe HS and all patients with significant anemia suffering from growth failure, skeletal changes, extramedullary hematopoietic tumors, and leg ulcers.[30] Whether patients with moderate HS and compensated, asymptomatic anemia should have a splenectomy remains controversial. In this group, splenectomy should be considered on a case-by-case basis. Patients with mild HS and well-compensated hemolysis can be managed expectantly, deferring splenectomy unless clinically indicated.[10] Management of patients with mild-to-moderate HS and gallstones is also controversial, as new treatments for cholelithiasis, including laparoscopic cholecystectomy, endoscopic sphincterotomy, and extracorporal choletripsy, lower the risk of treating this complication.

When splenectomy is indicated, laparoscopic splenectomy is the method of choice, resulting in less postoperative discomfort, shorter hospitalization, and decreased costs.[43,44] Partial splenectomy has been advocated for infants and young children with significant anemia associated, with HS and it may be of benefit in typical HS patients.[45,46] In young children, the goal of partial splenectomy is to ameliorate the hemolytic anemia while maintaining residual splenic immune function. Prior to splenectomy, patients should be immunized with vaccines against *Pneumococcus*, *Haemophilus influenzae* type b, and meningococcus.[30,47]

HEREDITARY ELLIPTOCYTOSIS, HEREDITARY PYROPOIKILOCYTOSIS, AND RELATED DISORDERS
Introduction

The hereditary elliptocytosis (HE) syndromes are a heterogeneous group of disorders characterized by the presence of elliptical-shaped erythrocytes on peripheral blood smear.[48,49] Clinical manifestations range from the asymptomatic carrier state to severe, transfusion-dependent hemolytic anemia. HE occurs worldwide in all racial and ethnic groups. It is much more common in areas of endemic malaria, particularly in people of African and Mediterranean ancestry, presumably because elliptocytes confer some resistance to malaria.[50] The worldwide incidence of HE has been estimated to be 1 case in 2000 to 4000 individuals, with the incidence of HE approaching 1 case in 100 people in parts of Africa.[49,51] The true incidence of HE is unknown, as many affected patients are asymptomatic.

Hereditary pyropoikilocytosis (HPP) is an uncommon severe hemolytic anemia characterized by erythrocyte morphology reminiscent of that seen in patients after a thermal burn (**Fig. 4**).[52] There is a strong association between HE and HPP, with one-third of family members of HPP patients exhibiting typical HE.[49,52,53] Thus not surprisingly, HPP occurs predominantly in patients of African descent. Many HPP patients suffer from severe hemolytic anemia in infancy that gradually improves, evolving toward typical HE later in life.

The principal defect in HE/HPP erythrocytes is mechanical weakness or fragility of the erythrocyte membrane skeleton due to defects in various membrane proteins,[4] including α- and β-spectrin, protein 4.1, and glycophorin C. Most cases of HE and HPP are caused by defects in spectrin, the principal structural protein of the erythrocyte membrane skeleton. Spectrin integrity is dependent on the self-association of heterodimers of α- and β-spectrin[54,55] into mature spectrin molecules that are critical for membrane stability and erythrocyte shape and function.[56]

HE is inherited in an autosomal-dominant pattern with rare cases of de novo mutations.[57,58] Mutations in the regions of spectrin where the α- and β-spectrin chains

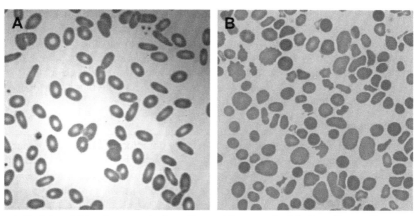

Fig. 4. Peripheral blood smears in hereditary elliptocytosis. (*A*) Hereditary elliptocytosis. Smooth, cigar-shaped elliptocytes are seen. (*B*). Hereditary pyropoikilocytosis. Pronounced microcytosis, poikilocytosis, fragmentation of erythrocytes, and elliptocytes are seen.

self-associate cause the majority of cases of HE/HPP. Most of these mutations are missense mutations at residues critical for spectrin function.[55] In contrast to HS, the HE/HPP syndromes, while also heterogeneous, have been associated with distinct spectrin mutations in persons of similar genetic backgrounds, suggesting a founder effect for these mutations.[59]

Clinical Manifestations

Clinical manifestations of the HE syndromes vary widely, from asymptomatic carriers to patients with severe, transfusion-dependent anemia. Most HE patients are completely asymptomatic. The diagnosis of HE is typically made incidentally during testing for unrelated conditions. The erythrocyte life span is normal in most patients. Symptomatology may vary between members of the same family, attributed to modifier alleles influencing spectrin expression.

Approximately 10% of HE patients and nearly all HPP patients suffer from compensated hemolysis with mild-to-moderate anemia. These patients are homozygotes or compound heterozygotes for defects inherited from each of the parents. Hemolytic HE and HPP patients have clinical features similar to HS including pallor, jaundice, anemia, and gallstones. Hemolysis and anemia are exaggerated in infancy. Elliptocytes are rare on peripheral smear before 6 months of age.

Laboratory Findings

The laboratory findings in HE are heterogeneous:

- Typical HE: varying numbers of elliptocytes on peripheral smear, no anemia or hemolysis
- Hemolytic HE: elliptocytes and fragmented cells on peripheral smear, normocytic anemia, reticulocytosis, markers of hemolysis, abnormal EMA binding, or incubated osmotic fragility
- HPP: elliptocytes and fragmented cells on peripheral smear, microcytic anemia, reticulocytosis, markers of hemolysis, abnormal EMA binding, or incubated osmotic fragility[52,60]

The only laboratory finding in typical HE is the presence of elliptocytes on peripheral blood smear (see **Fig. 4**). These normochromic, normocytic elliptocytes number from a few percent to 100%. In hemolytic HE and HPP, there is anemia, reticulocytosis, hyperbilirubinemia, elevated lactate dehydrogenase (LDH), and other findings of hemolysis. In these conditions, elliptocytes, fragmented cells, and rare ovalocytes, spherocytes, and stomatocytes may be found. In addition to the peripheral blood smear findings found in hemolytic HE, bizarre-shaped cells with fragmentation or budding, poikilocytes, pyknocytes, and microspherocytes are seen in HPP (see **Fig. 4**).[52] The MCV in HPP is frequently very low, 50 to 65 fL. EMA binding or incubated osmotic fragility testing is abnormal in hemolytic HE and HPP.[61]

Imaging Studies

In hemolytic HE and HPP, splenomegaly is typically detected on abdominal ultrasound examination or radionuclide scanning. Cholelithiasis may be detected on abdominal ultrasound.

Differential Diagnosis

Conditions with elliptocytes on peripheral smear include the megaloblastic anemias, the hypochromic microcytic anemias (iron deficiency anemia and thalassemia), myelodysplasic syndromes, and myelofibrosis. In these conditions, elliptocytes generally number less than one-third of erythrocytes. History and additional laboratory testing usually clarify the diagnosis of these disorders.

Complications

Complications in hemolytic HE and HPP are similar to those in HS.

Treatment

Treatment is rarely required for patients with typical HE.[49] In cases of severe HE and HPP, red blood cell transfusions may be required. Splenectomy has been curative. Many experts apply the same indications for splenectomy in HS to patients with symptomatic HE or HPP. After splenectomy, patients with HE or HPP experience resolution of anemia and improvement in clinical symptoms.

SUMMARY

Disorders of the erythrocyte membrane should be considered when evaluating a child with hemolytic anemia. Family history, past medical history, and physical examination findings may all provide important clues to the diagnosis. Initial laboratory testing should include a complete blood count, peripheral blood smear, reticulocyte count, and either EMA binding or incubated osmotic fragility testing. Patients should be monitored expectantly for complications associated with their disease. Splenectomy is curative in most patients with membrane-linked hemolytic anemia. Once considered routine, careful consideration should be given to the risks and benefits of splenectomy before undertaking the procedure.

REFERENCES

1. Da Costa L, Galimand J, Fenneteau O, et al. Hereditary spherocytosis, elliptocytosis, and other red cell membrane disorders. Blood Rev 2013. [Epub ahead of print]. http://dx.doi.org/10.1016/j.blre.2013.04.003.
2. Perrotta S, Gallagher PG, Mohandas N. Hereditary spherocytosis. Lancet 2008; 372:1411–26.
3. Eber S, Lux SE. Hereditary spherocytosis–defects in proteins that connect the membrane skeleton to the lipid bilayer. Semin Hematol 2004;41:118–41.
4. Mohandas N, Gallagher PG. Red cell membrane: past, present, and future. Blood 2008;112:3939–48.
5. Lusher JM, Barnhart MI. The role of the spleen in the pathoophysiology of hereditary spherocytosis and hereditary elliptocytosis. Am J Pediatr Hematol Oncol 1980;2:31–9.
6. Safeukui I, Buffet PA, Deplaine G, et al. Quantitative assessment of sensing and sequestration of spherocytic erythrocytes by the human spleen. Blood 2012; 120:424–30.
7. Gallagher PG. Update on the clinical spectrum and genetics of red blood cell membrane disorders. Curr Hematol Rep 2004;3:85–91.
8. Miraglia del Giudice E, Francese M, Nobili B, et al. High frequency of de novo mutations in ankyrin gene (ANK1) in children with hereditary spherocytosis. J Pediatr 1998;132:117–20.
9. Miraglia del Giudice E, Lombardi C, Francese M, et al. Frequent de novo monoallelic expression of beta-spectrin gene (SPTB) in children with hereditary spherocytosis and isolated spectrin deficiency. Br J Haematol 1998;101:251–4.

10. Eber SW, Armbrust R, Schroter W. Variable clinical severity of hereditary spherocytosis: relation to erythrocytic spectrin concentration, osmotic fragility, and autohemolysis. J Pediatr 1990;117:409–16.

11. Rocha S, Costa E, Catarino C, et al. Erythropoietin levels in the different clinical forms of hereditary spherocytosis. Br J Haematol 2005;131:534–42.

12. Agre P, Asimos A, Casella JF, et al. Inheritance pattern and clinical response to splenectomy as a reflection of erythrocyte spectrin deficiency in hereditary spherocytosis. N Engl J Med 1986;315:1579–83.

13. Agre P, Casella JF, Zinkham WH, et al. Partial deficiency of erythrocyte spectrin in hereditary spherocytosis. Nature 1985;314:380–3.

14. Agre P, Orringer EP, Bennett V. Deficient red-cell spectrin in severe, recessively inherited spherocytosis. N Engl J Med 1982;306:1155–61.

15. Delhommeau F, Cynober T, Schischmanoff PO, et al. Natural history of hereditary spherocytosis during the first year of life. Blood 2000;95:393–7.

16. Christensen RD, Henry E. Hereditary spherocytosis in neonates with hyperbilirubinemia. Pediatrics 2010;125:120–5.

17. Ribeiro ML, Alloisio N, Almeida H, et al. Severe hereditary spherocytosis and distal renal tubular acidosis associated with the total absence of band 3. Blood 2000;96:1602–4.

18. Whitfield CF, Follweiler JB, Lopresti-Morrow L, et al. Deficiency of alpha-spectrin synthesis in burst-forming units—erythroid in lethal hereditary spherocytosis. Blood 1991;78:3043–51.

19. Delaunay J, Nouyrigat V, Proust A, et al. Different impacts of alleles alphaLEPRA and alphaLELY as assessed versus a novel, virtually null allele of the SPTA1 gene in trans. Br J Haematol 2004;127:118–22.

20. Guarnone R, Centenara E, Zappa M, et al. Erythropoietin production and erythropoiesis in compensated and anaemic states of hereditary spherocytosis. Br J Haematol 1996;92:150–4.

21. Michaels LA, Cohen AR, Zhao H, et al. Screening for hereditary spherocytosis by use of automated erythrocyte indexes. J Pediatr 1997;130:957–60.

22. Brugnara C, Mohandas N. Red cell indices in classification and treatment of anemias: from M.M. Wintrobes's original 1934 classification to the third millennium. Curr Opin Hematol 2013;20:222–30.

23. Cynober T, Mohandas N, Tchernia G. Red cell abnormalities in hereditary spherocytosis: relevance to diagnosis and understanding of the variable expression of clinical severity. J Lab Clin Med 1996;128:259–69.

24. Hassoun H, Vassiliadis JN, Murray J, et al. Characterization of the underlying molecular defect in hereditary spherocytosis associated with spectrin deficiency. Blood 1997;90:398–406.

25. Jarolim P, Murray JL, Rubin HL, et al. Characterization of 13 novel band 3 gene defects in hereditary spherocytosis with band 3 deficiency. Blood 1996;88:4366–74.

26. King MJ, Smythe JS, Mushens R. Eosin-5-maleimide binding to band 3 and Rh-related proteins forms the basis of a screening test for hereditary spherocytosis. Br J Haematol 2004;124:106–13.

27. Bianchi P, Fermo E, Vercellati C, et al. Diagnostic power of laboratory tests for hereditary spherocytosis: a comparison study in 150 patients grouped according to molecular and clinical characteristics. Haematologica 2012;97:516–23.

28. King MJ, Zanella A. Hereditary red cell membrane disorders and laboratory diagnostic testing. Int J Lab Hematol 2013;35:237–43.

29. D'Alcamo E, Agrigento V, Sclafani S, et al. Reliability of EMA binding test in the diagnosis of hereditary spherocytosis in Italian patients. Acta Haematol 2011; 125:136–40.

30. Bolton-Maggs PH, Langer JC, Iolascon A, et al. Guidelines for the diagnosis and management of hereditary spherocytosis—2011 update. Br J Haematol 2012; 156:37–49.

31. King MJ, Telfer P, MacKinnon H, et al. Using the eosin-5-maleimide binding test in the differential diagnosis of hereditary spherocytosis and hereditary pyropoikilocytosis. Cytometry B Clin Cytom 2008;74:244–50.

32. Smith J, Rahilly M, Davidson K. Extramedullary haematopoiesis secondary to hereditary spherocytosis. Br J Haematol 2011;154:543.

33. Rabhi S, Benjelloune H, Meziane M, et al. Hereditary spherocytosis with leg ulcers healing after splenectomy. South Med J 2011;104:150–2.

34. Young NS. Hematologic manifestations and diagnosis of parvovirus B19 infections. Clin Adv Hematol Oncol 2006;4:908–10.

35. Lefrere JJ, Courouce AM, Girot R, et al. Six cases of hereditary spherocytosis revealed by human parvovirus infection. Br J Haematol 1986;62:653–8.

36. Delamore IW, Richmond J, Davies SH. Megaloblastic anaemia in congenital spherocytosis. Br Med J 1961;1:543–5.

37. Baird RN, Macpherson AI, Richmond J. Red-blood-cell survival after splenectomy in congenital spherocytosis. Lancet 1971;2:1060–1.

38. Schilling RF. Risks and benefits of splenectomy versus no splenectomy for hereditary spherocytosis—a personal view. Br J Haematol 2009;145:728–32.

39. Crary SE, Ramaciotti C, Buchanan GR. Prevalence of pulmonary hypertension in hereditary spherocytosis. Am J Hematol 2011;86:E73–6.

40. Hayag-Barin JE, Smith RE, Tucker FC Jr. Hereditary spherocytosis, thrombocytosis, and chronic pulmonary emboli: a case report and review of the literature. Am J Hematol 1998;57:82–4.

41. Schilling RF, Gangnon RE, Traver MI. Delayed adverse vascular events after splenectomy in hereditary spherocytosis. J Thromb Haemost 2008;6:1289–95.

42. Casale M, Perrotta S. Splenectomy for hereditary spherocytosis: complete, partial or not at all? Expert Rev Hematol 2011;4:627–35.

43. Wood JH, Partrick DA, Hays T, et al. Contemporary pediatric splenectomy: continuing controversies. Pediatr Surg Int 2011;27:1165–71.

44. Rescorla FJ, Engum SA, West KW, et al. Laparoscopic splenectomy has become the gold standard in children. Am Surg 2002;68:297–301 [discussion: 301–2].

45. Rice HE, Oldham KT, Hillery CA, et al. Clinical and hematologic benefits of partial splenectomy for congenital hemolytic anemias in children. Ann Surg 2003; 237:281–8.

46. Buesing KL, Tracy ET, Kiernan C, et al. Partial splenectomy for hereditary spherocytosis: a multi-institutional review. J Pediatr Surg 2011;46:178–83.

47. Grace RF, Mednick RE, Neufeld EJ. Compliance with immunizations in splenectomized individuals with hereditary spherocytosis. Pediatr Blood Cancer 2009; 52:865–7.

48. Dhermy D, Garbarz M, Lecomte MC, et al. Hereditary elliptocytosis: clinical, morphological and biochemical studies of 38 cases. Nouv Rev Fr Hematol 1986;28:129–40.

49. Gallagher PG. Hereditary elliptocytosis: spectrin and protein 4.1R. Semin Hematol 2004;41:142–64.

50. Dhermy D, Schrevel J, Lecomte MC. Spectrin-based skeleton in red blood cells and malaria. Curr Opin Hematol 2007;14:198–202.

51. Glele-Kakai C, Garbarz M, Lecomte MC, et al. Epidemiological studies of spectrin mutations related to hereditary elliptocytosis and spectrin polymorphisms in Benin. Br J Haematol 1996;95:57–66.

52. Zarkowsky HS, Mohandas N, Speaker CB, et al. A congenital haemolytic anaemia with thermal sensitivity of the erythrocyte membrane. Br J Haematol 1975;29:537–43.

53. Costa DB, Lozovatsky L, Gallagher PG, et al. A novel splicing mutation of the {alpha}-spectrin gene in the original hereditary pyropoikilocytosis kindred. Blood 2005;106:4367–9.

54. Gaetani M, Mootien S, Harper S, et al. Structural and functional effects of hereditary hemolytic anemia-associated point mutations in the alpha spectrin tetramer site. Blood 2008;111:5712–20.

55. Ipsaro JJ, Harper SL, Messick TE, et al. Crystal structure and functional interpretation of the erythrocyte spectrin tetramerization domain complex. Blood 2010; 115:4843–52.

56. Morrow JS, Rimm DL, Kennedy SP, et al. Of membrane stability and mosaics: the spectrin cytoskeleton. In: Hoffman J, Jamieson J, editors. Handbook of physiology. London: Oxford; 1997. p. 485–540.

57. Coetzer T, Lawler J, Prchal JT, et al. Molecular determinants of clinical expression of hereditary elliptocytosis and pyropoikilocytosis. Blood 1987;70:766–72.

58. Coetzer T, Palek J, Lawler J, et al. Structural and functional heterogeneity of alpha spectrin mutations involving the spectrin heterodimer self-association site: relationships to hematologic expression of homozygous hereditary elliptocytosis and hereditary pyropoikilocytosis. Blood 1990;75:2235–44.

59. Gallagher PG. Red cell membrane disorders. Hematology Am Soc Hematol Educ Program 2005;13–8.

60. Coetzer TL, Palek J. Partial spectrin deficiency in hereditary pyropoikilocytosis. Blood 1986;67:919–24.

61. King MJ, Jepson MA, Guest A, et al. Detection of hereditary pyropoikilocytosis by the eosin-5-maleimide (EMA)-binding test is attributable to a marked reduction in EMA-reactive transmembrane proteins. Int J Lab Hematol 2011;33: 205–11.

Sickle Cell Disease in Childhood
From Newborn Screening Through Transition to Adult Medical Care

Charles T. Quinn, MD, MS[a,b,*]

KEYWORDS

- Sickle cell disease • Genetics • Diagnosis • Pathophysiology • Treatment • Survival

KEY POINTS

- SCD affects the entire body, beginning in very early infancy, and a multidisciplinary team is needed to care for children with SCD.
- Some forms of SCD-related morbidity, such as overt stroke, are decreasing owing to prognostic and therapeutic advancements.
- Primary prevention of organ injury is an important focus of current research.
- Almost all children born with SCD in developed nations now survive to adulthood, but the transition to adult medical care is a high-risk period for death.

INTRODUCTION

Sickle cell disease (SCD) is the name for a group of genetic blood disorders caused by sickle hemoglobin (Hb S). The 2 key features of SCD are chronic hemolytic anemia and vaso-occlusion. Although it is fundamentally a blood disease, SCD affects the entire body, and the pathophysiology begins in very early infancy. Pediatricians and family practitioners are crucial partners in the multidisciplinary team that is required to manage children with SCD. This article provides a broad overview of SCD in childhood, focusing on common complications and current treatments. Special attention is given to the results of important clinical trials that have changed the management of SCD.

Funding Sources: Research funding from NHLBI, Eli Lilly and Co, MAST Therapeutics, Inc.
Conflict of Interest: Former advisory board member for Apotex Corporation.
[a] Division of Hematology, Cincinnati Children's Hospital Medical Center, MC 11027, 3333 Burnet Avenue, Cincinnati, OH 45229, USA; [b] Department of Pediatrics, University of Cincinnati College of Medicine, 231 Albert Sabin Way, Cincinnati, OH 45229, USA
* Division of Hematology, Cincinnati Children's Hospital Medical Center, MC 11027, 3333 Burnet Avenue, Cincinnati, OH 45229.
E-mail address: charles.quinn@cchmc.org

HEMOGLOBIN, GENETICS, AND BASIC PATHOPHYSIOLOGY

Hb is the oxygen-carrying protein in blood. It is a tetramer of 4 proteins, 2 α-globins and 2 β-globins. Each globin has an associated oxygen-binding heme group. The α-globins and β-globins are encoded by genes on different chromosomes. The Hb S mutation (β^S) is a single nucleotide substitution in the sixth codon of the β-globin gene (*HBB*). This yields a protein with a hydrophobic valine residue, instead of the normal hydrophilic glutamic acid at the sixth position, that is prone to polymerization on deoxygenation.

Heterozygosity for β^S, called sickle cell trait, occurs frequently in individuals of African ancestry (sub-Saharan, equatorial Africa), but it also occurs commonly in the eastern provinces of Saudi Arabia, central India, and parts of the Mediterranean. It is now found throughout the world due to migration. Heterozygosity for β^S provides some protection against severe malarial infection, which is the generally accepted explanation for the maintenance of this balanced polymorphism. The inheritance of SCD is often referred to as autosomal recessive. However, one can consider β^S to be inherited in an autosomal codominant fashion, because even a single β^S gene is expressed and produces phenotypic changes in the Hb profile (and rare clinical complications). Moreover, homozygous inheritance (β^S/β^S) or compound heterozygosity with certain other mutant β-globins, such as Hb C (β^S/β^C), produce different types of SCD (**Table 1**).

The polymerization of Hb S within red blood cells (RBCs) ("sickling") on deoxygenation underlies all the pathophysiology of SCD. As Hb S-containing RBCs traverse the circulation undergoing cycles of oxygenation and deoxygenation, rigid polymers of Hb S repeatedly form and damage the RBC membrane, drastically shortening the RBC life span. RBCs also become dehydrated, relatively inflexible, and abnormally adhesive. Consequently, they are prone to adhere to the endothelium of blood vessels, in concert with leukocytes and platelets, impeding the flow of blood. This microvascular obstruction, called vaso-occlusion, leads to ischemia, infarction, and ischemia-reperfusion injury of multiple organs and tissues. This pathophysiology produces an ongoing inflammatory response and endothelial dysfunction. Some complications of SCD can be considered to be primarily a consequence of either hemolysis or vaso-occlusion. For example, chronic hemolysis predisposes to bilirubinate cholelithiasis, whereas vaso-occlusive ischemia and infarction of bone marrow is thought to cause the acute painful event ("crisis"), the hallmark of SCD. The pathophysiology of SCD is more complex than a simple "log jam" model of vaso-occlusion by irreversibly sickled RBCs (**Fig. 1**).

FORMS OF SCD AND DIAGNOSIS

The most common and severe form of SCD is the homozygous state for β^S, called sickle cell anemia (Hb SS). Other forms of SCD result from coinheritance of β^S with one of several other abnormal β-globin genes. The most common interacting variants include Hb C and several β^+-thalassemia and β^0-thalassemia mutations. These compound heterozygous states produce types of SCD called sickle-hemoglobin C disease (Hb SC), sickle-β^+-thalassemia (Hb Sβ^+), and sickle-β^0-thalassemia (Hb Sβ^0). In general, Hb SS and Hb Sβ^0 are the most severe forms of SCD, and they may be clinically indistinguishable. In comparison, Hb SC and Hb Sβ^+ are usually less severe. **Table 1** provides an overview of these common forms of SCD.

In the United States and many other developed nations, SCD is usually diagnosed by universal newborn screening for hemoglobinopathies, which involves Hb separation techniques on extracted material from dried blood spots. Initial newborn

Table 1
Common types of sickle cell disease

Genotype	Abbreviation	Name	Typical Peripheral Blood Findings in Untreated SCD				
			Main Hbs Present	Hb (g/dL)	MCV[b] (fL)	Reticulocytes (%)	Severity[a]
β^S/β^S	Hb SS	Sickle cell anemia[c]	S	6–9	Normal	10–25	+++
β^S/β^0	Hb Sβ⁰	Sickle-β⁰-thalassemia	S	6–9	Decreased	10–25	+++
β^S/β^C	Hb SC	Sickle-Hb C disease	S, C	9–12	Usually normal	5–10	++
β^S/β^+	Hb Sβ⁺	Sickle-β⁺-thalassemia	S, A	10–13	Decreased	2–10	+

Abbreviations: Hb, hemoglobin; Hbs, hemoglobins; MCV, mean cell volume; SCD, sickle cell disease.

[a] A population-based generalization that may not apply to the individual (the number of plus signs corresponds to the overall degree of severity of the disease).

[b] Coinheritance of α-thalassemia trait, which is common, will produce microcytosis in Hb SS and Hb SC.

[c] Because they may be clinically indistinguishable, some use the term sickle cell anemia to apply to both Hb SS and Hb Sβ⁰.

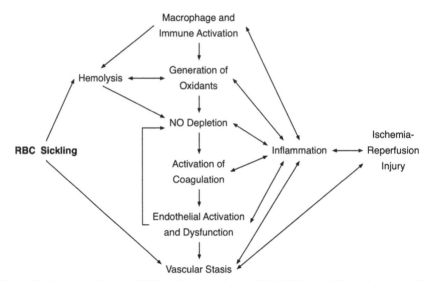

Fig. 1. The initiating factor of SCD pathophysiology is RBC sickling, which leads to hemolysis and vascular stasis. Ischemia-reperfusion injury is the end result of multiple, complex pathophysiologic interactions. (*Modified from* Hebbel RP. Reconstructing sickle cell disease: a data-based analysis of the "hyperhemolysis paradigm" for pulmonary hypertension from the perspective of evidence-based medicine. Am J Hematol 2011;86(2):123–54; with permission.)

screening test results should be confirmed by follow-up studies. Genetic testing is increasingly used for this purpose. Beyond the newborn period, the diagnosis of SCD is made by careful consideration of the complete blood count, peripheral blood morphology, and some combination of Hb separation techniques, family studies, and genetic testing.

The typical blood counts in the common types of SCD are shown in **Table 1**. The presence of irreversibly sickled cells (ISCs) is pathognomonic for SCD. ISCs are commonly seen in Hb SS and Hb Sβ^0 but are rare or absent in Hb SC and Hb Sβ^+. So, the absence of ISCs does not exclude the diagnosis of SCD. Target cells are common in Hb SC, Hb Sβ^0, and Hb Sβ^+. Microcytosis is a feature of Hb Sβ^0 and Hb Sβ^+ (and sometimes Hb SC), but it also occurs when α-thalassemia is independently coinherited with Hb SS or Hb SC.

The mainstay of the diagnosis of SCD, whether at birth or later in life, is an Hb separation technique, such as high-pressure liquid chromatography (HPLC), isoelectric focusing (IEF), or citrate agar electrophoresis. These techniques determine the presence and relative proportions of the different types of Hb present in RBC hemolysates (see **Table 1**). Two different techniques, such as HPLC followed by IEF, should be used to confirm the presence of an abnormal Hb, because different Hb molecules may comigrate in one but not another technique. Hb F will also be present in variable amounts in SCD, as well as small amounts of Hb A$_2$. Sickle Hb solubility testing (eg, Sickledex) is an inadequate diagnostic test because it cannot distinguish sickle trait from SCD. Simple electrophoresis (in cellulose acetate) is usually no longer performed.

Genetic testing is increasingly used to make the initial diagnosis or to confirm a diagnosis of SCD. Different techniques are used to detect point mutations, small deletions or insertions, and large deletions or rearrangements. It is necessary to know which particular technique is being used for the genetic diagnosis of a patient, because each technique has limitations that affect the reliability of the findings.

CLINICAL SCENARIOS AND COMPLICATIONS OF SCD
The Newborn and Infant

The first few months of life are asymptomatic, because affected newborns and very young infants still make a significant amount of fetal Hb (Hb F), which inhibits the polymerization of Hb S and protects against SCD. As Hb F declines over the first few months, there is a commensurate rise in Hb S (instead of the normal Hb A). This period of protection afforded by Hb F usually lasts about 3 months, allowing for newborn screening and early intervention. Universal newborn screening for hemoglobinopathies is performed in all US states (it is important to remember that immigrants may not have had newborn screening). Infants identified to have SCD, or at least those with Hb SS and Hb Sβ⁰, should be prescribed prophylactic penicillin to prevent early fatal pneumococcal sepsis (**Box 1**). Splenic dysfunction (hyposplenism) begins as early as 3 months of age, so prophylactic penicillin should be started by then. Children with SCD require extra vaccinations as well (see **Box 1**). Anemia is usually seen by 6 months of age, and it becomes more severe over the next several months to years. Dactylitis and splenic sequestration can occur in the first year of life, but most other overt complications tend to begin after 1 year of age.

Hemolytic Anemia

The rate of hemolysis in SCD usually exceeds the rate at which new RBCs can be produced by the bone marrow, resulting in anemia despite ongoing reticulocytosis.

Box 1
Penicillin prophylaxis and immunizations

Pencillin Prophylaxis

  For children with Hb SS and Hb Sβ⁰

    Begin at 1–2 months of age

    Age <3 years: penicillin V potassium 125 mg by mouth twice a day

    Age 3–5 years: penicillin V potassium 250 mg by mouth twice a day

    Continue until at least 5 years of age

    May continue past 5 years for pneumococcal sepsis, surgical splenectomy, or parental preference

  For children with Hb SC and Hb Sβ⁺

    Hyposplenism occurs years later than in Hb SS

    Practice varies by center

    Consider starting at age 4–5 years of age or for a history of pneumococcal sepsis or surgical splenectomy

Immunizations

  For all forms of SCD

    The 23-valent pneumococcal polysaccharide vaccine (PPV-23): Ages 2 and 5 years (consider reimmunization at 5-year intervals)

    4-valent meningococcal conjugate vaccine (MCV-4): Age 2 years (consider re-immunization at 5-year intervals)

    Influenza vaccine: yearly

    The normal vaccine series of childhood that includes the 13-valent pneumococcal conjugate vaccine (PCV-13), the *H. influenzae* type b and hepatitis B virus vaccines

RBC life span in Hb SS may be as short as 12 days (compared with the normal 120 days). The degree of anemia varies by the genotype of SCD. **Table 1** shows the typical "baseline" or "steady-state" Hb concentrations; that is, when the patient is not experiencing an acute illness or complication. Because it is chronic, most children are reasonably well compensated physiologically for their anemia, even if severe (eg, 6–7 g/dL). Chronic scleral icterus and a systolic ejection murmur are common and expected findings in patients with moderate to severe anemia, especially Hb SS and Hb Sβ^0. Unconjugated hyperbilirubinemia and an elevated lactate dehydrogenase concentration are also expected. Generally, the degree of chronic anemia itself is not an indication for transfusion in children. A minority of children have symptomatic chronic anemia that interferes with daily activities or quality of life, for whom hydroxyurea therapy or chronic transfusions should be considered. Folic acid supplements are often recommended to prevent depletion of folate stores and megaloblastic "crises," but this is probably unnecessary for most children with SCD in developed countries where many foods are fortified with folate. The 2 classic causes of acute, severe exacerbations of chronic anemia are the transient aplastic crisis and acute splenic sequestration (**Table 2**), discussed individually later in this article. Less severe acute exacerbations of chronic anemia occur during other complications or with concurrent illnesses.

Hyposplenism, Fever, and Sepsis

Children with SCD are at very high risk of invasive pneumococcal disease (300–500 times higher than the general population) because of loss of splenic filtrative function due to infarction (resulting in functional hyposplenism). Typical forms of pneumococcal disease in SCD include bacteremia, sepsis, meningitis, and pulmonary infection. Hyposplenism is detectable by 3 months of age in Hb SS and Hb Sβ^0, so it is necessary to begin prophylactic penicillin before then to prevent fatal pneumococcal sepsis (see **Box 1**).[1] The standard recommendation is to stop prophylactic penicillin at age 5 years in Hb SS and Hb Sβ^0, based on the results of a randomized clinical trial.[2] The routine administration of prophylactic penicillin to infants and young children with Hb SC disease may not be necessary, because hyposplenism does not begin until after 4 years of age.[3] Immunizations are especially important for children with SCD (see **Box 1**). Fatal pneumococcal sepsis is now rare in children with SCD in the United

Table 2		
Acute severe anemia in sickle cell disease: splenic sequestration versus transient aplastic crisis		
	Acute Splenic Sequestration[a]	**Transient Aplastic Crisis[a]**
Spleen	Acutely enlarged	Not palpable or not acutely enlarged
Reticulocytes	Increased from baseline	Inappropriately low[b]
NRBCs	Present	Absent[b]
Platelets	Decreased (Hypersplenism)	Normal or increased[c]
Transfusion	May need *rapid* transfusion for hypovolemic shock	May need *slow/small volume* transfusion to prevent fluid overload and heart failure

Abbreviation: NRBC, nucleated red blood cell.

  [a] Parvovirus infection can trigger acute splenic sequestration, so a patient can have simultaneous sequestration and aplasia. Thus, the typical features listed may not always be present or discriminative.

  [b] If a patient presents in the recovery phase of aplastic crisis, then the reticulocyte and NRBC counts will be increased (see text).

  [c] Parvovirus can sometimes cause multilineage cytopenias, so the platelet count may be decreased (see text).

States and United Kingdom (and other developed nations),[4,5] but pneumococcal disease has not been eradicated. Vigilance is still required for all febrile illnesses, especially because of the recent emergence of nonvaccine serotypes of *Streptococcus pneumoniae*, as well as sepsis in children older than 5 years with SCD.[6,7]

Accordingly, high fever (eg, >101–101.5°F) is a medical emergency in patients with SCD, because it can be the first sign of bacteremia. Patients and caregivers need to present promptly to medical attention. Febrile patients should be promptly evaluated with careful attention to cardiopulmonary status and identification of possible sites of infection. After obtaining a complete blood count and a blood culture, a broad-spectrum parenteral antibiotic (eg, ceftriaxone) should be given without delay. Most children with SCD and fever do not need to be hospitalized.[8] Inpatient management is needed for septic or toxic-appearing children and should be strongly considered for those who have high-risk features, such as very young age (<6 months), concomitant pulmonary disease, blood counts that are significantly different from baseline, missed doses of prophylactic penicillin, or uncertainty of follow-up. Follow-up of both the patient and the results of the blood culture are required for outpatient management.

Splenic Sequestration

Before involution is complete, the spleen is prone to sequestration (trapping of RBCs within the splenic sinusoids). Splenic sequestration typically occurs between 1 and 4 years of age, but much earlier presentation is possible. Splenic involution is usually complete by 5 years of age in Hb SS and Hb Sβ^0, so sequestration is uncommon thereafter. In acute splenic sequestration, the spleen becomes acutely engorged with blood sequestered from the systemic circulation. This leads to potentially severe anemia, hypovolemia, and possibly shock. Sequestration usually develops without warning, so it is important for both parents and health care professionals to be able to detect splenomegaly and the signs and symptoms of acute severe anemia to prevent death. Not all sequestration is severe and life threatening; transfusion is usually reserved for symptomatic or severe anemia. Acute splenic sequestration needs to be differentiated from the transient aplastic crisis, because the approach to transfusion can differ (see **Table 2**). In severe sequestration, the initial transfusion of packed RBCs (PRBCs) may need to be given rapidly to correct hypovolemic shock. Subsequent transfusions, if needed, should be given cautiously and in smaller volumes because of the potential for autotransfusion of sequestered blood that could lead to hyperviscosity. Splenectomy should be considered for severe or recurrent acute splenic sequestration.

In Hb SC and Hb Sβ$^+$, splenic involution is delayed, and sequestration occurs in older children and adults. Splenic sequestration in older individuals is often quite painful because of concomitant infarction. The use of hydroxyurea and chronic transfusions can delay the course of splenic involution, so preservation or "regrowth" of splenic tissue (but not proper splenic immune function) and sequestration can also occur in older children with Hb SS and Hb Sβ^0.

Transient Aplastic Crisis

Human parvovirus (B19) infects RBC precursors in the bone marrow and temporarily impairs the production of new RBCs (erythroblastopenia and reticulocytopenia). In the healthy host, parvovirus infection does not cause anemia because of the long life span of normal RBCs. However, in SCD and other forms of chronic hemolytic anemia (ie, conditions with a shortened RBC life span), parvovirus causes anemia that can be severe. This transient anemia is called the aplastic crisis. Jaundice decreases during aplastic crisis, because the red cell mass has greatly decreased, providing a clue from the history. Spontaneous recovery begins about 1 week after the onset of reticulocytopenia due to antibody-mediated clearance of the virus, heralded by an outpouring of nucleated RBCs followed shortly by reticulocytosis. If a patient presents in this early recovery phase, rather than the reticulocytopenic phase, the anemia and reticulocytosis can be confused with splenic sequestration or an acutely increased hemolytic rate. The need for RBC transfusion depends on the severity of anemia and the clinical status of the patient. Parvovirus aplastic crisis does not recur due to long-lasting humoral immunity.

Parvovirus infection of immunocompetent individuals classically produces isolated RBC aplasia. However, it may cause transient hypoplasia of multiple blood cell lines, including pancytopenia, which may be confusing and lead to unnecessary workup.[9] The acute anemia of the aplastic crisis also needs to be differentiated from acute splenic sequestration, because transfusion therapy can differ (see **Table 2**). The anemia of aplastic crisis develops progressively over the course of a week, so there is physiologic compensation, including increased blood volume and cardiac output. As such, patients with aplastic crisis may be euvolemic or mildly hypervolemic, and rapid transfusion of PRBCs or intravenous fluid boluses may precipitate heart failure. Strong consideration should be given to slow transfusion of PRBCs in small, sequentially administered aliquots (eg, each over 4 hours).

Painful Events and Bony Complications

Dactylitis, or hand-foot syndrome, is one of the earliest physical manifestations of SCD. Vaso-occlusive ischemia and infarction of the metacarpals and phalanges produces painful and often symmetric swelling of the hands, feet, or both. About 30% of children with Hb SS will have dactylitis in the first 3 years of life. Two-thirds of cases occur between 6 months and 2 years of age, and it is unusual beyond 5 years.

Acute SCD pain is typically multifocal and often regional or bilaterally symmetric. It has both nociceptive and neuropathic characteristics. Abdominal pain, the cause of which is unclear, occurs in about one-third of painful events. Fever, especially low grade, occurs in 40% of episodes of uncomplicated pain. With the exception of dactylitis, painful events often have no associated physical signs, like edema or erythema, or overt evidence of inflammation, like joint effusions or leukocytosis. Objective signs occur only 15% of the time, so it is important to believe a patient's report of pain despite a nonspecific history and physical examination. Antecedents of pain, some of which can be avoided, include infection, dehydration, and cooling of the skin. However, most painful episodes are unpredictable and occur without known triggers. Most children with SCD do not have frequent hospitalizations for pain (on average <1 per year). Mild to moderate pain is often managed at home with prompt use of oral analgesics and hydration.

The treatment of painful events is primarily supportive (**Box 2**). A combination of a nonsteroidal anti-inflammatory drug (NSAID) and opiate analgesics, titrated to effect, can usually provide adequate relief. Once the pain begins to resolve, analgesia can usually be decreased quickly. The complete resolution of a painful event may take as long as a week or two, with complete convalescence occurring at home. Transfusion is not indicated for uncomplicated painful events. There is still no abortive therapy for painful events; however, a number of trials of different drugs that target blood rheology, blood cell adhesion, or inflammation are currently under way.

SCD predisposes to osteomyelitis, which is thought to result from secondary infection of ischemic or avascular bone. Differentiating osteomyelitis from painful events is sometimes challenging, because both can cause bony tenderness and joint effusions.

> **Box 2**
> **Principles of supportive care for hospitalized children with sickle cell disease**
>
> Acute Painful Episodes
>
> Pharmacologic analgesia (nonsteroidal anti-inflammatory drugs [NSAIDs] and opiates) that is individualized to the patient and the degree of pain. Avoid overtreatment and undertreatment of pain.
>
> Nonpharmacological methods to decrease pain, such as warm compresses, relaxation, and massage.
>
> Correct any dehydration and maintain normal hydration. Avoid overhydration, which can precipitate acute chest syndrome (ACS).
>
> Incentive spirometry to prevent ACS.
>
> Vigilance for the development of fever and ACS.
>
> Laxative therapy for opiate-related constipation.
>
> Anti-pruritic therapy for opiate-related pruritus.
>
> ACS
>
> Supplemental oxygen for hypoxemia or increased work of breathing.
>
> Correct any dehydration and maintain normal hydration. Avoid overhydration, which can cause pulmonary edema.
>
> Adequate analgesia to prevent respiratory splinting. Inadequate or excessive analgesia can lead to hypoventilation and atelectasis.
>
> Empiric antibiotic therapy for S pneumoniae, Mycoplasma, and Chlamydia—commonly a cephalosporin and a macrolide.
>
> Incentive spirometry.
>
> Bronchodilator therapy for asthma or asthmalike signs and symptoms.
>
> Surgery and Anesthesia
>
> *Preoperative:* For elective surgeries and procedures, the patient should be in the baseline state of health, well hydrated, and free of infection and acute pulmonary disease.
>
> *Intraoperative:* careful attention to the physiologic status of the patient and prevention of hypoxemia, acidemia, hypotension, hypovolemia, and hypothermia.
>
> *Post-operative:* Adequate analgesia to prevent respiratory splinting. Inadequate or excessive analgesia can lead to hypoventilation/atelectasis and ACS.
>
> Incentive spirometry to prevent ACS.
>
> Maintain normal hydration. Avoid overhydration, which can cause pulmonary edema and ACS.
>
> Supplemental oxygen until the patient is fully awake and breathing normally.

Imaging studies may not be discriminative, because sterile bony infarction and osteomyelitis often produce similar findings on radiographs, radionuclide scans, and magnetic resonance imaging (MRI). Clinical features that increase the likelihood of osteomyelitis over an uncomplicated painful event are a single focus of pain, fever, and bacteremia.[10] However, painful events are far more common (50 times more common) than osteomyelitis in SCD, so the pretest probability of osteomyelitis always needs to be considered. Special imaging and biopsy of bone are best reserved for patients for whom there is high clinical suspicion of osteomyelitis. Empiric therapy should be directed against *Salmonella* and *Staphylococcus*, which are the most common causes of osteomyelitis in SCD. Specific therapy is given once an organism is identified.

Avascular necrosis (AVN) can occur as early as 5 years of age, but is most commonly diagnosed in the third decade of life in the United States. The most common site of AVN is the femoral heads, but it also occurs in the proximal humerus and other bones. Pain in the hips or knees should prompt the consideration of AVN. Plain radiographs are often sufficient to make the diagnosis, but MRI may be needed to detect early disease or to plan surgery. No therapy is needed for incidentally detected, asymptomatic AVN. Symptomatic AVN is managed with long-acting NSAIDs (eg, naproxen) and physical therapy. Some patients may require surgery.

Pulmonary Complications

Acute chest syndrome (ACS) refers to a spectrum of acute pulmonary illness in a person with SCD.[11] ACS is the second most common cause of hospitalization in SCD, and it is now the most common cause of death due to SCD. Diagnostic criteria vary, but most definitions specify a new radiographic pulmonary infiltrate and some combination of fever, chest pain, and signs or symptoms of pulmonary disease, such as tachypnea, dyspnea, cough, or hemoptysis. ACS has many antecedents or triggers, including infection, pulmonary fat embolism or thromboembolism, hypoventilation/atelectasis, bronchospasm, and inflammation of any cause. ACS is common in young children in whom it is associated with viral respiratory infections and is often self-limited. The death rate is lower in children than adults. ACS will not be apparent in 30% to 60% of patients at the time of hospitalization, yet ACS often develops in children hospitalized for treatment of other conditions, such as a painful event, or after surgery. Therefore, ACS should be an anticipated complication and prevented when possible (see **Box 2**).

Management of ACS is primarily supportive (see **Box 2**). Unfortunately, there are no randomized controlled trials that compare upfront transfusion (yes or no) or mode of transfusion (simple vs exchange) for established ACS. With this important caveat in mind, simple transfusion of RBCs should be considered for hypoxemia or acute exacerbation of anemia, whereas exchange transfusion should be performed for hypoxemia despite oxygen supplementation, widespread (bilateral, multilobar) pulmonary infiltrates, or rapid clinical deterioration. Corticosteroids can shorten the duration and severity of ACS but can also precipitate "rebound" painful events.[12,13] It is reasonable to use corticosteroids for patients with asthma when it is otherwise indicated (eg, an exacerbation of asthma with ACS) or for rapidly progressive or severe ACS with the intent of preventing or limiting mechanical ventilation.

Asthma is a common diagnosis in children and adults with SCD. This additional diagnosis is associated with an increased frequency of ACS and painful events and a higher risk of death. There is phenotypic overlap between ACS and acute exacerbation of asthma, so clearly differentiating the two is not always possible. There is evidence that asthma and SCD can be separate, comorbid conditions and also evidence that SCD may have asthmalike features.[14] It is prudent to evaluate for asthma when suspected, based on respiratory signs or symptoms, but also when a patient has frequent episodes of pain or ACS. Although there are no appropriate randomized trials to best inform management, good control of asthma or asthmalike pathology might decrease the frequency of ACS and the severity of SCD in general.[14]

Pulmonary hypertension in SCD has been the focus of much recent research and debate. Echocardiography is used as a screening test to estimate pulmonary artery pressure, and a tricuspid regurgitant jet velocity (TRJV) greater than 2.5 m/s is consistent with elevated pressure. A high TRJV is associated with early mortality in adults[15] but not in children.[16] The benefit of screening for elevated pulmonary artery pressures has not been established for children.

Neurologic Complications

The brain is affected in a number of ways in SCD, both structurally and functionally. Without primary prevention (discussed later in this article), overt stroke occurs in 11% of children with Hb SS by 18 years of age (**Fig. 2**), with a peak yearly incidence of about 1% between 2 and 9 years of age. Stroke is much less common in Hb SC and Hb Sβ+. Transient ischemic attacks (TIAs) may be premonitory. Stroke may be an isolated event or occur in conjunction with another complication of SCD, such as ACS, aplastic crisis, or priapism. Most overt strokes in children are ischemic and are associated with occlusive cerebral arterial vasculopathy in large intracranial vessels (see **Fig. 2**B). Hemorrhagic strokes occur with increasing frequency in young adulthood. Suspicion of a neurologic event (overt stroke or TIA) requires emergent neuroimaging. Initial computed tomography to assess for hemorrhage can be considered, especially for patients with severe headache, prior stroke, or known vasculopathy (eg, moya moya vessels), but MRI and MR angiography (MRI/MRA) are needed to define the timing and location of any ischemia or infarction and assess the cerebral arteries. A critical component of the management of acute overt stroke is transfusion. Initial exchange transfusion is associated with a lower risk of recurrent stroke than initial simple transfusion. Patients who have an associated medical event, such as ACS, at the time of stroke also seem to have a lower risk of recurrent stroke. Chronic transfusion therapy to maintain the Hb S lower than 30% decreases the chance of recurrent overt stroke from 60% to 90% to about 20% (see the section on Chronic Transfusions later in this article).

Abnormally increased transcranial Doppler (TCD) blood flow velocities identify children with Hb SS at highest risk of overt stroke. TCD detects dynamic or fixed cerebral arterial stenosis that can be the antecedent of overt stroke (see **Fig. 2**). An abnormal TCD status confers about a 10% risk of stroke per year for 3 years after the test. The Stroke Prevention Trial in sickle cell anemia (STOP trial) showed that chronic transfusions decreased the rate of first stroke in children with abnormal TCD by 92%

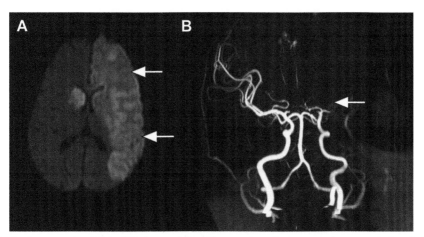

Fig. 2. Overt stroke. (*A*) A diffusion-weighted image that shows extensive acute ischemia in the left cerebral hemisphere (*arrows*) as well as in the right basal ganglia in a child with Hb SS. (*B*) MRA showing complete occlusion of the proximal middle cerebral artery (*arrow*).

compared with observation.[17] Therefore, screening (TCD) should be performed at least annually for children of age 2 to 16 years with Hb SS or Hb Sβ[0] to direct the initiation of chronic transfusion therapy for primary stroke prophylaxis. A follow-up study (STOP 2) showed that discontinuation of transfusions after 30 months resulted in a high rate of reversion to abnormal TCD velocities and stroke.[18] So, outside of a clinical trial, transfusions still need to be continued indefinitely. In the decade since the publication of the STOP study (1999–2009), the mean annual incidence of hospitalization for overt stroke in children with SCD in the United States has decreased by 45%.[19] Although this is clearly an important advance in the care of children with SCD, most children with abnormal TCD velocities will not actually have a stroke (if untreated) and chronic transfusion therapy is burdensome (see section on chronic transfusions later in this article), so further progress is needed.

Silent cerebral infarction (SCI) is more common than overt stroke, occurring in up to 37% of children with Hb SS or Hb Sβ[0] by 18 years of age (**Fig. 3**).[20] By definition, SCI produces no motor or sensory deficits, so it must be identified by screening MRI of the brain. SCI is associated with neurocognitive impairment, poor school performance, and increased risk for subsequent overt stroke. Low Hb concentration and high (relative) systolic blood pressure are risk factors for SCI.[21] The medical management of SCI is not yet defined. A newly recognized covert brain lesion, the acute silent cerebral ischemic event (ASCIE), occurs 40 times more frequently than initial SCI.[22,23] Acute anemic events appear to dramatically increase the risk of ASCIE.[23] A fraction of ASCIEs appear to be transient; others evolve into typical, permanent SCI. Anemia itself also affects neuropsychological function, and children commonly have academic and behavioral difficulties that cannot readily be explained by brain lesions alone. Neuropsychiatric testing, psychological counseling and support, and school intervention programs are key components of comprehensive SCD care.

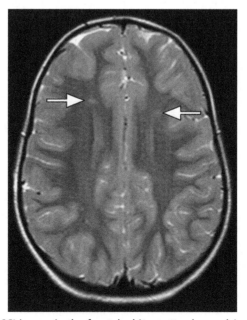

Fig. 3. SCI. Bilateral SCI is seen in the frontal white matter (*arrows*) in a child with Hb SS.

Renal and Genitourinary Complications

The hypoxic, acidic, and hyperosmolar environment of the renal medulla promotes RBC sickling and vaso-occlusion. Repeated vaso-occlusion eventually destroys the vasa recta, leading to inability to maximally concentrate the urine. This is the first renal manifestation of SCD, often occurring before 1 year of age. The urinary concentrating defect results in fixed urinary output (polyuria) and predisposes to dehydration and nocturia or enuresis. Renal ischemia also causes papillary necrosis and microscopic or gross hematuria. Ischemic medullary interstitial fibrosis is thought to promote glomerular hyperfiltration and hypertrophy, which can eventually result in focal segmental glomerular sclerosis, renal insufficiency, and even renal failure. Proteinuria is a marker of glomerular disease, and patients are increasingly prescribed angiotensin-converting enzyme inhibitors and angiotensin receptor blockers to decrease proteinuria with the hope of preventing progression to renal failure. Definitive clinical trial results are lacking for this indication, but a multicenter study of losartan is ongoing (clinicaltrials.gov: NCT01479439).

Priapism is an unwanted, painful erection of the penis. It occurs in all SCD genotypes but is far more common in Hb SS. It can occur as young as 3 years of age, and 90% of males with Hb SS will have at least one episode by 20 years. At the onset of priapism, patients should urinate, drink water, and take a warm shower to promote detumescence. Immediate-release oral pseudoephedrine can be given at home to terminate priapism along with oral analgesics for pain. For prolonged priapism ($\geq$4 hours), patients should seek urgent medical attention. Intravenous hydration and pseudoephedrine (or another vasoactive agent) should be administered if not taken recently by the patient. Aspiration and irrigation of the corpora cavernosa, which can be performed at the bedside, produces rapid detumescence and is the treatment of choice for prolonged priapism.[24] Acute transfusion for priapism is likely ineffective, and exchange transfusion has been associated with stroke. Surgical shunts should be avoided, if possible, to preserve erectile function.

Hepatobiliary Complications

SCD predisposes to cholelithiasis with bilirubinate or pigment gallstones. The prevalence of gallstones is about 10% in children 2 to 4 years of age, increasing to more than 50% in adults. Cholelithiasis and cholecystitis should be considered in the differential diagnosis of abdominal pain in patients with SCD. Symptomatic cholelithiasis and cholecystitis are managed the same way in SCD as in other patients. The caveat is that the patient with SCD must be properly prepared and carefully managed to minimize surgical and anesthetic complications, such as ACS (see **Box 2**). The liver, itself, can be affected in a number of ways by SCD, but consistent terminology has not been established. Acute complications include acute hepatic sequestration, right upper quadrant syndrome, hepatocellular necrosis with hepatic failure, and intrahepatic cholestasis. Cholestasis, even extreme, may appear "benign" and self-limited, but it may be associated with hepatic dysfunction or multiorgan failure. Biliary obstruction should always be excluded.

Surgery and Anesthesia

Patients with SCD are prone to complications after general anesthesia, especially ACS and painful events. This has been attributed to alterations in pH, oxygenation, blood flow, blood volume, and temperature that may promote polymerization of deoxyhemoglobin, blood cell adhesion, and vaso-occlusion. Postoperative respiratory splinting and atelectasis also contribute. ACS may occur in 10% of patients after surgery.

Risk factors include the type of surgery, such as thoracic or intra-abdominal operations, and a history of pulmonary disease, such as ACS or asthma. Principles of perioperative management, including adequate analgesia and aggressive pulmonary support, are shown in **Box 2**.

Two randomized trials showed that preoperative transfusion can prevent postoperative complications. The first trial showed that a single simple transfusion to a total Hb concentration of 10 g/dL was as effective as an aggressive regimen to decrease the Hb S to 30% or less (by exchange transfusion or multiple simple transfusions).[25] However, there was not a randomized, no-transfusion study arm. The second, recent trial randomized patients with SCD undergoing low-risk or medium-risk surgery to transfusion or not.[26] The trial was stopped early because of an excess of complications in the no-transfusion arm. Mostly Hb SS patients who had medium-risk surgery were included. A reasonable conclusion is that preoperative simple transfusion should be offered to patients with Hb SS having medium-risk surgery, and considered for other genotypes and low-risk surgery. Of note, exchange transfusion may be better for prolonged surgery, procedures in which regional blood flow is compromised, or when hypothermia is used. Patients with existing pulmonary or cardiac disease may also fare better following exchange transfusion. Patients with Hb SC or Hb Sβ+ may need exchange transfusion to prevent hyperviscosity because of their relatively high baseline Hb concentration. Lower-risk procedures, such as myringotomy, herniorrhaphy, and circumcision, may not require preoperative transfusion.[27] Transfusion may also not be needed for imaging under anesthesia.

DISEASE-MODIFYING THERAPIES
Hydroxyurea

Hydroxyurea has multiple beneficial effects for patients with SCD, and it is still the only approved medication for prevention of complications in SCD (for adults). Hydroxyurea increases the production of Hb F, which inhibits the polymerization of Hb S, and this is believed to be the principal mechanism of action of the drug. Hydroxyurea also lowers the leukocyte and platelet counts and improves blood rheology, thereby decreasing the propensity for vaso-occlusion. Hydroxyurea reduces the frequency of painful events, ACS, and transfusions by about 50% in adults. Smaller, mostly nonrandomized studies in children have shown similar effects. There is now suggestive evidence that hydroxyurea therapy decreases mortality in adults[28] and children.[29] Side effects are mostly mild, and include dose-related, reversible leukopenia and thrombocytopenia. Hydroxyurea does not appear to increase the risk of malignancy or impair growth.

When first introduced into clinical practice, clinicians waited to prescribe hydroxyurea until a patient manifested some arbitrary degree of disease "severity." Hydroxyurea is now being used increasingly for less rigidly defined indications. Indeed, some hematologists now advocate that a diagnosis of Hb SS or Hb Sβ0 itself is an indication for hydroxyurea therapy and recommend it be offered to children with Hb SS or Hb Sβ0 as young as 9 months of age, regardless of clinical severity, to reduce SCD-related complications (eg, pain, dactylitis, ACS, and anemia).

Hydroxyurea might provide primary prevention of SCD-related organ injury if the medication is started in very early life, but no high-quality clinical evidence yet supports this. The Pediatric Hydroxyurea Phase III Clinical Trial (BABY HUG) trial randomized young children (9–18 months) to a fixed dose of hydroxyurea or placebo for 2 years with the goal of preservation of splenic and renal function.[30] The study failed on its co-primary end points; that is, no differences were observed between the hydroxyurea and placebo arms. Secondary analyses suggested that hydroxyurea did decrease the frequency of dactylitis, other painful events, ACS, and the need for transfusion. Another primary prevention trial is now under way, the Hydroxyurea to Prevent Brain Injury in Sickle Cell Disease (clinicaltrials.gov: NCT01389024) trial, which randomizes children with Hb SS or Hb Sβ^0, 12 to 48 months of age, who have no evidence of overt or covert cerebrovascular disease to hydroxyurea or placebo. The primary outcome is a composite of abnormally increased cerebral arterial blood flow velocity (measured by TCD), SCI, or overt stroke. This critically important trial should be completed before hydroxyurea is routinely offered clinically for primary prevention of central nervous system injury.

There is also hope that hydroxyurea can be given instead of chronic transfusions for the prevention of stroke in high-risk patients. A randomized controlled trial (the SWiTCH study; clinicaltrials.gov: NCT00122980) of continued chronic transfusions versus hydroxyurea for long-term, secondary stroke prevention was stopped early due to futility, and there was an excess of recurrent strokes in the hydroxyurea arm compared with continued transfusions (7 vs 0).[31] The advanced baseline cerebral vasculopathy in many SWiTCH patients may have reduced the effectiveness of hydroxyurea, but the conclusion of the study is that chronic transfusions and chelation remain the best therapy for secondary stroke prevention. A follow-up trial (the TWiTCH study, clinicaltrials.gov: NCT01425307) is currently under way to compare hydroxyurea and chronic transfusions for primary stroke prevention in children with abnormal TCD velocities (and no overt stroke or severe cerebral vasculopathy on MRA).

Hydroxyurea has been used to treat patients with other SCD genotypes, such as Hb SC, but the published experience is limited to case series that provide modest evidence for efficacy of hydroxyurea. There is a theoretical concern that hydroxyurea might increase the frequency of painful events in some patients with Hb SC, perhaps because of increased blood viscosity due to a higher Hb concentration (in patients without baseline severe anemia), but this could be offset by the decrease in RBC adhesion and improvement in blood rheology.

Chronic Transfusions

Chronic transfusions are a prophylactic, disease-modifying therapy that involve regular, usually monthly, transfusions of PRBCs to suppress substantially the percentage of Hb S in peripheral blood and minimize the degree of chronic anemia. The most common indications are primary and secondary prophylaxis of overt stroke, for which the duration of chronic transfusion therapy is indefinite. The role of chronic transfusions for the prevention progressive SCI is currently being studied in the Silent Infarct Transfusion Trial (clinicaltrials.gov: NCT00072761). Chronic transfusions are also offered for other recurrent and severe SCD-related complications, either for a short period (eg, 6 months to 1 year) or indefinitely.

The usual goal of chronic transfusions is to maintain the pretransfusion Hb S <30% with a nadir pretransfusion Hb concentration of 9 to 10 g/dL. After 3 to 5 years of chronic transfusions for prophylaxis of stroke without recurrent neurologic events, some physicians "liberalize" the transfusion regimen to maintain the Hb S lower than 50%. Complications of transfusions include iron overload (and the need for chelation therapy), alloimmunization, autoantibody formation, and transfusion-transmitted infections. Blood may be administered by simple transfusion, partial exchange transfusion, or automated erythrocytapheresis. Exchange techniques may offer the long-term advantage of delaying the accumulation of iron. Up to 30% of patients with SCD who are repeatedly transfused will become alloimmunized to RBC antigens (especially C, E, and Kell). Extended antigen matching can decrease the frequency of alloimmunization.

Hematopoietic Stem Cell Transplantation

Hematopoietic stem cell transplantation (HCST) is the only cure for SCD, and more than 500 transplants for SCD have been reported to international registries. In North America, the most common indication is stroke or cerebrovascular disease, but transplantation is also offered for other recurrent and severe SCD-related complications. Widespread use of HSCT is limited by the lack of suitable related donors and concerns about the toxicities of the procedure. HSCT is safest with an HLA-matched sibling donor (without SCD), but only 10% will have such a donor. Regimen-related mortality for myeloablative HSCT using an HLA-matched sibling donor is about 5%, with a concomitant 5% to 10% risk of graft rejection and 5% to 10% risk of chronic graft versus host disease. There may be additional late effects of transplantation (eg, infertility, cardiovascular, endocrine). Of course, all these risks need to be considered in the context of the lifelong risk of SCD itself. All patients and families with SCD should be aware of the potential of HSCT. It is also reasonable to perform tissue typing on all full siblings to know if there is a matched sibling donor. The procedure should be performed only in centers with experience in HSCT for SCD and, ideally, as part of a clinical research study. The use of alternative donors and reduced intensity conditioning is an area of ongoing study to expand access to HSCT, but these procedures should be performed only on a prospective research protocol.

DISEASE SEVERITY AND PROGNOSTICATION

Hb SS and Hb Sβ^0 are more severe forms of SCD than Hb SC and Hb Sβ^+ (see **Table 1**). However, even within individual genotypes, there is a broad range of disease severity. The concentration of Hb F is the main (but not the only) determinant of this variability. Hb F modulates disease severity by inhibiting the polymerization of Hb S in a "dose-dependent" manner. The coinheritance of α-thalassemia can modify the phenotype of Hb SS by decreasing hemolytic rate and risk of stroke. However, there is some evidence that α-thalassemia may increase the frequency of painful episodes and AVN. Thus, α-thalassemia can modify the phenotype of Hb SS in both favorable and unfavorable ways.

Except for the successful prediction and prevention of overt stroke using screening TCD programs, it remains difficult to identify young children with Hb SS who are at highest risk of adverse outcomes before irreversible organ damage occurs. A promising predictive model was developed based on the occurrence of dactylitis, severe anemia, and leukocytosis in very young children,[32] but it was not validated in an independent cohort.[33] Ongoing research using broad genetic approaches and sophisticated statistical modeling might benefit future children.

SURVIVAL AND TRANSITION TO ADULT MEDICAL CARE

With current multidisciplinary care in an experienced SCD center, almost all children (>95%) born with SCD in developed nations now survive to adulthood.[4,5] The remarkable improvement in survival over the past 4 decades (**Fig. 4**) is the additive result of a variety of interventions, including newborn screening, prophylactic penicillin, immunizations against Haemophilus influenzae type b and S pneumoniae, advances in supportive care, and the increased use of disease-modifying treatments (hydroxyurea, chronic transfusions, and stem cell transplantation).

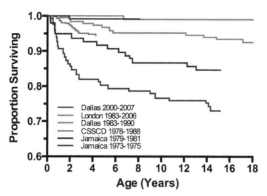

Fig. 4. Improvements in survival for children with Hb SS and Hb Sβ⁰. Overall survival curves spanning 4 decades are shown for large SCD cohorts in the United States, United Kingdom, and Jamaica. (*Data from* Quinn CT, Rogers ZR, McCavit TL, et al. Improved survival of children and adolescents with sickle cell disease. Blood 2010;115:3447–52.)

The burden of mortality in SCD has now shifted to adults, and the transition to adult medical care is a high-risk period for death.[4] There are a number of possible explanations for this vulnerability, including a flawed interface between pediatric and adult medical care in general and the gradual accumulation of SCD-related chronic organ injury during childhood that becomes manifest in young adulthood. Long-term survival estimates (beyond childhood) are less accurately known, but are estimated to be more than 50 years. Individuals with Hb SC and Hb Sβ⁺ have survival estimates that approximate the general population.

SUMMARY

SCD affects the entire body, beginning in very early infancy. A multidisciplinary team is required to manage children with SCD. Thanks to prognostic and therapeutic advancements, some forms of SCD-related morbidity in childhood, such as overt stroke, are decreasing. Primary prevention of organ injury is an important focus of current research. Fortunately, almost all children now born with SCD in developed nations survive to adulthood, but the transition to adult medical care is a high-risk period for death.

REFERENCES

1. Gaston MH, Verter JI, Woods G, et al. Prophylaxis with oral penicillin in children with sickle cell anemia. N Engl J Med 1986;314(25):1593–9.
2. Falletta JM, Woods GM, Verter JI, et al. Discontinuing penicillin prophylaxis in children with sickle cell anemia. Prophylactic Penicillin Study II. J Pediatr 1995; 127(5):685–90.
3. Lane PA, O'Connell JL, Lear JL, et al. Functional asplenia in hemoglobin SC disease. Blood 1995;85(8):2238–44.
4. Quinn CT, Rogers ZR, McCavit TL, et al. Improved survival of children and adolescents with sickle cell disease. Blood 2010;115(17):3447–52.
5. Telfer P, Coen P, Chakravorty S, et al. Clinical outcomes in children with sickle cell disease living in England: a neonatal cohort in East London. Haematologica 2007;92(7):905–12.

6. McCavit TL, Quinn CT, Techasaensiri C, et al. Increase in invasive *Streptococcus pneumoniae* infections in children with sickle cell disease since pneumococcal conjugate vaccine licensure. J Pediatr 2011;158(3):505–7.

7. McCavit TL, Xuan L, Zhang S, et al. Hospitalization for invasive pneumococcal disease in a national sample of children with sickle cell disease before and after PCV7 licensure. Pediatr Blood Cancer 2012;58(6):945–9.

8. Wilimas JA, Flynn PM, Harris S, et al. A randomized study of outpatient treatment with ceftriaxone for selected febrile children with sickle cell disease. N Engl J Med 1993;329(7):472–6.

9. Cauff BE, Quinn CT. Transient parvovirus-associated hypoplasia of multiple peripheral blood cell lines in children with chronic hemolytic anemia. Pediatr Blood Cancer 2008;50(4):861–4.

10. Berger E, Saunders N, Wang L, et al. Sickle cell disease in children: differentiating osteomyelitis from vaso-occlusive crisis. Arch Pediatr Adolesc Med 2009; 163(3):251–5.

11. Quinn CT, Buchanan GR. The acute chest syndrome of sickle cell disease. J Pediatr 1999;135(4):416–22.

12. Bernini JC, Rogers ZR, Sandler ES, et al. Beneficial effect of intravenous dexamethasone in children with mild to moderately severe acute chest syndrome complicating sickle cell disease. Blood 1998;92(9):3082–9.

13. Quinn CT, Stuart MJ, Kesler K, et al. Tapered oral dexamethasone for the acute chest syndrome of sickle cell disease. Br J Haematol 2011;155(2):263–7.

14. Field JJ, DeBaun MR. Asthma and sickle cell disease: two distinct diseases or part of the same process? Hematology Am Soc Hematol Educ Program 2009; 2009(1):45–53.

15. Gladwin MT, Sachdev V, Jison ML, et al. Pulmonary hypertension as a risk factor for death in patients with sickle cell disease. N Engl J Med 2004;350(9): 886–95.

16. Lee MT, Small T, Khan MA, et al. Doppler-defined pulmonary hypertension and the risk of death in children with sickle cell disease followed for a mean of three years. Br J Haematol 2009;146(4):437–41.

17. Adams RJ, McKie VC, Hsu L, et al. Prevention of a first stroke by transfusions in children with sickle cell anemia and abnormal results on transcranial Doppler ultrasonography. N Engl J Med 1998;339(1):5–11.

18. Adams RJ, Brambilla D, Optimizing Primary Stroke Prevention in Sickle Cell Anemia (STOP 2) Trial Investigators. Discontinuing prophylactic transfusions used to prevent stroke in sickle cell disease. N Engl J Med 2005;353(26):2769–78.

19. McCavit TL, Xuan L, Zhang S, et al. National trends in incidence rates of hospitalization for stroke in children with sickle cell disease. Pediatr Blood Cancer 2013;60(5):823–7.

20. Bernaudin F, Verlhac S, Arnaud C, et al. Impact of early transcranial Doppler screening and intensive therapy on cerebral vasculopathy outcome in a newborn sickle cell anemia cohort. Blood 2011;117(4):1130–40.

21. DeBaun MR, Sarnaik SA, Rodeghier MJ, et al. Associated risk factors for silent cerebral infarcts in sickle cell anemia: low baseline hemoglobin, sex, and relative high systolic blood pressure. Blood 2012;119(16):3684–90.

22. Quinn CT, McKinstry RC, Dowling MM, et al. Acute silent cerebral ischemic events in children with sickle cell anemia. JAMA Neurol 2013;70(1):58–65.

23. Dowling MM, Quinn CT, Plumb P, et al. Acute silent cerebral ischemia and infarction during acute anemia in children with and without sickle cell disease. Blood 2012;120:3891–7.

24. Rogers ZR. Priapism in sickle cell disease. Hematol Oncol Clin North Am 2005; 19:917–28.
25. Vichinsky EP, Haberkern CM, Neumayr L, et al. A comparison of conservative and aggressive transfusion regimens in the perioperative management of sickle cell disease. N Engl J Med 1995;333(4):206–13.
26. Howard J, Malfroy M, Llewelyn C, et al. The Transfusion Alternatives Preoperatively in Sickle Cell Disease (TAPS) study: a randomised, controlled, multicentre clinical trial. Lancet 2013;381(9870):930–8.
27. Fu T, Corrigan NJ, Quinn CT, et al. Minor elective surgical procedures using general anesthesia in children with sickle cell anemia without pre-operative blood transfusion. Pediatr Blood Cancer 2005;45(1):43–7.
28. Voskaridou E, Christoulas D, Bilalis A, et al. The effect of prolonged administration of hydroxyurea on morbidity and mortality in adult patients with sickle cell syndromes: results of a 17-year, single-center trial (LaSHS). Blood 2010;115(12): 2354–63.
29. Lopes de Castro Lobo C, Pinto JF, Nascimento EM, et al. The effect of hydroxcarbamide therapy on survival of children with sickle cell disease. Br J Haematol 2013;161(6):852–60.
30. Wang WC, Ware RE, Miller ST, et al. Hydroxycarbamide in very young children with sickle-cell anaemia: a multicentre, randomised, controlled trial (BABY HUG). Lancet 2011;377(9778):1663–72.
31. Ware RE, Helms RW, SWiTCH Investigators. Stroke with transfusions changing to hydroxyurea (SWiTCH). Blood 2012;119(17):3925–32.
32. Miller ST, Sleeper LA, Pegelow CH, et al. Prediction of adverse outcomes in children with sickle cell disease. N Engl J Med 2000;342(2):83–9.
33. Quinn CT, Lee NJ, Shull EP, et al. Prediction of adverse outcomes in children with sickle cell anemia: a study of the Dallas Newborn Cohort. Blood 2008;111(2): 544–8.

Thalassemias

Alissa Martin, MD, Alexis A. Thompson, MD, MPH*

KEYWORDS

- Thalassemia • Iron overload • Hemoglobinopathies • Anemia

KEY POINTS

- The thalassemia syndromes are a heterogeneous group of disorders characterized by variable degrees of hemolysis, chronic anemia, and ineffective erythropoiesis.
- Because more patients are living longer, disease- and treatment-related complications are becoming more common.
- Optimal and safe transfusion support, iron chelation, noninvasive iron assessments, and stem cell therapies provide new tools for effective management of thalassemia.

INTRODUCTION/HISTORY

The thalassemia syndromes are a group of inherited hemoglobinopathies that result from significantly reduced or absent synthesis of normal hemoglobin. The type of thalassemia is based on the defective globin gene involved; patients with affected β-globin genes have β-thalassemia, and those with affected α-globin genes have α-thalassemia. Patients with thalassemia have widely variable clinical presentations, ranging from nearly asymptomatic to severe anemia requiring lifelong blood transfusions with complications in multiple organ systems. The mainstay of therapy for thalassemia remains red blood cell transfusion, which then necessitates iron chelation. This article focuses on the diagnosis and clinical manifestations of thalassemia.

EPIDEMIOLOGY

Although thalassemia is rare in the United States, an estimated 5% of the world's populations carry at least one variant globin allele.[1] In general, these conditions are inherited in an autosomal recessive pattern. Numerous studies have confirmed that red blood cells in thalassemia carriers are less susceptible to invasion by *Plasmodium falciparum*, thus conferring a survival advantage in malaria-endemic regions.[2] The prevalence of thalassemia is highest in geographic regions that historically were most affected by malaria, including the Mediterranean, sub-Saharan Africa, the Middle

The authors have no relevant financial relationships to disclose.

Division of Hematology/Oncology, Ann and Robert H. Lurie Children's Hospital of Chicago, 225 East Chicago Avenue, Box #30, Chicago, IL 60611, USA

* Corresponding author.

E-mail address: a-thompson@northwestern.edu

East, the Asian-Indian subcontinent, and Southeast Asia. Resources available in many regions have substantially improved patient survival over time.[3] In 1973, fewer than 2% of patients with thalassemia were older than 25 years; today that cohort represents 36% of patients with thalassemia in the United States. Immigration has also contributed to the ethnic diversity of the thalassemia population in the United States.[4]

α-THALASSEMIA

α-Thalassemia is caused by absent or decreased production of α-globin chains. The α gene locus contains paired alleles (αα/αα) on chromosome 16. Clinical severity varies based on the number of alleles affected and also on the type of genetic mutation.[5] Deletional defects involving the α-globin gene locus can be from nonhomologous recombination or other mechanisms that either completely or at least partially delete both α-globin chains. Nondeletional mutations result in reduced production of α-globin and, in some cases, varying amounts of structurally aberrant α-globins that are associated with a more severe clinical phenotype.

Persons with one mutated allele are silent carriers (αα/α-). Patients with α-thalassemia trait have 2 deletions (αα/–) on the same chromosome (*cis*) or on opposite (α-/α-) chromosomes (*trans*.). The arrangement of these anomalies have important implications on reproduction. Inheritance of 2 mutant α alleles in *cis* from one parent, combined with a single mutation from a parent who is a silent carrier, may result in a clinically significant condition involving 3 of 4 genes in the offspring. α-Thalassemia involving all 4 α genes typically has a severe clinical phenotype, often causing intrauterine anemia and hydrops fetalis.[6]

Hemoglobin H (HbH) disease is caused by mutations of 3 of the 4 alleles, with compound heterozygosity for α^+ and α^0 mutations. In fetal development, the excess γ chains form homotetramers (γ_4), also called *Hb Bart's*, which are detectable transiently at birth. Later, excess β-globin chains form β_4 homotetramers (HbH), which are unstable and precipitate in developing red cells. The globin chain imbalance contributes to ineffective erythropoiesis and local intracellular oxidative damage in circulating red blood cells and shortened red cell life span. Most patients with HbH disease are not transfusion-dependent but may require transfusion support for infections and other oxidative stresses.[7,8]

The most common nondeletional form of HbH disease is HbH Constant Spring. The Constant Spring α-globin mutation results in the elongation of 3′ mRNA sequences, abnormally elongated α-globin chains, and reduced globin production from the unaffected allele.[8] Intracellular precipitation of oxidized chains of hemoglobin Constant Spring damages red cell membranes, which causes hemolysis and a more severe anemia. Unlike most other forms of HbH disease, patients with HbH Constant Spring are often transfusion-dependent.

β-THALASSEMIA

The β-globin locus on chromosome 11 includes genes that encode γ-, δ-, and β-globins, which pair with α-globin chains to create fetal hemoglobin (HbF), hemoglobin A_2, and normal adult hemoglobin (HbA), respectively. Hundreds of β-globin gene mutations cause β-thalassemia, involving both coding and intervening (noncoding) DNA sequences. The disease severity, or degree of transfusion dependence, correlates with the degree of α-globin chain excess.[9] Patients usually present with anemia as early as the first 6 months of life when HbF production declines,[10] or they can present in early childhood with symptoms such as abdominal distention, hepatosplenomegaly from extramedullary hematopoiesis, irritability, jaundice, and poor growth.

Operationally, β-thalassemia can be described based on blood transfusion requirements. *Thalassemia major* describes patients who require regular blood transfusions, usually more than 8 to 12 times per year. *Thalassemia intermedia* describes patients who can, under normal circumstances, maintain an adequate hemoglobin concentration and require red cell transfusions fewer than 8 times per year, or only in times of physiologic stress.

Hemoglobin E (HbE)/β-thalassemia is a β-thalassemia subtype that deserves special mention. It has been estimated that half of all patients worldwide with clinically severe thalassemia actually have the HbE/β-thalassemia genotype.[11] It is also the most common form of β-thalassemia now detected on newborn screening in some parts of the United States. HbE is a structural β-globin variant that results in both decreased β-globin chain synthesis and production of a structurally abnormal β^E-globin that has impaired interactions with α-globin. When coinherited with a β-thalassemia mutation, HbE/β-thalassemia results in a phenotype that is extremely variable, ranging from full transfusion dependence to only requiring occasional transfusions during times of physiologic stress, such as during acute febrile illnesses.

PATHOPHYSIOLOGY

Normally, α-globin production begins during fetal development and is constant throughout later life. γ-Globin is turned on during early embryonic development to create HbF ($\alpha_2\gamma_2$), which typically declines in the first 6 months after birth. β-Globin production begins in late gestation to create HbA ($\alpha_2\beta_2$), which reaches adult levels by 1 year of life.

The fundamental derangement that underpins thalassemia syndromes is globin synthesis imbalance, and often it is the relative excess of a given chain that is most destructive. In β-thalassemia, the reduced production of β-globin chains leads to decreased amounts of HbA per cell, and interaction of the relative excess α-globin chains with the red cell membrane causes hemolysis and premature intramedullary cell death. This ineffective erythropoiesis is compounded by sequestration of defective red cells in the spleen. In the absence of transfusion therapy, severe anemia over time contributes to growth retardation and high-output cardiac failure in thalassemia, and tissue hypoxia stimulates increased erythropoietin production and marrow expansion that causes bony deformities and fractures. Increased intestinal iron absorption and regular red cell transfusions contribute to parenchymal iron deposition. Excess tissue iron causes cirrhosis, cardiac dysfunction, and endocrinopathies.

DIAGNOSIS OF THALASSEMIA

The complete blood cell (CBC) count, including hemoglobin and red cell indices, and reticulocyte count are useful screening studies for thalassemia. Most patients with thalassemia will have microcytosis and hypochromia. The red blood cell count may be relatively elevated. The peripheral blood smear shows many bizarrely shaped, fragmented, microcytic red cells and may reveal red blood cell inclusion bodies (globin chains) after supravital staining.

Hemoglobin electrophoresis or high-performance liquid chromatography (HPLC) can be diagnostic for β-thalassemia, with predominant HbF, low or absent HbA, and elevated HbA_2. HbE may also be detected in patients with HbE/β-thalassemia. For patients with HbH disease or other forms of α-thalassemia, HPLC can detect elevated Hb Bart's at birth, HbH later in life, and Hb Constant Spring variants. In general, DNA-based testing is essential for a definitive diagnosis of α-thalassemia, and should be used for confirmatory testing in patients with suspected β-thalassemia.

COMPLICATIONS OF THALASSEMIA
Growth Impairment

Children with thalassemia are at risk for growth failure from chronic anemia, and a hypermetabolic state from high-volume ineffective erythropoiesis.[12] Nutritional deficiencies, chelation toxicity, and iron-induced endocrinopathies also contribute to suboptimal linear growth and weight gain. Pubertal development may also be delayed because of iron loading and/or severe anemia.

Bone Abnormalities

Marked erythroid expansion can cause significant bony abnormalities in patients with thalassemia, particularly those with β-thalassemia.[12,13] Radiographic abnormalities in untreated patients can become marked after the first year of age.[14] Long bones show cortical thinning with expansion of the medullary space, and become prone to pathologic fractures. Skull findings are classic, with marked widening of the diploic space and a resultant "hair on end" appearance (**Fig. 1**). Other skeletal findings include failed pneumatization of maxillary sinuses and maxillary overgrowth that contributes to the classic thalassemic facies, widening of the ribs, and squared vertebral bodies.

Osteopenia, osteoporosis, and related complications are prevalent in patients with β-thalassemia major and thalassemia intermedia.[15] Low bone mass can begin in childhood with an imbalance between osteoblastic bone formation and osteoclastic bone resorption. By adulthood, up to 50% of patients with β-thalassemia major have osteoporosis.[14,16,17] Up to 40% of patients will have at least one pathologic bone fracture. The cause of decreased bone mineral density in patients with thalassemia is multifactorial, including delayed sexual maturation, deficiencies of insulin-like growth factor 1 (IGF-1), and growth hormone, and direct toxic effects of iron on osteoblasts.

Endocrinopathies

Hypogonadotropic hypogonadism is common in adults with thalassemia, with reported rates upward of 50%.[3,12,18] Iron toxicity has been implicated as a major contributor to hypogonadism and impaired fertility from pituitary, hypothalamic, and, to a lesser degree, gonadal iron deposition.[19] Hypothyroidism and diabetes are also prevalent complications because of iron-induced tissue injury. Although

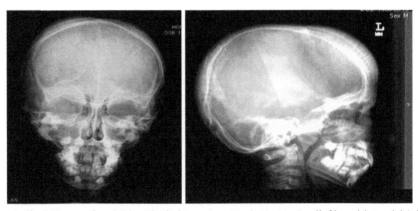

Fig. 1. Skull X-rays of a child with thalassemia, anterior-posterior (*left*) and lateral (*right*) views. Note expansion of the medullary space which is most prominent in the frontal and parietal regions with associated "hair on end" appearance.

uncommon in thalassemia, hypoparathyroidism can be associated with impaired calcium metabolism and suboptimal responses to vitamin D supplementation.

Prevention is the best treatment for bone disease and other endocrinopathies in thalassemia. This entails adequate transfusion and chelation to prevent chronic anemia and iron loading, and adequate vitamin D and calcium intake, particularly during skeletal development. Hormone replacement therapy improves quality of life and alleviates manifestations of hypogonadism, and may improve bone mineral density in patients with thalassemia. Insulin and thyroid hormone are often needed to manage diabetes and hypothyroidism. Treatment of osteoporosis with bisphosphonates can improve bone density.[13]

Splenomegaly and Hypersplenism

Splenic enlargement in thalassemia may be caused by extramedullary hematopoiesis and sequestration of defective red blood cells. Splenomegaly is particularly problematic in patients who are inadequately transfused, and may result in leukopenia, thrombocytopenia, and exacerbation of anemia from hypersplenism. Splenectomy alone may be sufficient to control anemia and obviate transfusions in thalassemia intermedia, and may be indicated for patients with β-thalassemia major whose transfusion requirements are higher than expected.[20]

Hypercoagulability

Several factors lead to an overall hypercoagulable state in patients with thalassemia. The altered physiology of the red cell membrane makes the cells more rigid and more likely to aggregate. Splenectomy may increase the susceptibility to thrombosis in chronic hemolytic anemias (not just thalassemia). In patients who have undergone splenectomy, thrombin generation is increased and protein C and S are decreased, further contributing to the prothrombotic state. Chronic activation of platelets and altered vascular endothelial physiology occur in thalassemia major after splenectomy, and in patients with thalassemia intermedia regardless of history of splenectomy.[21]

Pulmonary Hypertension

Increased pulmonary arterial pressure has been increasingly described as a cause of morbidity and mortality in thalassemia.[22] Contributing factors may include activation of the coagulation system, platelets, and endothelial cells, and inflammation. Risk seems to be higher with increasing age and in patients who have undergone splenectomy, particularly those with thalassemia intermedia. Echocardiography is the most commonly used test to detect elevated regurgitant tricuspid jet velocity as a marker for increased pulmonary artery pressure. Antiplatelet agents (aspirin and dipyridamole); pulmonary vasodilators, such as prostaglandins and endothelin receptor antagonists; and phosphodiesterase type 5 inhibitors have been used with varying success to manage pulmonary hypertension in thalassemia and related conditions.

TREATMENT FOR THALASSEMIA

The only curative treatment for thalassemia is stem cell transplantation. The mainstay of long-term management is red cell transfusion, but the resultant iron overload causes severe complications.

Transfusion Therapy

The primary treatment for severe thalassemia remains red blood cell transfusion. The decision to begin a transfusion regimen is based largely on clinical assessment and the impact of chronic anemia on a patient's life, including factors such as impaired growth, bony deformities, and fatigue. In most patients with β-thalassemia major, transfusions are initiated before 1 year of age. Specific transfusion goals may differ among treatment centers, but in general, transfusion regimens should target a pre-transfusion hemoglobin of 9 to 10 g/dL. Maintaining this hemoglobin level suppresses endogenous erythropoietin levels and reduces marrow expansion and extramedullary hematopoiesis. Measuring linear growth and weight gain are important in determining if the transfusion regimen is adequate. Most patients will require 10 to 20 mL/kg of packed red blood cells every 2 to 4 weeks, for a total of approximately 200 mL/kg/y.

HbF Induction

HbF may be important in ameliorating symptoms of β-thalassemia intermedia, because increased γ-globin production decreases the relative excess of α chains and increases total hemoglobin levels.[23] Three main classes of medications have been investigated for efficacy in increasing HbF, although clinical experience in thalassemia still lags behind that in sickle cell disease.

Hydroxyurea

Despite success in treating sickle cell disease, hydroxyurea has not been extensively studied in thalassemia and results have not been as consistent. Hydroxyurea does not seem to have the same positive effects on red cell morphology and deformability in thalassemia. However, some evidence suggests that hydroxyurea may diminish phosphatidylserine expression on red cell membranes in some patients with thalassemia, which can prolong erythrocyte survival and decrease hypercoagulability.[23] Hydroxyurea may rarely decrease transfusion requirements in patients with thalassemia major. Combinations of hydroxyurea with other agents, such as recombinant erythropoietin, improve total hemoglobin levels in some patients with non–transfusion-dependent thalassemia.[24]

DNA methylation inhibitors

Repression of γ-globin genes in adult red blood cells involves DNA methylation and other epigenetic changes. Demethylating agents, such as 5-azacytidine, resulted in a rapid increase in γ-globin synthesis with increased total hemoglobin levels in single patients and small case series; however, concerns over potential mutagenicity and cytotoxicity limited its use clinically.[23,24] Decitabine (5-aza-2′-deoxycytadine) has a more favorable safety profile and resulted in increased total hemoglobin and absolute HbF levels in a small pilot study of patients with β-thalassemia intermedia.[23,25]

Short-chain fatty acids

Short-chain fatty acids can ameliorate anemia in non–transfusion-dependent thalassemia through inducing HbF production.[24] Sodium phenylbutyrate can result in increased levels of total hemoglobin and improved markers of ineffective erythropoiesis in patients with β-thalassemia. Isobutyramide has had variable effect on HbF levels but no change in markers of ineffective erythropoiesis. Clinical trials with other short-chain fatty acids are either underway or currently being planned for both thalassemia and other hemoglobinopathies.

Stem Cell Transplantation

Hematopoietic stem cell transplantation (HSCT) using HLA-matched related donor stem cells has become part of conventional treatment for thalassemia.[26] Early studies of HSCT in thalassemia identified hepatomegaly, portal fibrosis, and poor chelation history as patient characteristics that, when incorporated into the Pesaro classification, predict overall survival, thalassemia-free survival, and graft rejection.[27] Patients with no adverse features (class 1) had a probability of thalassemia-free survival of 87%. Class 2 patients with at least 1 adverse feature had an 85% thalassemia-free survival and class 3 patients with 2 or more adverse features had a 53% thalassemia-free survival. With modifications in the conditioning regimen used, the probability of thalassemia-free survival in class 3 patients has improved.[28] Additional risk factors that favor superior HSCT outcomes using multivariate analysis include young age (<7 years), limited iron burden, and minimal comorbidities, such as hepatic dysfunction.[29] Results of HSCT using alternative donors and reduced intensity or nonmyeloablative conditioning may expand the availability of this treatment option while preserving fertility.[30]

Splenectomy

Although removal of the spleen can alleviate anemia in non–transfusion-dependent thalassemia, splenectomy is now used less frequently in both thalassemia intermedia and major.[31] In addition to the potential infectious complications, increasing evidence supports that patients who undergo splenectomy are at increased risk for thrombotic events. Thrombin generation is increased and protein C and S are decreased in these patients, further contributing to this prothrombotic state. Platelet counts are also

---

Box 1
Recommended thalassemia comprehensive care assessments

Monthly assessments

- CBC count
- Serum ferritin
- Comprehensive metabolic panel
- Urinalysis

Annual assessments

- Cardiac T2-star (T2*) magnetic resonance imaging (MRI) (>age 10 years)
- Liver iron measurement (R2* MRI or FerriScan)
- Bone mineral density
- Hearing
- Vision

Annual laboratory screening

- Fasting serum glucose
- Free T4, thyroid-stimulating hormone
- Parathyroid hormone
- Luteinizing hormone, follicle-stimulating hormone, estradiol/testosterone
- Ionized calcium
- Vitamin D
- IGF-1, IGF binding protein-3
- Vitamin C
- Trace elements: zinc, copper, selenium
- Viral studies (human immunodeficiency virus, hepatitis A, B, C)

higher in patients after splenectomy, but this is not necessarily associated with increased clotting tendency.[21] Patients should receive pneumococcal, meningococcal, and *Haemophilus influenzae* vaccines before splenectomy and should take lifelong penicillin for prophylaxis.

MANAGEMENT/OBSERVATION OF PATIENTS WITH THALASSEMIA

Patients should have regular comprehensive visits to evaluate the most common and important complications of disease. In addition to CBC and reticulocyte counts, age-appropriate laboratory studies should be performed to evaluate endocrine function and nutritional deficiencies, and to screen for chelation-related toxicities. Bone density measurements and noninvasive imaging for tissue iron burden provide important information and opportunities for intervention. Recommended assessments are summarized in **Box 1**.

SUMMARY

The thalassemia syndromes are a heterogeneous group of disorders characterized by a variable degree of hemolysis, chronic anemia, and ineffective erythropoiesis. Because more patients are living longer, disease- and treatment-related complications are becoming more common. Optimal and safe transfusion support, iron chelation, noninvasive iron assessments, and stem cell therapies provide new tools for effective management of thalassemia.

REFERENCES

1. Weatherall DJ. The definition and epidemiology of non-transfusion-dependent thalassemia. Blood Rev 2012;26(Suppl 1):S3–6.
2. Taylor SM, Parobek CM, Fairhurst RM. Haemoglobinopathies and the clinical epidemiology of malaria: a systematic review and meta-analysis. Lancet Infect Dis 2012;12(6):457–68.
3. Borgna-Pignatti C, Rugolotto S, De Stefano P, et al. Survival and complications in patients with thalassemia major treated with transfusion and deferoxamine. Haematologica 2004;89(10):1187–93.
4. Vichinsky EP, MacKlin EA, Waye JS, et al. Changes in the epidemiology of thalassemia in North America: a new minority disease. Pediatrics 2005;116(6):e818–25.
5. Higgs DR, Gibbons RJ. The molecular basis of alpha-thalassemia: a model for understanding human molecular genetics. Hematol Oncol Clin North Am 2010;24(6):1033–54.
6. Vichinsky E. Complexity of alpha thalassemia: growing health problem with new approaches to screening, diagnosis, and therapy. Ann N Y Acad Sci 2010;1202:180–7.
7. Lal A, Goldrich ML, Haines DA, et al. Heterogeneity of hemoglobin H disease in childhood. N Engl J Med 2011;364(8):710–8.
8. Chui DH, Fucharoen S, Chan V. Hemoglobin H disease: not necessarily a benign disorder. Blood 2003;101(3):791–800.
9. Rund D, Rachmilewitz E. Beta-thalassemia. N Engl J Med 2005;353(11):1135–46.
10. Manca L, Masala B. Disorders of the synthesis of human fetal hemoglobin. IUBMB Life 2008;60(2):94–111.
11. Vichinsky E. Hemoglobin e syndromes. Hematology Am Soc Hematol Educ Program 2007;79–83.

12. Vogiatzi MG, Macklin EA, Trachtenberg FL, et al. Differences in the prevalence of growth, endocrine and vitamin D abnormalities among the various thalassaemia syndromes in North America. Br J Haematol 2009;146(5):546–56.
13. Toumba M, Skordis N. Osteoporosis syndrome in thalassaemia major: an overview. J Osteoporos 2010;2010:537673.
14. Perisano C, Marzetti E, Spinelli MS, et al. Physiopathology of bone modifications in beta-Thalassemia. Anemia 2012;2012:320737.
15. Vogiatzi MG, Macklin EA, Fung EB, et al. Bone disease in thalassemia: a frequent and still unresolved problem. J Bone Miner Res 2009;24(3):543–57.
16. Haidar R, Musallam KM, Taher AT. Bone disease and skeletal complications in patients with beta thalassemia major. Bone 2011;48(3):425–32.
17. Jensen CE, Tuck SM, Agnew JE, et al. High prevalence of low bone mass in thalassaemia major. Br J Haematol 1998;103(4):911–5.
18. Thuret I, Pondarre C, Loundou A, et al. Complications and treatment of patients with beta-thalassemia in France: results of the National Registry. Haematologica 2010;95(5):724–9.
19. Tsironi M, Karagiorga M, Aessopos A. Iron overload, cardiac and other factors affecting pregnancy in thalassemia major. Hemoglobin 2010;34(3):240–50.
20. Cohen A, Gayer R, Mizanin J. Long-term effect of splenectomy on transfusion requirements in thalassemia major. Am J Hematol 1989;30(4):254–6.
21. Cappellini MD, Musallam KM, Poggiali E, et al. Hypercoagulability in non-transfusion-dependent thalassemia. Blood Rev 2012;26(Suppl 1):S20–23.
22. Morris CR, Vichinsky EP. Pulmonary hypertension in thalassemia. Ann N Y Acad Sci 2010;1202:205–13.
23. Musallam KM, Taher AT, Cappellini MD, et al. Clinical experience with fetal hemoglobin induction therapy in patients with beta-thalassemia. Blood 2013;121(12): 2199–212 [quiz: 2372].
24. Taher AT, Musallam KM, Karimi M, et al. Contemporary approaches to treatment of beta-thalassemia intermedia. Blood Rev 2012;26(Suppl 1):S24–27.
25. Olivieri NF, Saunthararajah Y, Thayalasuthan V, et al. A pilot study of subcutaneous decitabine in beta-thalassemia intermedia. Blood 2011;118(10):2708–11.
26. Smiers FJ, Krishnamurti L, Lucarelli G. Hematopoietic stem cell transplantation for hemoglobinopathies: current practice and emerging trends. Pediatr Clin North Am 2010;57(1):181–205.
27. Lucarelli G, Galimberti M, Polchi P, et al. Bone marrow transplantation in patients with thalassemia. N Engl J Med 1990;322(7):417–21.
28. Sodani P, Gaziev D, Polchi P, et al. New approach for bone marrow transplantation in patients with class 3 thalassemia aged younger than 17 years. Blood 2004; 104(4):1201–3.
29. Sabloff M, Chandy M, Wang Z, et al. HLA-matched sibling bone marrow transplantation for beta-thalassemia major. Blood 2011;117(5):1745–50.
30. Bernardo ME, Piras E, Vacca A, et al. Allogeneic hematopoietic stem cell transplantation in thalassemia major: results of a reduced-toxicity conditioning regimen based on the use of treosulfan. Blood 2012;120(2):473–6.
31. Thompson AA, Cunningham MJ, Singer ST, et al. Red cell alloimmunization in a diverse population of transfused patients with thalassaemia. Br J Haematol 2011;153(1):121–8.

Evaluation and Treatment of Transfusional Iron Overload in Children

Hannah M. Ware, Janet L. Kwiatkowski, MD, MSCE*

KEYWORDS

- Transfusion • Iron overload • Chelation • Magnetic resonance imaging

KEY POINTS

- Regular red cell transfusions lead to progressive iron accumulation that causes liver, heart, and endocrine organ toxicity.
- Transfusional iron burden is monitored with serum ferritin levels and liver and cardiac magnetic resonance imaging.
- Three different chelators are available for clinical use in the United States: deferoxamine, deferasirox, and deferiprone.
- Trends in iron burden, transfusional iron intake, patient/family preferences, adverse effect profiles, and adherence are factors to consider in individualizing chelation plans.

INTRODUCTION

Transfusions are increasingly being used in the management of blood disorders in children. Regular red cell transfusions have been used to alleviate the severe anemia and suppress ineffective erythropoiesis in patients with thalassemia major for many years, and are increasingly being used in the management of children with sickle cell disease (SCD). In SCD, the goal of regular transfusions generally is to reduce the hemoglobin S level to less than 30% to 50% to prevent or treat disease complications, such as stroke. An estimated 1000 to 2000 individuals with thalassemia and 100,000 individuals with SCD live in the United States,[1] and therefore patients with SCD account for a larger proportion of transfused individuals. Other hematologic disorders treated with transfusions include bone marrow failure syndromes, such as Diamond-Blackfan anemia (DBA), and hemolytic anemias, such as pyruvate kinase deficiency.

The monitoring and treatment guidelines for transfusional iron overload generally have been derived from the experience with patients with thalassemia and are described herein. However, differences in transfusional iron loading and its clinical

Division of Hematology, Department of Pediatrics, Children's Hospital of Philadelphia, University of Pennsylvania, 34th Street, Civic Center Boulevard, Philadelphia, PA 19104, USA
* Corresponding author. Children's Hospital of Philadelphia, 3501 Civic Center Boulevard, Colket Building, Room 11024, Philadelphia, PA 19104.
E-mail address: kwiatkowski@email.chop.edu

Pediatr Clin N Am 60 (2013) 1393–1406
http://dx.doi.org/10.1016/j.pcl.2013.09.003
0031-3955/13/$ – see front matter © 2013 Elsevier Inc. All rights reserved.

manifestations between patients with thalassemia and other blood disorders are becoming better understood. These differences and the implications for clinical management are discussed where applicable.

HOW TRANSFUSIONS LEAD TO IRON OVERLOAD

Typical regular transfusion regimens involve the administration of 10 to 15 mL/kg of packed red blood cells every 3 to 5 weeks. Each milliliter of pure packed red cells (hematocrit 100%) contains just more than 1 mg of iron. Humans do not have the physiologic ability to excrete excess iron, and therefore chronic red cell transfusion therapy leads to progressive iron accumulation. Chelation therapy is necessary to prevent iron accumulation and/or to remove excess iron. In children with SCD, exchange transfusion also may be used, which limits transfusional iron loading and may obviate the need for chelation.[2]

TOXICITY OF IRON

Free iron is toxic; therefore, iron is usually bound to proteins within the body. For example, iron in plasma is bound to transferrin, a transport protein. However, transferrin becomes saturated in iron overload states, leading to the presence of non–transferrin-bound iron (NTBI) forms.[3] Labile plasma iron (LPI), a form of NTBI, is taken up into cells and causes oxidative damage. The heart, liver, and endocrine organs are most susceptible to iron-related injury.

Cardiac toxicity, including congestive heart failure and atrial and ventricular arrhythmias, is the leading cause of death related to iron overload in patients with thalassemia major.[4] Iron-related heart disease generally does not become evident until the teen years in patients with thalassemia who are poorly chelated.[5] Furthermore, iron-associated cardiac disease is uncommon in transfused individuals with SCD, even at older ages.[6] However, children with DBA and sideroblastic anemias may be at risk for iron-related heart disease at younger ages.[7]

Hepatic toxicity from iron overload includes inflammation, fibrosis, and cirrhosis.[8] It is important to vaccinate children against hepatitis A and B viruses and to counsel against alcohol abuse to avoid exposure to additional hepatotoxins. Iron also damages endocrine organs, leading to growth failure, growth hormone deficiency, delayed puberty,[9] hypogonadotropic hypogonadism, impaired glucose metabolism and insulin-dependent diabetes mellitus, osteopenia, hypothyroidism, and hypoparathyroidism.[5] In a registry of North American patients with thalassemia, almost half of patients in the 16- to 24-year-old age group had developed endocrinopathies.[5] Iron-associated endocrinopathies are less common in patients with SCD than in those with thalassemia, but may occur at earlier ages in patients with DBA.[7,10] Good control of iron burden in children is important because organ damage likely results from cumulative exposure to iron.

EVALUATION OF IRON OVERLOAD

Several different tests can be used to monitor the degree of iron overload. Measured with a simple blood test, the serum ferritin level is the easiest and least expensive test to obtain. Although the ferritin level correlates with total body iron burden in patients receiving chronic transfusions,[11] the utility of the test is limited because infection, inflammation, and ascorbate deficiency can either raise or lower serum ferritin levels, altering the ability to accurately predict iron stores. In particular, the serum ferritin may not correlate well with the degree of transfusional iron loading in patients with SCD.[12] Ferritin levels also do not predict cardiac iron loading accurately.[13]

The liver iron concentration (LIC) correlates well with total iron burden in transfusion associated iron overload,[14] and levels greater than 15 mg of iron per gram (Fe/g) dry weight (dw) of liver are associated with increased morbidity and mortality.[15] However, LIC does not adequately predict cardiac iron levels due to differential rates of iron loading and unloading in these organs.[16,17] Before the validation of noninvasive imaging techniques, liver biopsy was considered the best method for determining LIC.[18] Biopsy also enables direct assessment of histology, which is helpful in assessing tissue injury from iron, infections such as hepatitis C, and chelator-related toxicity. However, the risks of the procedure limit its acceptability to patients and providers, and noninvasive imaging techniques have superseded liver biopsy for the estimation of liver iron.

The superconducting quantum interference device (SQUID) is one noninvasive technique for estimating LIC,[19] but given that few SQUID scanners exist worldwide, the use of this technique is impractical for many patients. Magnetic resonance imaging (MRI) is more widely available, and liver iron estimation by R2 and R2* techniques correlates well with LIC determined by biopsy.[20,21] The presence of iron in hepatocytes or cardiomyocytes causes the tissues to darken more rapidly on MRI than non–iron-loaded tissue. R2 and R2* represent the rate of tissue relaxation (darkening), and the values typically are converted into milligrams of Fe/g dw tissue on clinical reports. MRI has now become the primary monitoring tool for both liver and cardiac iron.[22]

The ability to estimate cardiac iron using T2* MRI techniques has revolutionized the care of patients with transfusional iron overload. Cardiac T2* can predict the risk of developing heart disease, allowing intensification of therapy that may prevent this outcome. T2*, the reciprocal of R2* (1000/R2*), reflects the half-life of tissue darkening, and thus lower values are worse.[23] Cardiac T2* greater than 20 ms is normal, white values less than 10 ms indicate severe cardiac iron loading. In one multicenter cohort study, 98% of patients who developed heart failure had T2* less than 10 ms in the year prior.[13] Patients with cardiac T2* less than 6 ms were at highest risk, with a 47% chance of developing heart failure within a year of the T2* study. In addition, most (83%) cardiac arrhythmias occurred with T2* values less than 20 ms. Thus, cardiac T2* values that decrease to less than 20 ms indicate the presence of cardiac iron loading and a need for better chelation.

Abnormal cardiac T2* is uncommon in children with thalassemia in the first decade of life, but increased cardiac iron was reported to be detectable in 24% of children between 9.5 and 15.0 years old and 36% of children 15 to 18 years old in one study.[24] Regularly transfused patients with SCD have a lower risk of cardiac iron loading, even at older ages.[6] Therefore, beginning cardiac T2* surveillance around 10 years old in children with thalassemia major is generally recommended, whereas monitoring in children with SCD often may be postponed until the teen years. In contrast, chronically transfused children with DBA may be at increased risk for early cardiac disease,[7] and T2* monitoring beginning at 5 years old may be warranted.

MRI also may detect iron loading in endocrine organs. Abnormal pancreatic iron levels (R2* >100 MHz) are associated with an increased risk of glucose dysregulation,[25] and pituitary iron loading and volume loss are associated with an increased risk of hypogonadism.[26] These MRI techniques need to be studied further and currently are not in widespread clinical use.

GOALS OF IRON CHELATION

Chelation therapy is used to limit iron loading from ongoing transfusions and to remove excess accumulated iron. Chelators also bind and detoxify NTBI forms and protect susceptible organs from oxidative injury. Chelation therapy can prevent and reverse iron-associated cardiac disease, and with aggressive chelation, some endocrinopathies may improve.[27,28]

Chelation therapy should be started in children 2 years of age or older, after 1 to 2 years of chronic transfusions, and when the serum ferritin level is greater than 1000 ng/mL on 2 separate measurements obtained when the child is well. Chelation therapy is dosed to maintain the liver and cardiac iron in an acceptable range and to match ongoing transfusional iron intake; with increasing transfusional iron intake, higher doses of chelator are needed.[29] Target ranges for LIC and cardiac T2* results are shown in **Fig. 1**. Traditionally, the goal has been to keep the LIC between 2 and 7 mg/g dw, ferritin between 500 and 1500 ng/mL, and cardiac T2* greater than 20 ms. Some centers have shown improvement in endocrinopathies and other iron-related toxicities in adult patients using more aggressive chelation regimens to achieve normal body iron stores.[28,30] This approach has not been studied in growing children.

PHARMACOLOGIC STRATEGIES

Three chelators are currently approved by the FDA, each with varying properties.

Deferoxamine

Deferoxamine was the only available chelator for more than 30 years. The drug has poor oral bioavailability and a short half-life[31]; thus, deferoxamine is given as a continuous infusion of 25 to 40 mg/kg given over 8 to 12 hours, 5 to 7 days per week either subcutaneously or intravenously. Daily administration of higher doses (50–60 mg/kg/d) over longer durations of up to 24 hours often is used for patients with evidence of

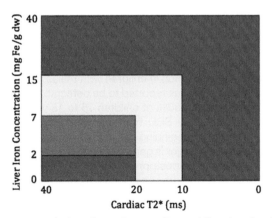

Fig. 1. Chelation recommendations for various cardiac and liver iron levels. The green area indicates optimal liver and cardiac iron levels; current chelation can be continued. The gray area indicates low iron stores with an increased risk of chelator toxicity. Children should be monitored closely for chelator-associated toxicities, and chelator dose should be reduced if these occur. The yellow area shows moderate cardiac and liver iron burden, with concern for an increased risk of iron-associated toxicity. If the iron levels are not improving from prior studies, adherence should be addressed and/or chelation intensified. The red area denotes iron levels that are unacceptably high; adherence should be addressed and chelation intensified. Combination chelation should be considered because of the increased risk of cardiac morbidity and mortality.

significant cardiac iron loading (cardiac T2* <10 ms) or iron-related cardiac toxicity. Deferoxamine induces both urinary and fecal iron excretion.[32] This chelator effectively removes hepatic and cardiac iron[27,33] and can prevent, and even reverse, iron-related cardiac complications.[34,35]

Adverse effects associated with the use of deferoxamine are described in **Table 1**. Some adverse effects, including audiologic, ophthalmologic, and growth and bone toxicities, are dose-related and may be minimized through adjusting the deferoxamine dose based on the degree of iron loading.[36–39] In addition, deferoxamine often is not started until 3 years of age, and lower doses (25–30 mg/kg/d) are used in young children to minimize side effects. Acute neurotoxicity and pulmonary toxicity have been reported with doses of 10 to 20 mg/kg/h, and these high doses generally are not recommended.[40,41]

Deferiprone

Deferiprone (Ferriprox, ApoPharma, Inc, Toronto, Canada) has been in clinical use in Europe and other countries for more than a decade. The drug received FDA approval in late 2011 for patients with transfusion-dependent thalassemia for whom treatment with another chelator has failed. Deferiprone has good oral bioavailability but a short half-life.[42] The typical daily dose is 75 to 100 mg/kg in 3 divided doses orally.

Iron excretion with deferiprone is primarily urinary.[43] Although serum ferritin levels and LIC improve in some patients taking deferiprone, others have experienced no change or even an increase in these values with treatment.[44] Using higher doses of deferiprone (up to 100 mg/kg/d) may improve ferritin levels and LIC in poor responders.[45,46] Importantly, deferiprone is particularly effective at cardiac iron removal. Retrospective analyses have shown better cardiac T2* values and reduced cardiac morbidity and mortality among patients receiving deferiprone compared with deferoxamine.[47,48] A prospective randomized study confirmed that deferiprone improves cardiac T2* and left ventricular function better than deferoxamine.[49]

Common adverse effects of deferiprone and monitoring recommendations are described in **Table 1**. The most concerning side effects are neutropenia and agranulocytosis, occurring in 6.2% and 1.7% of patients, respectively.[50] Most cases of agranulocytosis occur within the first year of treatment, although a few cases have developed later.[51,52] Patients with underlying bone marrow failure syndromes, such as DBA, may be at higher risk.[53,54] Neutropenia generally resolves with discontinuation of the drug; rechallenge is not recommended for patients who develop agranulocytosis.[51]

Deferasirox

Deferasirox (ICL670, Exjade, Novartis Pharma Stein AG, Stein, Switzerland) was approved for use in the United States in 2005. The drug is supplied as orally dispersible tablets that must be dissolved in a large glass of water or juice and taken once daily.[55] The drug is recommended to be taken on an empty stomach, 30 minutes before a meal. Administration with fatty food increases the bioavailability of the drug,[55] but if the requirement for fasting impedes adherence, administration with a low-fat meal can be considered. The typical dose of deferasirox for the treatment of transfusional iron overload is 20 to 40 mg/kg/d. Iron excretion with this drug is primarily fecal, and therefore not easily measurable.

Deferasirox at doses of 20 to 30 mg/kg/d reduces LIC and ferritin levels comparable to deferoxamine.[33] However, 22% to 44% of patients treated with deferasirox at doses greater than 30 mg/kg/d do not experience satisfactory iron balance, which may be related to individual differences in drug bioavailability, adherence, or other

Table 1
Chelator adverse effects, monitoring, prevention, and treatment recommendations

Chelator	Adverse Effect	Monitoring	Prevention	Treatment
DFO	Local reaction	Examine infusion sites at each visit	Rotate infusion sites; use more dilute concentration of DFO	For severe reactions, may consider addition of hydrocortisone to infusion
	Audiologic: tinnitus, high-frequency hearing loss	Audiologic examination annually	Maintain ratio of DFO (mean dose in mg/kg/day)/ferritin <0.025; limit exposure to loud noises, such as high volume on headphones	Hold/reduce dose
	Ophthalmologic: visual loss and/or changes in visual acuity, color vision changes, retinal opacities and pigment changes, delayed visual evoked potentials, optic neuritis	Ophthalmologic examination annually	Maintain ratio of DFO (mean dose in mg/kg/day)/ferritin <0.025	Hold/reduce dose
	Bony deformities	Growth velocity and seated height twice yearly; consider knee radiographs	Avoid use in children <3 y; administer low doses (25–30 mg/kg/d) to growing children	Hold/reduce dose
	Increased risk of infection with Yersinia, Klebsiella	Blood cultures if indicated	Hold DFO with unexplained fever	Antibiotic therapy if cultures positive
	Neurotoxicity	Neurologic examination	Avoid very high doses	Hold/reduce dose
	Pulmonary toxicity	NA	Avoid very high doses	Hold/reduce dose

Drug	Toxicity	Monitoring	Prevention	Management
DFP	Neutropenia (ANC 500 to <1500 × 10⁹/L) and agranulocytosis (ANC <500 × 10⁹/L)	Complete blood cell count with white blood cell differential weekly and with febrile events	Avoid concomitant use of medications that may cause cytopenias; avoid use in children with history of unexplained neutropenia or bone marrow failure syndromes	Hold drug GCSF may be administered in setting of neutropenia/agranulocytosis and infection
	GI symptoms	Query for nausea, vomiting, diarrhea	Increase dose gradually	Administer with food Supportive care (eg, antiemetic) Symptoms often improve with continued drug administration
	Arthralgia and arthropathy	Routine joint examinations; for arthralgia or arthropathy of large joints persisting after discontinuing DFP, consider radiograph or MRI	NA	Supportive care (eg, nonsteroidal anti-inflammatory agents); hold/reduce dose if persistent symptoms
	Elevated hepatic enzymes	Hepatic enzymes at least quarterly	NA	Generally resolves without dose adjustment Hold/reduce dose if persists
	Decreased plasma zinc	Plasma zinc concentration at least annually	NA	Zinc supplementation
DFX	Audiologic: high-frequency hearing loss	Audiologic examination annually	Avoid high doses in children with low iron burden; limit exposure to loud noises	Hold/reduce dose

(continued on next page)

Table 1
(continued)

Chelator	Adverse Effect	Monitoring	Prevention	Treatment
	Ophthalmologic: cataracts, lenticular opacities, retinal disorders, elevations in intraocular pressure	Ophthalmologic examination annually	Avoid high doses in children with low iron burden	Hold/reduce dose
	Rash	Physical examination	NA	For mild or moderate, may continue current dose; For more severe, may hold and then restart drug at lower dose; Short course of oral steroids may be considered
	GI symptoms	Query for nausea, vomiting, diarrhea, abdominal pain	Patients with lactose intolerance may experience more GI symptoms because of presence of lactose in drug manufacturing	Supportive care (eg, Lactaid or antidiarrheal agent); Reduce dose; Divide dose (twice daily); Symptoms may improve over time
	Elevated hepatic enzymes; rare reports of hepatic failure	Hepatic enzymes and bilirubin 2 wk after starting DFX and then monthly	NA	Hold for transaminase that are consistently rising or >5x upper limit; Reduce dose; discontinue if hepatic failure
	Nephrotoxicities: elevated creatinine, proteinuria, renal Fanconi syndrome	Creatinine, urinalysis, electrolytes monthly	NA	Hold/reduce dose if creatinine abnormal or persistent proteinuria; Hold for Fanconi syndrome and discontinue if recurs with rechallenge
	GI bleeding	Monitor for dark or bloody stools	Avoid concomitant use of steroids, nonsteroidal anti-inflammatory medications, and anticoagulants if possible	Hold drug; Gastroenterology referral
	Cytopenias	Monitor complete blood count at least quarterly	NA	Hold drug

Abbreviations: ANC, absolute neutrophil count; DFO, deferoxamine; DFP, deferiprone; DFX, deferasirox; GCSF, granulocyte colony-stimulating factor; GI, gastrointestinal; NA, not applicable.
Data from Refs.[50,73,74]

factors.[56–58] Giving the drug in 2 divided doses, rather than once daily, improved iron excretion in some poor responders.[56,58]

Treatment with deferasirox improves cardiac T2* in patients with abnormal studies and prevents new cardiac iron accumulation in patients with prior normal cardiac T2*.[59] However, patients who have very high liver iron levels may not respond as well.[60] In contrast to deferiprone,[49] deferasirox has not been shown to improve left ventricular ejection fraction.[59,60] The utility of deferasirox in patients with abnormal heart function is not yet known.

The adverse effect profile of deferasirox is shown in **Table 1**. Gastrointestinal disturbances have been reported to occur less commonly in children younger than 16 years (15.8%) compared with older patients (29.1%).[61] Nephrotoxicity includes mild elevations in serum creatinine levels and intermittent proteinuria.[33] In one single-center retrospective review of 10 children, the glomerular filtration rate declined by 20% after deferasirox was started.[62] Several cases of proximal renal tubular dysfunction leading to electrolyte abnormalities (Fanconi syndrome) have been reported in children and adults receiving deferasirox.[63,64] This toxicity has been noted both in the setting of acute illness and in otherwise well patients, and was reversible with discontinuation of the drug.

EVALUATION/ADJUSTMENT

Patients who are receiving chelation therapy need close monitoring to ensure optimal treatment. The volume of red cells administered should be recorded to assess transfusional iron intake. Serum ferritin levels should be obtained at least quarterly to follow trends in iron loading. Liver and cardiac MRI scans generally are obtained annually. Guidelines for maintaining optimal iron levels on chelation therapy are provided in **Fig. 1**. In general, when the cardiac T2* decreases to less than 20 ms, and especially less than 10 ms, or when the LIC is higher than 7 mg/g dw and not improving, better chelation is needed.

When iron burden is too high, several strategies can be used to improve chelation. First, patients and parents should be queried about adherence, and any obstacles should be addressed. Methods for improving adherence include giving the child choices about how to take the chelator, making the routine for taking the chelator fun, and creating a reward system to encourage taking the chelator.[65] In older children and adolescents, parental involvement in chelator administration may improve adherence.[66] Chelator dose can be increased if the patient is not currently taking the maximal dose. Chelation agents may also be switched. Finally, the addition of a second chelator can be considered, especially if iron burden is at very concerning levels (LIC >15 mg/g dw or cardiac T2* <10 ms) or if adverse effects prevent dose escalation.

COMBINATION CHELATION THERAPY

Treatment with more than one chelator should be considered if the patient has poorly controlled iron burden, experiences dose-limiting chelator toxicity, or has difficulty taking a chelator (eg, deferoxamine) on a daily basis. Most published data of dual chelation involve treatment of patients in their teens and older.

The most extensively studied chelator combination is that of deferiprone and deferoxamine. Both serum ferritin levels and LIC significantly improved with this chelator combination.[67,68] Combination deferoxamine and deferiprone is currently recommended for patients with iron-related cardiac disease, because this regimen has shown superior improvement in cardiac T2*, left ventricular ejection fraction, and cardiac function compared with deferoxamine monotherapy.[67]

Few data on the combination of deferoxamine and deferasirox are currently available. In one pilot study of 22 subjects with transfusion-dependent thalassemia and severe iron overload or iron-related organ dysfunction, both the serum ferritin levels and LIC improved after a year of combination treatment.[69] Cardiac T2* also improved in all 6 subjects with abnormal baseline values. Unexpected adverse effects were not reported. Additional safety and efficacy data are needed before clinical recommendations for combination therapy with deferasirox and deferoxamine can be made.

Similarly, only pilot data are available regarding combination therapy with the 2 oral chelators, deferasirox and deferiprone. Among 15 adult subjects with thalassemia major who had well-controlled iron burden at baseline, serum ferritin levels and LIC significantly improved after 12 to 24 months of combination therapy.[30] Rates of adverse effects were similar to those expected with monotherapy.[30] Further studies assessing the safety and efficacy of this drug combination in patients with high liver and/or cardiac iron loading and organ dysfunction are needed.

OTHER ORAL CHELATORS IN DEVELOPMENT

FBS0701 (SSP-004184) is a new oral chelator derived from desferrithiocin and modified to minimize nephrotoxicity. In an initial phase 2 study of FBS0701 in adults with transfusion-dependent anemias, the mean LIC rose with a dose of 16 mg/kg/d, and essentially was unchanged with a dose of 32 mg/kg/d.[70] Adverse effects included nausea, vomiting, abdominal pain, and diarrhea; nephrotoxicity was not evident. Data on cardiac iron removal are not yet available. Additional phase 2 studies in children and adults are ongoing.[71,72]

SUMMARY

Routine use of cardiac and hepatic MRI and trends in serum ferritin levels allow for close monitoring of organ-specific iron loading in children and teens receiving regular red cell transfusions. Chelation regimens should be adjusted based on trends in these iron levels, because timely changes may prevent the development of iron-related organ toxicity in at-risk children. Three iron chelators, deferoxamine, deferiprone, and deferasirox, are currently approved in the United States to treat iron overload. These drugs can be administered as monotherapy or in combination, although limited data are available for combinations other than deferiprone and deferoxamine, and on the use of combination therapy in young children. Iron burden, transfusional iron intake, adherence, and adverse effects should be assessed regularly, and the information should be used to tailor each child's chelation plan. For growing children, the risks of overchelation and chelator toxicity must be balanced with the risks of cumulative iron exposure.

REFERENCES

1. Hassell KL. Population estimates of sickle cell disease in the U.S. Am J Prev Med 2010;38(Suppl 4):S512–21.
2. Kim HC, Dugan NP, Silber JH, et al. Erythrocytapheresis therapy to reduce iron overload in chronically transfused patients with sickle cell disease. Blood 1994; 83(4):1136–42.
3. Piga A, Longo F, Duca L, et al. High nontransferrin bound iron levels and heart disease in thalassemia major. Am J Hematol 2009;84(1):29–33.
4. Zurlo MG, De Stefano P, Borgna-Pignatti C, et al. Survival and causes of death in thalassaemia major. Lancet 1989;2(8653):27–30.

5. Cunningham MJ, Macklin EA, Neufeld EJ, et al. Complications of beta-thalassemia major in North America. Blood 2004;104(1):34–9.
6. Wood JC, Tyszka M, Carson S, et al. Myocardial iron loading in transfusion-dependent thalassemia and sickle cell disease. Blood 2004;103(5):1934–6.
7. Roggero S, Quarello P, Vinciguerra T, et al. Severe iron overload in Blackfan-Diamond anemia: a case-control study. Am J Hematol 2009;84(11):729–32.
8. Jean G, Terzoli S, Mauri R, et al. Cirrhosis associated with multiple transfusions in thalassaemia. Arch Dis Child 1984;59(1):67–70.
9. Borgna-Pignatti C, De Stefano P, Zonta L, et al. Growth and sexual maturation in thalassemia major. J Pediatr 1985;106(1):150–5.
10. Fung EB, Harmatz PR, Lee PD, et al. Increased prevalence of iron-overload associated endocrinopathy in thalassaemia versus sickle-cell disease. Br J Haematol 2006;135(4):574–82.
11. Brittenham GM, Cohen AR, McLaren CE, et al. Hepatic iron stores and plasma ferritin concentration in patients with sickle cell anemia and thalassemia major. Am J Hematol 1993;42(1):81–5.
12. Kwiatkowski JL, Cohen AR, Garro J, et al. Transfusional iron overload in children with sickle cell anemia on chronic transfusion therapy for secondary stroke prevention. Am J Hematol 2011;87(2):221–3.
13. Kirk P, Roughton M, Porter JB, et al. Cardiac T2* magnetic resonance for prediction of cardiac complications in thalassemia major. Circulation 2009;120(20):1961–8.
14. Angelucci E, Brittenham GM, McLaren CE, et al. Hepatic iron concentration and total body iron stores in thalassemia major. N Engl J Med 2000;343(5):327–31.
15. Olivieri NF, Nathan DG, MacMillan JH, et al. Survival in medically treated patients with homozygous beta-thalassemia. N Engl J Med 1994;331(9):574–8.
16. Anderson LJ, Holden S, Davis B, et al. Cardiovascular T2-star (T2*) magnetic resonance for the early diagnosis of myocardial iron overload. Eur Heart J 2001;22(23):2171–9.
17. Chirnomas DS, Geukes-Foppen M, Barry K, et al. Practical implications of liver and heart iron load assessment by T2*-MRI in children and adults with transfusion-dependent anemias. Am J Hematol 2008;83(10):781–3.
18. Angelucci E, Baronciani D, Lucarelli G, et al. Needle liver biopsy in thalassaemia: analyses of diagnostic accuracy and safety in 1184 consecutive biopsies. Br J Haematol 1995;89(4):757–61.
19. Brittenham GM, Farrell DE, Harris JW, et al. Magnetic-susceptibility measurement of human iron stores. N Engl J Med 1982;307:1671–5.
20. St Pierre TG, Clark PR, Chua-anusorn W, et al. Noninvasive measurement and imaging of liver iron concentrations using proton magnetic resonance. Blood 2005;105(2):855–61.
21. Wood JC, Enriquez C, Ghugre N, et al. MRI R2 and R2* mapping accurately estimates hepatic iron concentration in transfusion-dependent thalassemia and sickle cell disease patients. Blood 2005;106(4):1460–5.
22. Kwiatkowski JL, Kim HY, Thompson AA, et al. Chelation use and iron burden in North American and British thalassemia patients: a report from the thalassemia longitudinal cohort. Blood 2012;119(12):2746–53.
23. Wood JC. Magnetic resonance imaging measurement of iron overload. Curr Opin Hematol 2007;14(3):183–90.
24. Wood JC, Origa R, Agus A, et al. Onset of cardiac iron loading in pediatric patients with thalassemia major. Haematologica 2008;93(6):917–20.
25. Noetzli LJ, Mittelman SD, Watanabe RM, et al. Pancreatic iron and glucose dysregulation in thalassemia major. Am J Hematol 2012;87:155–60.

26. Noetzli LJ, Panigrahy A, Mittelman SD, et al. Pituitary iron and volume predict hypogonadism in transfusional iron overload. Am J Hematol 2012;87:167–71.

27. Anderson LJ, Westwood MA, Holden S, et al. Myocardial iron clearance during reversal of siderotic cardiomyopathy with intravenous desferrioxamine: a prospective study using T2* cardiovascular magnetic resonance. Br J Haematol 2004;127(3):348–55.

28. Farmaki K, Tzoumari I, Pappa C, et al. Normalisation of total body iron load with very intensive combined chelation reverses cardiac and endocrine complications of thalassaemia major. Br J Haematol 2009;148(3):466–75.

29. Cohen AR, Glimm E, Porter JB. Effect of transfusional iron intake on response to chelation therapy in {beta}-thalassemia major. Blood 2008;111(2):583–7.

30. Farmaki K, Tzoumari I, Pappa C. Oral chelators in transfusion-dependent thalassemia major patients may prevent or reverse iron overload complications. Blood Cells Mol Dis 2011;47(1):33–40.

31. Lee P, Mohammed N, Marshall L, et al. Intravenous infusion pharmacokinetics of desferrioxamine in thalassaemic patients. Drug Metab Dispos 1993;21(4):640–4.

32. Pippard MJ, Letsky EA, Callender ST, et al. Prevention of iron loading in transfusion-dependent thalassaemia. Lancet 1978;1(8075):1178–81.

33. Cappellini MD, Cohen A, Piga A, et al. A phase 3 study of deferasirox (ICL670), a once-daily oral iron chelator, in patients with beta-thalassemia. Blood 2006;107(9):3455–62.

34. Brittenham GM, Griffith PM, Nienhuis AW, et al. Efficacy of deferoxamine in preventing complications of iron overload in patients with thalassemia major. N Engl J Med 1994;331(9):567–73.

35. Davis BA, Porter JB. Long-term outcome of continuous 24-hour deferoxamine infusion via indwelling intravenous catheters in high-risk beta-thalassemia. Blood 2000;95(4):1229–36.

36. Olivieri NF, Buncic JR, Chew E, et al. Visual and auditory neurotoxicity in patients receiving subcutaneous deferoxamine infusions. N Engl J Med 1986;314:869–73.

37. Chan YL, Pang LM, Chik KW, et al. Patterns of bone diseases in transfusion-dependent homozygous thalassaemia major: predominance of osteoporosis and desferrioxamine-induced bone dysplasia. Pediatr Radiol 2002;32(7):492–7.

38. De Sanctis V, Pinamonti A, DiPalma A, et al. Growth and development in thalassemia major patients with severe bone lesions due to desferrioxamine. Eur J Pediatr 1996;155(5):368–72.

39. Olivieri NF, Koren G, Harris J, et al. Growth failure and bony changes induced by deferoxamine. Am J Pediatr Hematol Oncol 1992;14(1):48–56.

40. Freedman MH, Grisaru D, Oliveri N, et al. Pulmonary syndrome in patients with thalassemia major receiving intravenous deferoxamine infusions. Am J Dis Child 1990;144(5):565–9.

41. Levine JE, Cohen A, MacQueen M, et al. Sensorimotor neurotoxicity associated with high-dose deferoxamine treatment. J Pediatr Hematol Oncol 1997;19(2):139–41.

42. Al-Refaie FN, Sheppard LN, Nortey P, et al. Pharmacokinetics of the oral iron chelator deferiprone (L1) in patients with iron overload. Br J Haematol 1995;89(2):403–8.

43. Collins AF, Fassos FF, Stobie S, et al. Iron-balance and dose-response studies of the oral iron chelator 1,2-dimethyl-3-hydroxypyrid-4-one (L1) in iron-loaded patients with sickle cell disease. Blood 1994;83(8):2329–33.

44. Addis A, Loebstein R, Koren G, et al. Meta-analytic review of the clinical effectiveness of oral deferiprone (L1). Eur J Clin Pharmacol 1999;55(1):1–6.
45. Wonke B, Wright C, Hoffbrand AV. Combined therapy with deferiprone and desferrioxamine. Br J Haematol 1998;103(2):361–4.
46. Taher A, Sheikh-Taha M, Sharara A, et al. Safety and effectiveness of 100 mg/kg/day deferiprone in patients with thalassemia major: a two-year study. Acta Haematol 2005;114(3):146–9.
47. Anderson LJ, Wonke B, Prescott E, et al. Comparison of effects of oral deferiprone and subcutaneous desferrioxamine on myocardial iron concentrations and ventricular function in beta-thalassaemia. Lancet 2002;360(9332):516–20.
48. Pignatti C, Cappellini MD, De Stefano P, et al. Cardiac morbidity and mortality in deferoxamine- or deferiprone-treated patients with thalassemia major. Blood 2006;107(9):3733–7.
49. Pennell DJ, Berdoukas V, Karagiorga M, et al. Randomized controlled trial of deferiprone or deferoxamine in beta-thalassemia major patients with asymptomatic myocardial siderosis. Blood 2006;107(9):3738–44.
50. Ferriprox [package insert]. Rockville, MD: ApoPharma, USA, Inc; 2012.
51. Ceci A, Baiardi P, Felisi M, et al. The safety and effectiveness of deferiprone in a large-scale, 3-year study in Italian patients. Br J Haematol 2002;118(1):330–6.
52. Cohen AR, Galanello R, Piga A, et al. Safety and effectiveness of long-term therapy with the oral iron chelator deferiprone. Blood 2003;102(5):1583–7.
53. Henter JI, Karlen J. Fatal agranulocytosis after deferiprone therapy in a child with Diamond-Blackfan anemia. Blood 2007;109(12):5157–9.
54. Hoffbrand AV, Bartlett AN, Veys PA, et al. Agranulocytosis and thrombocytopenia in patient with Blackfan-Diamond anaemia during oral chelator trial. Lancet 1989;2(8660):457.
55. Galanello R, Piga A, Cappellini MD, et al. Effect of food, type of food, and time of food intake on deferasirox bioavailability: recommendations for an optimal deferasirox administration regimen. J Clin Pharmacol 2008;48(4):428–35.
56. Chang HH, Lu MY, Liao YM, et al. Improved efficacy and tolerability of oral deferasirox by twice-daily dosing for patients with transfusion-dependent beta-thalassemia. Pediatr Blood Cancer 2011;56(3):420–4.
57. Chirnomas D, Smith AL, Braunstein J, et al. Deferasirox pharmacokinetics in patients with adequate versus inadequate response. Blood 2009;114(19):4009–13.
58. Pongtanakul B, Viprakasit V. Twice daily deferasirox significantly improves clinical efficacy in transfusion dependent thalassaemias who were inadequate responders to standard once daily dose. Blood Cells Mol Dis 2013;51(2):96–7.
59. Pennell DJ, Porter JB, Cappellini MD, et al. Efficacy of deferasirox in reducing and preventing cardiac iron overload in beta-thalassemia. Blood 2010;115(12):2364–71.
60. Wood JC, Kang BP, Thompson A, et al. The effect of deferasirox on cardiac iron in thalassemia major: impact of total body iron stores. Blood 2010;116(4):537–43.
61. Cappellini MD, Bejaoui M, Agaoglu L, et al. Iron chelation with deferasirox in adult and pediatric patients with thalassemia major: efficacy and safety during 5 years' follow-up. Blood 2011;118(4):884–93.
62. Dubourg L, Laurain C, Ranchin B, et al. Deferasirox-induced renal impairment in children: an increasing concern for pediatricians. Pediatr Nephrol 2012;27(11):2115–22.
63. Milat F, Wong P, Fuller PJ, et al. A case of hypophosphatemic osteomalacia secondary to deferasirox therapy. J Bone Miner Res 2012;27(1):219–22.

64. Yacobovich J, Stark P, Barzilai-Birenbaum S, et al. Acquired proximal renal tubular dysfunction in beta-thalassemia patients treated with deferasirox. J Pediatr Hematol Oncol 2010;32(7):564–7.

65. Mednick LM, Braunstein J, Neufeld E. Oral chelation: should it be used with young children? Pediatr Blood Cancer 2010;55(4):603–5.

66. Alvarez O, Rodriguez-Cortes H, Robinson N, et al. Adherence to deferasirox in children and adolescents with sickle cell disease during 1-year of therapy. J Pediatr Hematol Oncol 2009;31(10):739–44.

67. Tanner MA, Galanello R, Dessi C, et al. A randomized, placebo-controlled, double-blind trial of the effect of combined therapy with deferoxamine and deferiprone on myocardial iron in thalassemia major using cardiovascular magnetic resonance. Circulation 2007;115(14):1876–84.

68. Kattamis A, Ladis V, Berdousi H, et al. Iron chelation treatment with combined therapy with deferiprone and deferoxamine: a 12-month trial. Blood Cells Mol Dis 2006;36(1):21–5.

69. Lal A, Porter J, Sweeters N, et al. Combined chelation therapy with deferasirox and deferoxamine in thalassemia. Blood Cells Mol Dis 2013;50(2):99–104.

70. Neufeld EJ, Galanello R, Viprakasit V, et al. A phase 2 study of the safety, tolerability, and pharmacodynamics of FBS0701, a novel oral iron chelator, in transfusional iron overload. Blood 2012;119(14):3263–8.

71. Shire Development LLC. Pharmacokinetics of SSP-004184 in the treatment of chronic iron overload requiring chelation therapy. In: ClinicalTrials.gov [Internet]. Bethesda (MD): National Library of Medicine (US); 2000. Available at: http:// clinicaltrials.gov/ct2/results?term=NCT01604941. Accessed October 12, 2012. NLM Identifier NCT01604941.

72. Shire Development LLC. Safety, efficacy and pharmacokinetics of an oral iron chelator given for a year to pediatric patients with iron overload. In: ClinicalTrials.gov [Internet]. Bethesda (MD): National Library of Medicine (US); 2000. Available at: http://clinicaltrials.gov/ct2/results?term=NCT01363908. Accessed October 12, 2012. NLM Identifier NCT01363908.

73. EXJADE [package insert]. East Hanover, NJ: Novartis Pharmaceuticals Corporation; 2013.

74. DESFERAL [package insert]. East Hanover, NJ: Novartis Pharmaceuticals Corporation; 2011.

Developmental Hemostasis
Clinical Implications From the Fetus to the Adolescent

Julie Jaffray, MD[a], Guy Young, MD[b],*

KEYWORDS

- Developmental hemostasis • Neonatal • Children • Coagulation

KEY POINTS

- Developmental hemostasis is the evolution of the coagulation system from a fetus to an adolescent.
- The levels of procoagulant and anticoagulant protein levels differ substantially between infants and adults, and these differences affect both the ability to accurately diagnose and treat infants and children with hemostatic and thrombotic diseases.

INTRODUCTION

Hemostasis refers to the process by which ruptures in the wall of blood vessels are occluded by a fibrin clot and involves the interaction of the blood vessel wall, platelets, and coagulation proteins. In addition to preventing excessive bleeding, the fibrin clot provides the structure for wound repair. Developmental hemostasis describes the evolution of the coagulation system from fetal life to adolescence. The coagulation system, which includes both procoagulant and anticoagulant proteins, forms early in utero, although the levels of many of these proteins are different than those seen in normal adults. Many of these proteins exhibit levels that are far less than those seen in adults, although a few are, in fact, more than adult levels. Although much of the evolution to normal adult levels takes place within the first 6 months, some proteins do not reach normal adult levels until adolescence. The evolving changes in the functional level of the coagulation proteins lead to several challenges for the clinician. First,

[a] Department of Hematology/Oncology, Children's Hospital of Los Angeles, University of Southern California Keck School of Medicine, 4650 Sunset Boulevard, Mail Stop #54, Los Angeles, CA 90027, USA; [b] Department of Hematology/Oncology, Hemostasis and Thrombosis Center, Children's Hospital of Los Angeles, University of Southern California Keck School of Medicine, 4650 Sunset Boulevard, Mail Stop #54, Los Angeles, CA 90027, USA
* Corresponding author.
E-mail address: gyoung@chla.usc.edu

Pediatr Clin N Am 60 (2013) 1407–1417
http://dx.doi.org/10.1016/j.pcl.2013.08.003
0031-3955/13/$ – see front matter © 2013 Elsevier Inc. All rights reserved.
pediatric.theclinics.com

the changes make it more difficult to correctly diagnose a child with a disorder of coagulation. Second, the particularly rapid changes that occur during the neonatal period can affect the choice and monitoring of anticoagulant agents. Third, the changes create significant challenges for the clinical coagulation laboratory as it relates to establishing normal ranges for various laboratory assays. This article reviews the current data on the development of the coagulation system as it matures from early fetal life into the teenage years and explains how these changes impact the diagnosis and treatment of pediatric coagulation disorders.

HEMOSTASIS PHYSIOLOGY

A basic overview of the coagulation cascade is crucial to understanding developmental hemostasis. Damaged endothelium exposes tissue factor (TF) present in the subendothelium, which then activates the coagulation cascade,[1] consisting of multiple procoagulant proteins that interact together to lead to the formation of a fibrin clot. The procoagulant proteins, mostly known as factors, include fibrinogen and factors (F) II, V, VII, VIII, IX, X, XI, and XIII. Of note, there are several factors (FXIII, prekallikrein, and high-molecular-weight kininogen) in the so-called contact activation system that are not currently considered to be involved in hemostasis, although abnormal levels will result in an abnormal activated partial thromboplastin time (aPTT). In order to prevent excessive clotting, there exist several natural inhibitors to the procoagulant factors (also known as *natural anticoagulants*), including antithrombin (AT), α_2-macroglobulin (α_2-M), heparin cofactor II (HCII), protein C, protein S, and TF pathway inhibitor (TFPI).

The activation of the coagulation cascade results in the formation of large quantities of thrombin (FIIa) at the site of bleeding. Thrombin plays a pivotal role in the formation of the fibrin clot. It activates FV and FVIII, which are the main catalysts of the coagulation cascade resulting in the generation of even more thrombin. This large amount of thrombin leads to the conversion of the soluble protein fibrinogen into its insoluble form, fibrin, which forms the structure of the clot (**Fig. 1**). Thrombin also activates 2 proteins, FXIII and thrombin-activatable fibrinolysis inhibitor, both of which are critical to the formation of a stable clot that is resistant to fibrinolysis. Lastly, thrombin also activates platelets at the site of bleeding.

Thrombin plays the key role in its own downregulation by forming a complex with thrombomodulin that serves to activate protein C,[2,3] which, along with its cofactor, protein S, inactivates the catalysts FV and FVIII. The prohemostatic effect of thrombin remains local to the site of endothelial damage because any thrombin that remains in the circulation is quenched by AT.

HEMOSTASIS IN THE INFANT AND CHILD

At birth, an infant's coagulation system differs significantly from that of an adult. The levels of many of their procoagulant and natural anticoagulants are low; as a result, the screening coagulation tests, the aPTT and the prothrombin time (PT), are prolonged compared with adults. Some of the components of the hemostatic system even have fetal forms whose actions vary from the adult forms, such as protein C and fibrinogen.[4,5] These fetal forms have been shown to generate and regulate thrombin differently or to be synthesized at a different rate.

All coagulation factors are present at birth; but most coagulation factors do not reach typical adult levels until 6 months of age and some not until adolescence.[6–9] **Fig. 2** shows the evolution of the components of the coagulation system throughout fetal life. Because coagulation factors cannot cross the placenta,[10] the fetus starts

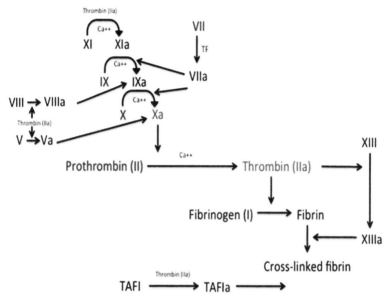

Fig. 1. Overview of the coagulation cascade showing procoagulant interactions. TF from the subendothelium activates the coagulation cascade, which causes interaction of multiple coagulation factors (II, V, VII, VIII, IX, X, XI and XIII) to form a fibrin clot. a, activated form of the factor; TAFI, thrombin activatable fibrinolysis inhibitor.

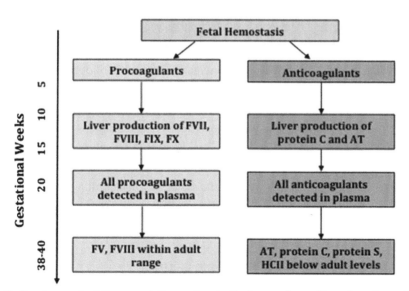

Fig. 2. Development of the coagulation system in the human fetus. (*Data from* Reverdiau-Moalic P, Delahousse B, Body G, et al. Evolution of blood coagulation activators and inhibitors in the healthy human fetus. Blood 1996;88:900–6; and Hassan HJ, Leonardi A, Chelucci C, et al. Blood coagulation factors in human embryonic-fetal development: preferential expression of the FVII/tissue factor pathway. Blood 1990;76:1158–64.)

to produce its own procoagulants and anticoagulants in the liver at about 5 weeks' gestation.[9–12] At 20 weeks' gestation, the coagulation factors can be measured in plasma, yet they are still at very low levels.[10] As a result of this process, premature infants have even lower levels of procoagulant and anticoagulant factors than term infants; but their levels quickly mature toward adulthood, with most components reaching near adult levels by 6 months of age.[6]

At birth, the only procoagulant factors that are within the adult range are fibrinogen, FV, and FVIII.[6,7] The vitamin K-dependent coagulant factors (II, VII, IX and X) and contact factors (XI, XII, prekallikrein), high-molecular-weight kininogen are approximately 50% of the adult values at birth. These factors rapidly increase in the first few weeks of life and overlap substantially with the adult range by 6 months of age, although the average values of most remain 20% lower until the teenage years. Prothrombin, which is the precursor to thrombin, is decreased by 20% throughout childhood.[8] FVIII levels are normal to high at birth, and von Willebrand factor levels are elevated until about 3 months of age.[6,7] Andrew and colleagues[6–8] created an extensive database of normal reference ranges for the human coagulation system in healthy term and preterm infants as well as children and adolescents. It should be noted that the levels in the Andrew publications are specific to the methodology for the assays performed in her laboratory; thus, specific values cannot be extrapolated to results from other laboratories. **Table 1** summarizes, in a qualitative fashion, the main differences of the coagulation system found between the developing child and adult.

Studies from ultrasound-guided umbilical sampling[10] have shown that between 19 and 30 weeks' gestation, the PT, aPTT, and thrombin clotting time (TCT) are all prolonged secondary to low levels of vitamin K–dependent factors, contact factors, FV, FVIII, and fibrinogen. These factors began to increase after the 34th week of gestation, but only FV and FVIII reached adults levels at birth.

The anticoagulants, AT and HCII, are 50% of adult values at birth and increase to adult levels by 3 months of age.[7,8,13] Protein C and S are even lower at birth; protein C, which starts out in a fetal form, remains markedly low until 6 months of age. Theoretically, to compensate for the low level of AT, another anticoagulant, α_2-M, is produced at levels that are increased over adult values at birth, are twice adult values at 6 months of age, and continue to be increased until the third decade of life.[7,8,13]

Andrew and colleagues[6–8] also compared components of the fibrinolytic system, which is involved in fibrin clot degradation, of children with adults. The levels of plasminogen, which is a pro-fibrinolytic, and $\alpha2$-antiplasmin, which is an anti-fibrinolytic, were similar to adults throughout childhood (after 1 year of age). Although the pro-fibrinolytic, tissues plasminogen activator (TPA), was found to be lower in children and the anti-fibrinolytic, plasminogen activator inhibitor, had increased levels in children.

Of note, the differences in the hemostatic system between children and adults may be important not only in hemostasis. Some of these coagulant proteins, such as TF and thrombomodulin, are also involved in angiogenesis, inflammation, and wound repair, which may be the driving force behind the coagulation system changes.[9,11]

COAGULATION TESTING IN THE INFANT AND CHILD

As a result of the developmental changes in hemostasis, the interpretation of commonly ordered laboratory tests is challenging. Andrew and colleagues[6–8] realized this problem, and along with studying proteins levels in patients from the premature infant to the teenager, they also created a well-referenced document of normal laboratory values for PT and aPTT, international normalized ratio (INR), and TCT. In

Table 1
Maturation of coagulation proteins from birth to adulthood

	Age					
	Birth	**1 mo**	**6 mo**	**1–5 y**	**11–16 y**	**Adult**
Procoagulants						
FII	Decreased	Decreased	Decreased[a]	Decreased[a]	Decreased[a]	**Adult**
FV	Decreased[a]	Decreased[a]	Decreased[a]	Decreased[a]	Decreased[a]	**Adult**
FVII	Decreased	Decreased[a]	Decreased[a]	Decreased[a]	Decreased[a]	**Adult**
FVIII	**Adult** ──→					
FIX	Decreased	Decreased	Decreased[a]	Decreased[a]	Decreased[a]	**Adult**
FX	Decreased	Decreased	Decreased[a]	Decreased[a]	Decreased[a]	**Adult**
FXI	Decreased	Decreased	Decreased[a]	**Adult**	Decreased[a]	**Adult**
FXII	Decreased	Decreased	Decreased[a]	**Adult**	Decreased[a]	**Adult**
FXIII	Decreased	**Adult** ──────────────────────────────────────→				
PK	Decreased	Decreased	Decreased[a]	**Adult** ──────────────────────→		
HMWK	Decreased	**Adult** ──────────────────────────────────────→				
Fibrinogen	**Adult** ──→					
Anticoagulants						
AT	Decreased	Decreased	Adult ──────────────────────────────→			
α2M	Increased	Increased	Increased	Increased	Increased	**Adult**
HCII	Decreased	Decreased	Increased	Decreased[a]	Decreased[a]	**Adult**
Protein C	Decreased	Decreased	Decreased	Decreased[a]	Decreased[a]	**Adult**
Protein S	Decreased	Decreased	Decreased[a]	**Adult**[b] ──────────────────────→		

Abbreviations: HMWK, high-molecular-weight-kininogen; PK, prekallikrein.
All values are compared with adult means and ranges.
   [a] Denotes values that are within the adult lower range but less than the adult mean.
   [b] Denotes values that are within the adult mean, but 15% of the values are less than the adult low range.
   Data from Refs.[6–8]

addition, Monagle and colleagues[13] also created reference ranges for PT, aPTT, INR, TCT, and D-dimer levels. A compilation of values from these 2 studies is shown in **Table 2**.

As can be seen from **Table 2**, the normal ranges for the PT/INR and aPTT, the 2 most commonly ordered coagulation assays, are different from the adult normal ranges throughout childhood. This information is particularly important because very few laboratories will provide age-related reference ranges, and often the clinician is faced with interpreting the results without a valid reference range. Furthermore, it

Table 2
Comparison of coagulation testing between the normal term infant or child and the adult

	Age					
Coagulation Tests	**Birth**	**1 mo**	**6 mo**	**1–5 y**	**11–16 y**	**Adults**
PT	1.15	0.95	0.99	0.97	0.99	1.0
aPTT	1.2	1.27	1.11	1.10	1.14	1.0
INR	1.2	0.95	0.95	0.96	0.97	1.0
TCT	1.12	1.17	1.22	0.84	0.81	1.0
D-dimer	8.17	1.22	1.22	1.39	1.50	1.0

Values represent the ratio between infant and child means compared with adult means. A ratio greater than 1 reflects a higher mean value in the infant/child compared with the adult mean.
   Data from Refs.[6–8,13]

should be noted that the reagents and instruments used to measure the PT and aPTT are highly variable between laboratories; thus, results cannot be compared across laboratories. The only truly valid reference range would be an age-matched range specific to the reagents and instruments used. This process is a costly and time-consuming process that few laboratories perform. The interpretation of these assays should always be done with caution particularly in neonates whereby the largest differences from adult norms occurs. Suffice it to say that the PT and aPTT in newborns are almost always prolonged compared with the adult reference range for a particular laboratory.

Besides the difficulty in interpreting the results of coagulation tests in neonates and children, there are also challenges in specimen procurement. Venipuncture in a small child can be difficult; without a free-flowing blood sample, the coagulation system can get activated before it comes into contact with the citrate anticoagulant in the tube, resulting in falsely elevated PT and aPTT results caused by consumption of clotting factors. Those samples that are drawn from heparinized catheters can be contaminated with heparin. An insufficient amount of blood can result in an appropriate citrate-to-blood ratio in the collection tube. Finally, samples from patients with inordinately low or high hematocrits can result in falsely elevated or falsely low values, respectively.[14]

PROTECTIVE MECHANISMS

Although infants have levels of coagulation proteins that are less than adults, the typical healthy infant has a much lower incidence of thrombosis without an increased incidence of bleeding.[13,15,16] Healthy neonates do not show easy bruising, do not demonstrate excessive bleeding with surgery, and have normal wound healing.[17] With respect to thrombosis, infants and children (healthy or sick) rarely develop thrombosis even with known prothrombotic genetic mutations.[18,19]

The main reason for the lack of excessive bleeding and thrombosis in neonates, despite the physiologically lower levels of both procoagulation and anticoagulant proteins, lies in the fact that although the levels are low, the reduction of both sets of proteins is balanced. For example, a low level of AT offsets the low level of prothrombin. This point can be demonstrated in studies using thromboelastography in which the clotting time and time to form a clot were shorter in preterm and term neonates than in adults despite a much lower level of prothrombin.[20] In another study, it was demonstrated that although neonates and children seem to produce less thrombin than adults, they may actually produce thrombin faster because of having less TFPI and less AT.[17]

Protective mechanisms have also been postulated in growing infants and children. As stated previously, infants are born with low levels of the anticoagulants AT and protein C and S but with α_2-M levels that are far greater than those seen in adults. α_2-M may even inhibit more thrombin that the other anticoagulants and is seen as a protective mechanism in children with AT deficiency. In children with AT deficiency, thrombotic symptoms typically do not appear until adolescence, when the levels of α_2-M normalize to adult levels.[21]

IMPACT OF DEVELOPMENTAL HEMOSTASIS IN THE CLINIC
Vitamin K Deficiency

Because of the immature coagulation system whereby the vitamin K–dependent factors (II, VII, IX, and X) are normally at about 50% of adult levels, neonates are especially susceptible to vitamin K–deficient bleeding (VKDB). Because vitamin K is poorly transferred across the placenta and there is very little vitamin K in breast milk,[22–24] newborns who do not receive vitamin K prophylaxis (see later discussion) can have extremely low levels of factors II, VII, IX, and X, which could result in severe bleeding symptoms.

Despite the low factor levels in the absence of vitamin K prophylaxis, VKDB is rare (4–7 cases per 10^5 births)[24]; however, when it does occur, it can be life threatening particularly if intracranial hemorrhage occurs. Mild cases of VKDB will manifest as a prolongation of the PT and, in more severe cases, prolongation of the aPTT. Newborns can present with bleeding at any site, with bruising often the most visible manifestation. There are categories of VKDB called early, classic, and late (**Table 3**). Early VKDB is seen in the first 24 hours of life and is usually seen in infants of mothers who have taken drugs that interfere with vitamin K metabolism (warfarin, anticonvulsants). Classic VKDB occurs in the first week of life and can be prevented with a small dose of vitamin K at birth. Late VKDB occurs at 3 to 8 weeks of life, is usually caused by inadequate absorption of vitamin K cholestasis, and may present with a serious bleeding episode, for example, an intracranial hemorrhage.

Hemophilia

Hemophilia (deficiencies of FVIII or FIX) is covered in detail in a separate article by Carcao and colleagues elsewhere in this issue, and will only be discussed here to the extent that it relates to developmental hemostasis. The hemophilias can present in the neonatal period with the typical symptoms, including oozing from venipuncture or heel stick, bruising, and excessive bleeding following circumcision. Less common symptoms include bleeding from the umbilical cord stump, intracranial hemorrhage, or bleeding from the gastrointestinal tract.[25] Because unaffected infants have levels of FVIII that are in the normal adult range at birth, making the diagnosis of hemophilia A (FVIII deficiency) is straightforward in the newborn period. However, making the accurate diagnosis of FIX deficiency can be challenging because physiologic levels of FIX are substantially less than the normal adult range. Severe FIX deficiency can often be confirmed in the neonate, but diagnosing a mild deficiency usually requires repeat testing at 6 months of age.

Table 3
Vitamin K deficiency classification

	Early	Classic	Late
Age	First 24 h	2–7 d	1–6 mo (even later)
Risk factors	Maternal use of drugs that interfere with vitamin K metabolism (warfarin, anticonvulsants)	None (all newborns are prone)	Disorders that interfere with vitamin K intake (cystic fibrosis, other GI fat malabsorption disorders, chronic antibiotic use, liver disease)
Bleeding sites	ICH, GI, umbilical stump, bruising	ICH, GI, umbilical stump, bruising	ICH, GI, mucocutaneous
Treatment	Recognition of drugs that can cause this and eliminating them from maternal use	Prevention with neonatal vitamin K administration	Parenteral vitamin K

Abbreviation: GI, gastrointestinal; ICH, intracranial hemorrhage.

With respect to rare congenital factor deficiencies, making the diagnosis in the neonatal period for those whose levels are within the adult range at birth (fibrinogen, FV, FXI, and FXIII) can be done, whereas diagnosing deficiencies of factors II, VII, X, or XI may not be possible because the normal ranges are low enough that they may overlap with the range found in the deficient state.[5]

Thrombosis

Most neonatal thrombosis is caused by the presence of central venous catheters; however, there are rare genetic disorders that can present in the neonatal period whose diagnosis is impacted by developmental hemostasis. Deficiencies of protein C and protein S, as well as AT, increase the susceptibility to developing a thrombotic event. Severe (usually homozygous) deficiencies of proteins C and S manifest at birth with purpura fulminans and can usually be diagnosed fairly easily because laboratory measurements usually demonstrate levels less than 5%[6,7,10,13]; however, heterozygotes or compound heterozygotes with less severe deficiencies are more difficult to diagnose because their levels will overlap with the normal neonatal ranges. Although such infants do not necessarily present in the neonatal period, for those who do, making an accurate diagnosis is challenging. Lastly, although there are little data to support the value of thrombophilia testing in newborns with thrombosis, such testing is not performed infrequently. Interpreting the results of such testing, particularly functional levels of proteins C and S and AT, is problematic. The physician reviewing such testing must understand the impact of developmental hemostasis on the results.[22,23] In general, abnormal results should not automatically lead to a diagnosis of a deficiency; but if the levels are less than adult norms, testing should be repeated after at least 6 months of age when they should normally reach adult levels.[6]

IMPACT OF DEVELOPMENTAL HEMOSTASIS ON ANTICOAGULATION MANAGEMENT

Besides the impact on making the correct diagnosis in a variety of coagulation disorders, developmental hemostasis also impacts the management of anticoagulation therapy in infants and children. First, it should be made clear that the target therapeutic ranges for children have been extrapolated from adult studies; although adjusting the dosing of anticoagulant medication in children to reach the desired adult standardized INR, aPTT, or anti-Factor Xa level is deemed necessary, correlation of these ranges with clinical outcomes has not been proven.

The most commonly used anticoagulants in children are unfractionated heparin, low-molecular-weight heparin (LMWH) (usually enoxaparin), and warfarin (**Fig. 3**). A full discussion of these agents is in another article by Goldenberg and colleagues elsewhere in this issue. More details can also be found in an article by Young.[26] Next, the authors discuss the impacts of developmental hemostasis on the management of infants who require these medications.

Heparin is given parentally as unfractionated heparin (UFH) or LMWH. It functions by binding to and potentiating the inhibitory effects of AT on thrombin and activated FX.[27] The use of heparin in the neonatal period is complicated by 2 issues, both of which result in the need for substantially higher dosing of heparin and LMWH in neonates. First, as discussed, neonates have a reduced amount of AT. Second, in children less than 1 year of age, there is increased heparin binding to non-AT proteins resulting in reduced binding to AT.[28]

Another complication of heparin therapy in neonates resulting from the effects of developmental hemostasis involves laboratory monitoring. The anticoagulant effect of UFH is usually monitored by the aPTT; as previously described, the normal aPTT

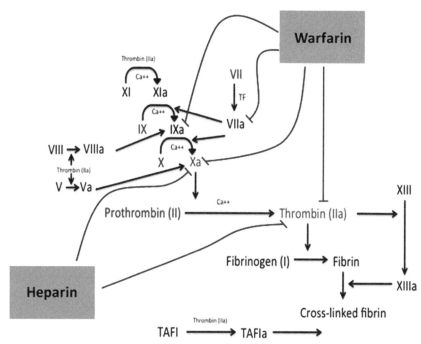

Fig. 3. The interaction of current anticoagulation medications with the components of the coagulation system. Warfarin inhibits the vitamin K carboxylation conversion cycle, thus decreasing the active forms of thrombin and factors VII, IX, and X. Heparin binds to thrombin and enhances the inhibition of thrombin and activated factor X.

levels in infants are elevated when compared with adults. Therefore, adjusting the heparin dose based on adult aPTT ranges may not be appropriate and can lead to an inappropriate level of anticoagulation.

Warfarin is an oral anticoagulant that competitively inhibits the vitamin K carboxylation conversion cycle, resulting in low plasma concentrations of functional factors II, VII, IX, X, which depend on γ–carboxylation for their biological activity.[29] Warfarin causes decreased thrombin generation, which then prolongs the PT and INR, although the extent of prolongation in children may not be comparable to adults. Studies have found that children taking warfarin make even less thrombin compared with adults because of the lower prothrombin and vitamin K–dependent coagulation factor levels.[30] When children are on warfarin, the thrombin that is generated is complexed to the anticoagulant α_2-M. Thus, there is actually increased inhibition of thrombin caused by α_2-M in children with similar INR values than adults, which suggests that children require lower intensities of warfarin for effective anticoagulation.[30] In young children (less than 1 year of age), higher doses of warfarin are required to achieve similar anticoagulant effectiveness as measured by the INR as an adult, which is caused, in part, by their intake of commercial milk formulas with high vitamin K concentrations that compete with warfarin.[5]

SUMMARY

Developmental hemostasis describes the dynamic development of the coagulation system, including both procoagulant and anticoagulant proteins, from the fetus to the adolescent. The levels and function of the coagulation proteins rapidly change as the child ages, thus creating a challenge for the pediatrician not only when it comes to diagnosing bleeding or thrombotic disorders but also as it applies to the management of anticoagulation. When presented with a child with a suspected bleeding or thrombotic disorder, the pediatrician should consider age-appropriate coagulation protein levels as well as screening test ranges when interpreting the test results. One must also consider the developing coagulation system when treating and monitoring a child with anticoagulant medications because the doses and the desired anticoagulant levels can be quite varied when treating a neonate versus a child or adult.

REFERENCES

1. Kuhle S, Male C, Mitchell L. Developmental hemostasis: pro- and anticoagulant systems during childhood. Semin Thromb Hemost 2003;29:329–38.
2. Andrew M. Developmental hemostasis: relevance to newborns and infants. In: Nathan D, Orkin S, editors. Nathan and Oski's hematology of infancy and childhood. 5th edition. Philadelphia: WB Saunders; 1998. p. 114–57.
3. Kamath P, Huntington JA, Krishnaswamy S. Ligand binding shuttles thrombin along a continuum of zymogen- and proteinase-like states. J Biol Chem 2010; 285:28651–8.
4. Ignjatovic V, Ilhan A, Monagle P. Evidence for age-related differences in human fibrinogen. Blood Coagul Fibrinolysis 2011;22:110–7.
5. Williams MD, Chalmers EA, Gibson BE. The investigation and management of neonatal haemostasis and thrombosis. Br J Haematol 2002;119:295–309.
6. Andrew M, Paes B, Milner R, et al. Development of the human coagulation system in the healthy premature infant. Blood 1988;72:1651–7.
7. Andrew M, Paes B, Milner R, et al. Development of the human coagulation system in the full-term infant. Blood 1978;70:165–72.
8. Andrew M, Vegh B, Johnston M, et al. Maturation of the hemostatic system during childhood. Blood 1992;80:1998–2005.
9. Manco-Johnson MJ. Development of hemostasis in the fetus. Thromb Res 2005; 115:55–63.
10. Reverdiau-Moalic P, Delahousse B, Body G, et al. Evolution of blood coagulation activators and inhibitors in the healthy human fetus. Blood 1996;88:900–6.
11. Menashi S, Aurousseau MH, Gozin D, et al. High levels of circulating thrombomodulin in human foetuses and children. Thromb Haemost 1999;81:906–9.
12. Hassan HJ, Leonardi A, Chelucci C, et al. Blood coagulation factors in human embryonic-fetal development: preferential expression of the FVII/tissue factor pathway. Blood 1990;76:1158–64.
13. Monagle P, Barnes C, Ignjatovic V, et al. Developmental haemostasis. Impact for clinical haemostasis laboratories. Thromb Haemost 2006;95:362–72.
14. Monagle P, Ignjatovic V, Savoia H. Hemostasis in neonates and children: pitfalls and dilemmas. Blood Rev 2010;24:63–8.
15. Andrew M. Developmental hemostasis: relevance to thromboembolic complications in pediatric patients. Thromb Haemost 1995;74:415–25.
16. Ignjatovic V, Mertyn E, Mongale P. The coagulation system in children: developmental and pathophysiological considerations. Semin Thromb Hemost 2011;37: 723–9.
17. Cvirn G, Gallistl S, Leschnik B, et al. Low tissue factor pathway inhibitor (Tfpi) together with low antithrombin allows sufficient thrombin generation in neonates. J Thromb Haemost 2003;1:263–8.

18. van Ommen CH, Heijboer H, Buller HR, et al. Venous thromboembolism in childhood: a prospective two-year registry in the Netherlands. J Pediatr 2001;139: 676–81.
19. Newall F, Wallace T, Crock C, et al. Venous thromboembolic disease: a single center case series study. J Paediatr Child Health 2006;42:803–7.
20. Strauss T, Levy-Shraga Y, Ravid B, et al. Clot formation of neonates tested by thromboelastography correlates with gestational age. Thromb Haemost 2010; 103:344–50.
21. Mitchell L, Piovella F, Ofosu F, et al. Alpha-2-macroglobulin may provide protection from thromboembolic events in antithrombin III-deficient children. Blood 1991;78:2299–304.
22. Lippi G, Franchini M, Montagnana M, et al. Coagulation testing in pediatric patients: the young are not just miniature adults. Semin Thromb Hemost 2007;33: 816–20.
23. Saxonhouse MA, Manco-Johnson MJ. The evaluation and management of neonatal coagulation disorders. Semin Perinatol 2009;33:52–65.
24. Shearer MJ. Vitamin K deficiency bleeding (Vkdb) in early infancy. Blood Rev 2009;23:49–59.
25. Chalmers EA. Haemophilia and the newborn. Blood Rev 2004;18:85–92.
26. Young G. New anticoagulants in children: a review of recent studies and a look to the future. Thromb Res 2011;127:70–4.
27. Hirsh J, Bauer KA, Donati MB, et al. Anticoagulants: American College of Chest Physicians evidence-based clinical practice guidelines (8th edition). Chest 2008; 133:141S–59S.
28. Ignjatovic V, Furmedge J, Newall F, et al. Age-related differences in heparin response. Thromb Res 2006;118:741–5.
29. Hirsh J, Dalen J, Anderson DR, et al. Oral anticoagulants: mechanism of action, clinical effectiveness, and optimal therapeutic range. Chest 2001;119:8S–21S.
30. Massicotte P, Leaker M, Marzinotto V, et al. Enhanced thrombin regulation during warfarin therapy in children compared to adults. Thromb Haemost 1998;80: 570–4.

Inherited Abnormalities of Coagulation
Hemophilia, von Willebrand Disease, and Beyond

Riten Kumar, MD, MSc[a], Manuel Carcao, MD, MSc, FRCP(C)[a,b,*]

KEYWORDS

- Hemostasis • Hemophilia • von Willebrand disease • Rare factor deficiency

KEY POINTS

- Hemostasis, the arrest of bleeding at the site of vascular injury has been traditionally divided into primary and secondary hemostasis.
- Primary hemostasis consists of vasoconstriction, platelet adhesion to the subendothelium via von Willebrand factor, platelet activation and aggregation with the eventual formation of a platelet plug.
- Secondary hemostasis involves serine protease zymogens (coagulation factors) and their cofactors which interact sequentially to form cross-linked fibrin which helps stabilize the initial platelet plug.
- Abnormalities of primary hemostasis classically present with mucocutaneous bleeding, whereas deficiency of coagulation factors involved in secondary hemostasis may manifest with joint and muscle bleeds.
- Hemophilia A (HA) and hemophilia B (HB), X-linked deficiencies of factors VIII (FVIII) and IX (FIX) respectively, are associated with significant morbidity.
- von Willebrand disease, encompassing both quantitative deficiency and qualitative defects of the von Willebrand factor, is thought to be the most common bleeding disorder in humans.

INTRODUCTION

Bleeding disorders are broadly classified into primary and secondary hemostatic defects (**Fig. 1**). Primary hemostatic disorders (disorders of platelets and von Willebrand factor [VWF]) mainly result in mucocutaneous bleeding symptoms such as epistaxis,

Disclosures: None.
[a] Division of Haematology/Oncology, Department of Paediatrics, Hospital for Sick Children, University of Toronto, 555 University Avenue, Toronto, Ontario M5G 1X8, Canada; [b] Child Health Evaluative Sciences, Research Institute, Hospital for Sick Children, University of Toronto, 555 University Avenue, Toronto, Ontario M5G 1X8, Canada
* Corresponding author.
E-mail address: manuel.carcao@sickkids.ca

Pediatr Clin N Am 60 (2013) 1419–1441
http://dx.doi.org/10.1016/j.pcl.2013.09.002   **pediatric.theclinics.com**
0031-3955/13/$ – see front matter © 2013 Elsevier Inc. All rights reserved.

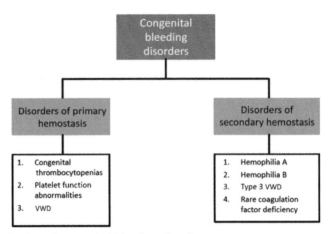

Fig. 1. Classification of congenital bleeding disorders.

menorrhagia, petechiae, easy bruising, and bleeding after dental and surgical interventions. Secondary hemostatic disorders (congenital or acquired deficiencies of coagulation factors) typically manifest with delayed, deep bleeding into muscles and joints. This article provides a generalized overview of the pathophysiology, clinical manifestations, laboratory abnormalities, and molecular basis of inherited abnormalities of coagulation with a focus on hemophilia, von Willebrand disease (VWD), and rare inherited coagulation disorders (RICD).

OVERVIEW OF HEMOSTASIS

Hemostasis, the arrest of bleeding from a site of vascular injury, is traditionally divided into primary and secondary hemostatic responses. Primary hemostasis begins immediately after endothelial damage and consists of 4 sequential and overlapping phases: (1) vasospasm, (2) platelet adhesion to the underlying collagen mediated by VWF, (3) platelet activation, and (4) platelet aggregation.[1–3] The end result of primary hemostasis is the formation of a platelet plug. Primary hemostasis is short lived; once the post-injury vasospasm abates and blood flow in the damaged vessel increases, the platelet plug may be rapidly sheared from the injured surface.[4] Secondary hemostasis involves a series of serine protease zymogens and their cofactors, which interact sequentially on phospholipid surfaces (platelets or damaged endothelial cells) and result in the formation of covalently cross-linked fibrin, which helps stabilize and reinforce the initial platelet plug.[5,6]

This sequential activation of serine protease zymogens is called the coagulation cascade. Historically, the coagulation cascade was divided into the intrinsic and extrinsic pathways, with the activated partial thromboplastin time (APTT) and prothrombin time/international normalized ratio (PT/INR) being used in clinical and laboratory settings to measure the integrity of the intrinsic and extrinsic pathways, respectively (**Fig. 2**).[7] Biologic advances over the past few decades have elaborated that *in vivo*, instead of occurring in pathways, the coagulation cascade occurs in distinct phases, namely, (1) initiation, (2) amplification, and (3) propagation.[4,8] The coagulation cascade is initiated when tissue factor (TF), released from the injured endothelial cells and monocytes binds to factor VII (FVII) to form the TF-activated FVII (FVIIa) complex. The TF-FVIIa complex, in turn, activates factor X (FX) and FIX. Activated FX (FXa) combines with

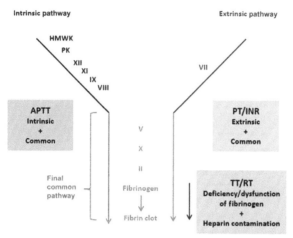

Fig. 2. Schematic representation of the coagulation cascade in-vitro. APTT, activated partial thromboplastin time; HMWK, high-molecular-weight kininogen; INR, international normalized ratio; PK, prekallikrein; PT, prothrombin time, RT, reptilase time; TT, thrombin time. (*Adapted from* Kamal AH, Tefferi A, Pruthi RK. How to interpret and pursue an abnormal prothrombin time, activated partial thromboplastin time, and bleeding time in adults. Mayo Clin Proc 2007;82(7):866; with permission.)

activated factor V (FVa) to form the FXa-FVa complex (the *prothrombinase complex*). The prothrombinase complex converts small amounts of prothrombin (FII) to thrombin (FIIa) (*initiation phase*). The amount of thrombin generated in the initiation phase is inadequate (2% of the total amount required) to generate sufficient amounts of fibrin to reinforce the initial platelet plug.[4] The primary role of this initial thrombin is to activate FV, FVIII, factor XI (FXI), and platelets through a positive feedback mechanism (**Fig. 3**) (*amplification phase*).

The amplification phase is followed by the propagation phase in which activated FIX (FIXa) binds with FVIIIa to form the FIXa-FVIIIa complex (the *tenase complex*). The tenase complex activates FX, which again associates with FVa (forming more prothrombinase complex), now leading to the generation of large amounts of thrombin—the so called *thrombin burst*. The thrombin generated catalyzes the conversion of fibrinogen to fibrin, which is covalently cross-linked in the presence of activated factor XIII (FXIIIa) to yield a stable clot. The propagation phase occurs on the surface of activated platelets. Contact factors of the intrinsic pathway (high-molecular-weight kininogen, prekallikrein, and factor XII) are not involved in the propagation phase, thus congenital deficiencies of these factors, although significantly prolonging the APTT, are not associated with bleeding. This article focuses on the main coagulation factor deficiencies and will not discuss disorders of platelets, which are discussed in another article appearing in this issue.

HEMOPHILIA
Introduction

HA and HB are X-linked, recessive, bleeding disorders caused by deficiency of blood coagulation factors FVIII and FIX, respectively. The incidence of HA is estimated to be 1 in 5000 males, whereas that of HB is 1 in 30,000 males.[9,10] Based on the coagulation factor activity level, hemophilia is classified into severe (<0.01 IU/dL), moderate (0.01–0.05 IU/dL), and mild (0.06–0.4 IU/dL). Overall, severe hemophilia accounts for

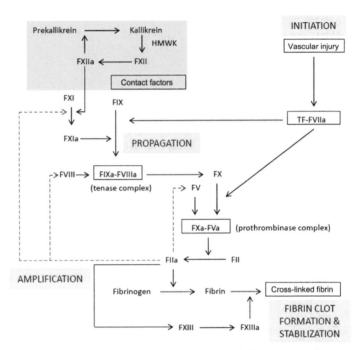

Fig. 3. Schematic representation of the coagulation cascade *in vivo*. Vascular injury initiates the coagulation cascade, via release of tissue factor. For the sake of clarity, calcium ions and phospholipids, 2 important cofactors for most coagulation reactions, have been omitted from this image. The red box indicates the contact factors, which plays a minimal role in activation of the coagulation cascade in vivo. The red dashed lines indicate the feedback amplification loops that follow the initial generation of small amounts of thrombin (FIIa).

40% or more of all hemophilia cases, although the distribution of the different severities of hemophilia varies; countries with more comprehensive national patient registries report a higher prevalence of mild hemophilia.[11,12] Patients with severe hemophilia typically develop spontaneous and recurrent bleeds, most commonly into joints (hemarthrosis) and muscles, whereas those with mild-moderate hemophilia tend to experience bleeding related to trauma or surgery.

Molecular Basis and Genetics

Both FVIII and FIX circulate in blood as inactive precursors that are activated at the time of vascular injury (see **Fig. 3**). FVIII is a protein cofactor with no intrinsic enzymatic activity, whereas FIX is a serine protease zymogen with an absolute requirement of FVIII as a cofactor.[13] On activation, FVIIIa and FIXa form the tenase complex, which activates FX. Thus, the basic biochemical abnormality in patients with hemophilia is the inability to activate FX and thereby generate thrombin and fibrin to stabilize the platelet clot. The inheritance pattern of hemophilia is elaborated in **Fig. 4**.

The genes for FVIII and FIX are located in the long arm of chromosome X at positions Xq28 and Xq27, respectively.[14,15] The FVIII gene spans 186 kb and consists of 28 exons. The FVIII precursor protein consists of 2351 amino acids, spaced out in 6 domains: (1) three A domains (A-1, A-2, and A-3), (2) a connecting B domain, and (3) two C-terminal domains (C-1 and C-2).[16,17] Intracellular proteolytic processing of FVIII involves cleavage at the Arg1689 site (at the B-A3 junction), which results in the formation of a heterodimer

Fig. 4. (*A*) In a mating between a hemophilia carrier woman and an unaffected man, 50% of the daughters will be carriers and 50% of sons will have hemophilia. (*B*) In a mating between an unaffected woman and a man with hemophilia, no son will be affected (having inherited the Y chromosome from the father) but all daughters will be carriers (having inherited the X chromosome from the father). Note: very rarely, females may have *true* hemophilia secondary to consanguinity in a hemophilic family, skewed inactivation of the normal X chromosome, or loss of part or all of the normal X chromosome (Turner syndrome).

consisting of an N-terminal heavy chain (A-1, A-2, and partially proteolyzed B domain) bound noncovalently to a C-terminal light chain (A-3, C-1, and C-2). This heterodimeric form of FVIII circulates in blood complexed with von Willebrand factor (VWF). Activation of FVIII by thrombin involves (1) release of FVIII by VWF and (2) excision of the remnant B domain.[17] The FIX gene is much smaller; it is 34 kb long and consists of 8 exons.[13,18] FIX consists of 416 amino acids and requires posttranslational, vitamin K-dependent, γ-glutamylcarboxylation to become physiologically active.

As of November 2012 more than 2000 unique mutations in the FVIII gene have been recorded in an international database (HAMSTeRS [The Hemophilia A Mutation, Structure, Test and Resource Site]; http://hadb.org.uk/). The most common mutation in HA, affecting nearly 45% of patients with severe disease, is an intron 22 inversion.[19,20] A similar database recording mutations for HB is accessible at http://www.umds.ac.uk/molgen/haemBdatabase. Inversion mutations are not seen in HB, and most patients ($\approx$70%) have missense mutations.[18] HB Leyden is a rare variant of HB that occurs secondary to point mutations in the promoter region of the FIX gene. Typically, patients with this mutation present with severe HB (FIX<0.01 IU/dL) in early childhood. However, postpuberty, increased androgen production results in increased FIX promoter activity and increased FIX production (eventually reaching $\approx$ 0.5 IU/dL), thereby correcting the hemophilia phenotype.[21]

Clinical Presentation and Diagnosis

About 50% to 70% of newborns with hemophilia have a family history of the disease.[16,22] Diagnosis of HA in this subcohort is usually made early in life by measuring the FVIII level on the cord blood. FIX levels, however, are physiologically low in the neonatal period (see **Table 1**), and a low FIX level in the cord blood, needs to be repeated at 6–12 months, before a diagnosis of HB can be confirmed. FIX levels increase throughout early childhood, and therefore, the ultimate classification of a patient's HB severity may change with aging, that is, a child labeled with moderate HB in the first year of life may ultimately be labeled as having mild HB. In the remaining 30% to 50% of patients without a positive family history, the diagnosis is usually made later in life, once the neonate or toddler is worked up for bleeding symptoms. Screening laboratory tests in patients with hemophilia usually demonstrate a prolonged APTT with a normal PT/INR value (see **Fig. 2**). Diagnosis can be confirmed by demonstrating a low or absent FVIII or FIX coagulant activity. This is typically measured in platelet-poor plasma using a functional clotting assay (usually a one-stage APTT-based assay), although some laboratories may use a two-stage or chromogenic substrate assay.[16] Of note, low FVIII and FIX activity levels do not always indicate hemophilia. A differential diagnosis of low plasma factor levels is elaborated in **Table 1**.

Clinical manifestations of HA and HB are identical, although there is some suggestion that HB may be milder than HA for the same level of factor activity.[23] Bleeding is the

Table 1
Differential diagnosis of low FVIII and FIX levels

Factor	Condition Associated with Low Factor Level	
FVIII	Type 3 VWD	• FVIII level usually ranges between 0.02 and 0.05 IU/dL • Associated reduction in VWF:Ag and VWF:RCo activity (see section on VWD for details)
FVIII	Type 2N VWD	• Caused by specific mutations in the VWF gene that result in reduced binding of FVIII by VWF • FVIII level usually range between 0.05 and 0.4 IU/dL; VWF:Ag and VWF:RCo activity are usually normal • Distinguished using the VWF:FVIII binding assay and/or genetic analysis
FVIII	Combined deficiency of FV and FVIII	• Very rare (1 in a million) • Generally causes FVIII levels in the 0.2 IU/dL range • Caused by mutations in genes encoding for intracellular transport protein (*LMAN1 and MCFD2*) • APTT and PT/INR are both prolonged
FVIII	Acquired hemophilia	• Very rare in children (0.045 in a million) • Associated with infection, penicillin antibiotics, and autoimmune conditions • Abnormal incubated mixing study • Bethesda assay or Nijmegen modification of Bethesda assay may be used to quantify inhibitor titer
FIX	Neonatal age	• FIX levels are low in healthy neonates • Low FIX levels in a newborn should be rechecked at 6–12 mo of age
FIX	Acquired vitamin K deficiency	• Liver disease, malabsorption, prolonged antibiotic use, and coumadin • Associated reduction in other Vitamin-K-dependent proteins (FII, FVII, FX)
FIX	Congenital deficiency of Vitamin-K-dependent clotting factors	• Mutations in *GGCX* or *VKOR* gene • Associated reduction in other Vitamin-K-dependent proteins (FII, FVII,FX)

Abbreviations: GGCX, γ-glutamylcarboxylase; LMAN1, lectin mannose-binding 1; MCFD2, multiple coagulation factor deficiency 2; VKOR, vitamin K epoxide reductase.

clinical hallmark of hemophilia, but the sites and pattern of bleeding vary significantly based on disease severity and age of patients.[16,24] Birth is thought to be the first hemostatic challenge for a newborn with hemophilia. In a large prospective study of 580 infants with hemophilia, enrolled in the Universal Data Collection of the Center for Disease Control and Prevention, 53% of infants with hemophilia had a bleeding episode by the age of 1 month.[25] Bleeding post circumcision accounted for almost half (47.9%) of the bleeds in the first month of life; this was followed by head bleeds (19.4%) and bleeding from heel sticks (10.4%).[25] Intracranial hemorrhage (ICH) remains the most serious complication of hemophilia in the immediate postnatal period and can result in severe morbidity or death. Recent studies have indicated that the rate of ICH in newborns with hemophilia (all severities) ranges from 1% to 4%, which is significantly higher than in newborns who do not have a bleeding disorder.[25–27] The optimal mode of delivery for a woman known to be a hemophilia carrier has been extensively debated.[28,29] However, it is clear that caesarean delivery does not completely eliminate the risk of ICH, and consequently, in most centers, the recommended mode of delivery remains an atraumatic, non–instrument-assisted vaginal delivery. In a prospective European study, assisted vaginal delivery with instrumentation was associated with a marked increased risk of head bleeds (odds ratio [OR], 8.84; 95% confidence interval [CI], 3.05–25.5), and it is generally accepted that instrumentation of any kind (forceps, vacuum extraction, or fetal scalp electrodes) should be avoided in infants born to known carriers of hemophilia.[26] For newborns with a clinical suspicion of an ICH, factor should be administered immediately and prior to imaging confirmation.[30] When the hemophilia subtype (HA vs HB) is not known, it may be appropriate to administer fresh frozen plasma (FFP) (10–15 mL/kg) while awaiting laboratory confirmation.[16] It is also recommended that intramuscular vitamin K should be avoided until the diagnosis of hemophilia is excluded, and oral vitamin K may be administered in the interim or once the diagnosis of hemophilia is confirmed.[30]

Bleeding from the oral mucous membranes becomes more common as infants with hemophilia grow older.[25] Other sites of bleeding that become apparent by 6 to 12 months of age include bleeding into joints (hemarthrosis), muscle bleeds, and bleeding from the gastrointestinal and urinary tracts. ICH remains a serious complication of hemophilia at all ages. In a nested case-control study of more than 10,000 patients with hemophilia, older than 2 years, 2% of patients had experienced an ICH with a 20% mortality rate.[31] High titer inhibitors (OR, 4.01; 95% CI, 2.40–6.71), prior ICH (OR, 2.62; 95% CI, 2.66–4.92), and severe hemophilia (OR, 3.25; 95% CI, 2.01–5.25) were found to be independent predictors of ICH.

Hemarthrosis is the clinical hallmark of severe hemophilia. Although all synovial joints are at potential risk, the most frequently affected are the knees, elbows, and ankles. Joint bleeds usually become apparent once the toddler starts bearing weight. The range of ages at which children experience a first joint bleed varies tremendously. In a Dutch study, the median age of first joint bleed was 1.8 years but the range was between 0.2 and 5.8 years.[32] This marked variation in the age at which children with severe hemophilia experience their first joint bleed reflects the considerable heterogeneity that exists in the bleeding phenotype of patients with severe hemophilia. Differences in levels of physical activity, structural integrity of joints, and coinheritance of pro-thrombotic conditions, particularly Factor V Leiden mutation, have been proposed as possible explanations for this heterogeneity.[16,33,34]

Bleeding into a joint results in synovial hypertrophy and inflammation (synovitis). A joint that undergoes repeated bleeds is referred to as a target joint. While the exact definition of a target joint is debatable, it usually refers to a joint that develops 3 or more bleeds in a period of 3 to 6 months.[16] A target joint may eventually develop hemophilic arthropathy, characterized by loss of joint space, cystic changes within the subchondral bone, osteoporosis, and atrophy of the surrounding muscles.[16,35] The final stage of hemophilic arthropathy is a deformed and dysfunctional joint, which may significantly compromise a patient's quality of life (**Fig. 5**).

Muscle hematomas, the second most common type of bleeding in patients with hemophilia account for 10% to 25% of all bleeds in this cohort.[36] Bleeding into the iliopsoas muscle, a large muscle in the pelvis, is particularly concerning because patients can lose a significant volume of blood into this muscle. Inadequate or delayed treatment of muscle hematomas may result in compartment syndrome, atrophy of tendons, myositis ossificans, and rarely hemophilic pseudotumors. Pseudotumors result from recurrent hemorrhage into an enlarging, encapsulated hematoma and may lead to pressure necrosis and destruction of adjacent structures.[37]

Clinical Management

General overview

Management of hemophilia is complex and requires a multi-disciplinary comprehensive care approach involving hematologists specialized in bleeding disorders, dedicated nurses, social workers, physiotherapists as well as the availability of dentistry, orthopedics, and psychology. It is recommended that all patients with hemophilia be followed in comprehensive hemophilia treatment centers able to provide such multidisciplinary care. Education of patients and primary care providers about risks of bleeding and related complications is important. Lifestyle modifications including avoidance of contact and collision sports, routine dental care to reduce the risk of gingival bleeding, avoidance of platelet-impairing medications (aspirin and nonsteroidal antiinflammatory drugs), and use of MedicAlert bracelets should be encouraged. Given the risk of exposure to blood-derived products, patients should be vaccinated against hepatitis B. Vaccinations for patients with hemophilia can, and ideally should, be given subcutaneously, using the smallest gauge needle, with local pressure applied for at least 5 minutes.

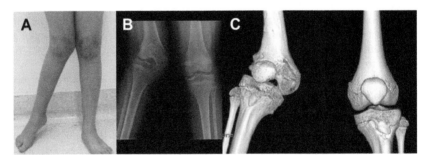

Fig. 5. A 12-year-old boy with severe hemophilia B had received minimal treatment for hemophilia before immigrating to Canada. At presentation to our clinic, he showed significant arthropathy of his right knee. (*A*) Photograph of the legs showing valgus deformity, limb length discrepancy, and loss of normal landmarks of the right knee with diffuse muscle wasting. (*B*) Radiograph of the legs shows valgus deformity, loss of joint space, osteopenia, and deformity of the medial femoral condyle and tibial plateau. (*C*) Preoperative computed tomography shows sclerosis and irregularity of the distal femoral physis and anterolateral physeal fusion at the distal femur growth plate (architecture of the left knee is relatively preserved). ([*A*] *Courtesy* of Ms Pamela Hilliard, BSc (PT), Department of Rehabilitation Services, Hospital for Sick Children.)

Management of acute bleeds

Factor replacement Treatment needs to be administered expeditiously in the case of acute bleeds to prevent both short-term complications and long-term disabilities.[38,39] Factor replacement therapy using FVIII and FIX concentrates forms the backbone of management for patients with severe hemophilia. These concentrates may be broadly divided into 2 categories: plasma-derived and recombinant concentrates. The dose of concentrate to be administered is calculated based on the hemophilia subtype, baseline factor activity, and desired increase in the factor level. Generally, 1 U/kg of administered FVIII increases the plasma FVIII coagulant activity by 0.02 IU/dL; whereas 1 U/kg of recombinant FIX increases the plasma FIX coagulant activity by approximately 0.008 IU/dL (the expected increase is 0.01 IU/dL when using plasma-derived FIX).[16] The half-life of FVIII is 8 to 12 hours and that of FIX is 12 to 24 hours.[40,41] Factor concentrates may be administered in bolus doses or through continuous infusion. Continuous infusion of factor prevents the peaks and troughs associated with bolus dosing and may be particularly useful in surgical and postsurgical settings.[24] A bolus dose of 50 U/kg of FVIII or FIX followed by an initial continuous infusion of 2 to 3 U/kg/h of FVIII or 4 to 8 U/kg/h of FIX is recommended with periodic measurement of factor levels to ensure that they are being maintained in the hemostatic range.[24,42,43] For mild-moderate hemorrhage, the targeted hemostatic range is 0.3 to 0.4 IU/dL for FVIII and 0.25 to 0.3 IU/dL for FIX, whereas for severe life-threatening hemorrhages, the target range is 1 IU/dL.[44] For details on the specific dose of factor used and duration of therapy, see article by Robertson and colleagues.[45]

Local measures Mild superficial bleeding symptoms in patients with mild-moderate hemophilia may be managed with local measures. Compression, use of gelatin sponge or gauge soaked in tranexamic acid may be tried for superficial wounds. Epistaxis may be managed by nasal packing and use of topical thrombin (eg, Thrombi-Gel, Evithrom) and fibrin sealant gel (Evicel).

Desmopressin Desmopressin (1-deamino-8-D-arginine-vasopressin; DDAVP), a synthetic analog of the antidiuretic hormone, vasopressin, exerts its procoagulant effect by causing the release of stored VWF and FVIII from Weibel-Palade bodies in endothelial cells into the plasma thus increasing (doubling or tripling) the circulating levels of FVIII and VWF.[46] Clinically meaningful response is usually seen only in patients with a baseline FVIII activity of more than 0.10 to 0.15 IU/dL.[47] DDAVP does not increase FIX levels and therefore is not useful in patients with HB. It is important to know *a priori* how a patient will respond to DDAVP before using it in a clinical setting. This information is usually obtained by administering the standard dose of 0.3 μg/kg (maximum 20 μg) of DDAVP intravenously/subcutaneously or intranasally (150 μg [for children weighing <50 kg] or 300 μg [for children weighing ≥50 kg]) and monitoring the FVIII and VWF response at 1 and 4 hours (DDAVP challenge test). Younger patients (eg, <3–5 years of age) often have a suboptimal response to DDAVP, and the DDAVP challenge should be repeated in patients who were assessed as nonresponders at a young age. For patients who respond, DDAVP may be used to treat minor bleeds and for prophylaxis before dental and minor surgical procedures. Peak FVIII levels are reached within 30 to 60 minutes after intravenous injection and 90 to 120 minutes after intranasal and subcutaneous administration. Side effects of DDAVP include fluid retention and hyponatremia, and patients should be advised to limit their fluid intake for 24 hours after DDAVP administration. For the same reason, DDAVP is avoided in children younger than 2 years. The ability of DDAVP to increase FVIII and VWF levels is lost after multiple doses.

Antifibrinolytic agents Lysine analogs, tranexamic acid (cyclokapron) and ε-amino-caproic acid (Amicar), are usually used in combination with other therapeutic modalities (FVIII or FIX concentrates or DDAVP). They are particularly useful in patients with epistaxis, gingival bleeding, and menorrhagia and may also be used for prevention of bleeding after minor surgical and dental procedures. Both agents can be used orally and intravenously. The dose of tranexamic acid is 15 to 25 mg/kg orally, taken 3 to 4 times a day (or 10 mg/kg intravenously every 8 hours). This drug is also available as a mouthwash (10 mL of a 5% solution taken 4 to 6 times a day), which if swallowed is equivalent to a dose of 500 mg. Common side effects are nausea and diarrhea, which are dose dependent. Antifibrinolytics are contraindicated in hematuria given the risk of clot formation within the renal collecting system.

Long-term management: prophylaxis versus episodic therapy

In the 1950s, Nilsson and colleagues[48] in Malmö, Sweden, observed that patients with moderate hemophilia rarely develop chronic arthropathy and disability.[49] They hypothesized that by prophylactically replacing FVIII/FIX concentrates on a regular basis, they could convert the phenotype of patients with severe hemophilia to a moderate one and thereby prevent recurrent hemarthrosis and arthropathy. Almost 25 years later, Professor Nilsson published data on 60 patients who had received prophylactic factor replacement for 2 to 25 years; and demonstrated that when prophylaxis was started early and administered regularly, patients with severe hemophilia had significantly reduced bleeding, excellent joint status, and were able to lead normal lives.[50] The superiority of prophylaxis (regular administration of factor to patients with hemophilia to prevent bleeding episodes) over on-demand therapy (administration of factor only at the time of an acute bleed) was demonstrated in a landmark randomized trial published by Manco-Johnson and colleagues[51] in 2007.

Prophylaxis is now the standard of care for patients with severe hemophilia in the developed world. Full-dose primary prophylaxis entails the administration of high doses of factor (25–40 U/kg), every other day for HA and twice a week for HB starting by 2 years of age and before the onset of joint damage.[38] The biggest disadvantage of this regimen is the need for frequent infusions of factor starting at a very young age, which leads to a high need for central venous access devices (CVADs). Although CVADs allow the early initiation of prophylaxis and home therapy, they are associated with a substantial rate of infections and thrombosis.[52] An alternative approach to starting very young children on full-dose prophylaxis is to instead use escalating dose/frequency prophylaxis. Such an approach starts patients on once-a-week infusions, then escalates them to twice-a-week prophylaxis, and finally moves them to full-dose prophylaxis. Some countries, notably Sweden, escalate all children quickly to full-dose prophylaxis regardless of whether these children are experiencing bleeds, whereas other groups, instead, only escalate patients if they experience what is judged to be an unacceptably high bleeding frequency (tailored prophylaxis).[53] A head-to-head comparison between tailored prophylaxis and full-dose prophylaxis has not been done.

The Future of Hemophilia Care

Long-acting factor concentrates

The management of hemophilia is likely to change with the development of longer acting FVIII and FIX concentrates.[54] Several companies, using different technologies (PEGylation, fusion to albumin or the Fc component of immunoglobulin), have already shown a 3- to 6-fold prolongation in the half-life of FIX. These products are still undergoing clinical trials, although preliminary data seem promising. Similar technologies are being used to develop long-acting FVIII concentrates, but so far, these technologies have only been able to result in a 1.5 to 1.7 prolongation of the half-life of FVIII.

Gene therapy

In 2011, the first successful results of gene therapy for HB were published.[55] Six patients with severe HB (FIX<0.01 IU/dL) were treated with 3 escalating dose levels of an adenovirus-associated virus vector expressing a codon-optimized human FIX gene. A transient elevation of liver enzymes observed in 2 patients treated with the highest vector dose was rapidly cleared with a short course of steroids. Other than this there was no acute toxicity observed over 6 to 16 months of follow-up. FIX coagulant activity trough levels of 0.02 to 0.11 IU/dL were observed in all patients, and 4 of 6 patients were able to discontinue prophylaxis. Further studies evaluating the safety and long-term efficacy of gene therapy are underway.

Inhibitors in Hemophilia

Development of inhibitors is currently the most serious complication of hemophilia. Inhibitors are neutralizing allo-antibodies that develop in 30% or more of patients with HA and about 2%to 5% of patients with HB.[56] These antibodies, which usually develop within the first 20 to 50 exposure days to factor, rapidly inactivate infused factor, rendering replacement therapy ineffective and are associated with significant morbidity. Risk factors for inhibitor development[16] include genetic factors such as family history of inhibitor, race, underlying mutation and polymorphisms in immune regulatory genes (interleukin-10, tumor necrosis factor-α, and cytotoxic T-lymphocyte antigen-4),[57,58] as well as acquired risk factors, for example, intense exposure to factor, particularly during surgery, hemorrhage, and vaccination. It is thought that these conditions act as *danger signals* to the immune system, resulting in upregulated immunity, and increase the risk of antibody development. The immunogenicity of recombinant versus plasma-derived factor concentrates has been a subject of intense debate.[38,59–61] A randomized prospective study (Survey of inhibitors in plasma-product exposed toddlers [SIPPETT trial]) is currently ongoing to address this issue.

Inhibitors levels are measured using the Bethesda assay and are quantified in Bethesda units (BU; 1 BU is the amount of antibody that inactivates 50% of factor after 2 hours of incubation at 37°C). A low-titer inhibitor is defined as less than 5 BU, and a high-titer inhibitor is defined as 5 BU or more. Management of inhibitors is complex and essentially includes 2 aspects:

1. Management and prevention of acute bleeds: acute bleeds in patients with low-titer inhibitors may be managed by giving high doses of FVIII or FIX. In patients with high-titer inhibitors, bypass agents (activated prothrombin complex concentrates [FEIBA] and/or recombinant FVIIa [NovoSeven]) may be used. In a prospective, randomized, open-label, crossover trial, both products were equally efficacious.[62] These bypass agents can also be used in a prophylactic manner to prevent bleeding.
2. Immune tolerance therapy: Permanent eradication of inhibitors can be achieved using immune tolerance induction (ITI). ITI entails the frequent administration of large doses of factor concentrate, and when successful, results in normalization of factor pharmacokinetics and subsequent improvement in the patient's quality of life. ITI has been mainly studied in HA inhibitor patients where success rates of 60% to 80% have been reported.[56] Different regimens of ITI have been reported. A recent randomized trial comparing low-dose (50 U/kg 3 times/wk) and high-dose (200 U/kg/ day) ITI showed similar efficacy, although high dose was associated with quicker success and less bleeding while on ITI.[16,63] Readers interested in learning details

about the diagnosis and management of inhibitors are referred to the following excellent reviews.[64,65]

VON WILLEBRAND DISEASE
Introduction

VWD is the most common inherited bleeding disorder in humans. Large, epidemiologic studies, measuring von Willebrand activity in healthy school children estimated the prevalence to be 1 in 100,[66,67] although the prevalence of clinically symptomatic VWD is probably closer to 1 in 1000.[68] VWD occurs secondary to a mild or severe quantitative deficiency (type 1 or type 3, respectively) or a qualitative defect (type 2) in VWF, a large, adhesive, multimeric glycoprotein. VWD is generally milder than hemophilia with most patients manifesting mucocutaneous bleeding symptoms and postoperative hemorrhage. VWF plays an important role in both the primary and secondary hemostatic pathways:

1. Platelet adhesion to the underlying subendothelium is mediated by VWF, which binds to platelet surface glycoprotein GPIb/IX/V.
2. Platelet aggregation is mediated by both VWF and fibrinogen, which bind to the platelet surface glycoprotein GPIIb/IIIa.
3. VWF binds and stabilizes FVIII in circulation, protecting it from degradation by activated protein C.

Molecular Basis and Genetics

The VWF gene, cloned in 1985, is located at the tip of the short arm of chromosome 12 at 12p13.3.[69,70] The gene spans 178 kb, consists of 52 exons, and codes for a protein consisting of 2813 amino acids.[71] VWF is synthesized in vascular endothelial cells and megakaryocytes and undergoes significant posttranslational modification including dimerization, sulfation, and glycosylation.[72] The final protein is either constitutively released from endothelial cells into plasma or stored in Weibel-Palade bodies of endothelial cells and then secreted into plasma in the setting of stress or bleeding. VWF produced in megakaryocytes is stored within platelet alpha granules. On activation of platelets, this VWF participates in hemostasis but is not secreted into plasma. When in circulation, the molecular weight of VWF ranges from 500 (short VWF multimers) to 20,000 (high-molecular-weight multimers) kDa depending on the extent of multimerization. Multimer size is an important determinant of the functional activity of VWF, as high-molecular-weight-VWF (HMW-VWF) is most physiologically active. The molecular weight of VWF is controlled by the metalloprotease enzyme, ADAMTS13 (a *d*isintegrin *a*nd *m*etalloprotease with *t*hrombospondin 1 motif, member *13*), which cleaves VWF between Tyr1605 and Met1606 residues in the A2 domain.[73]

The molecular basis of VWD has only recently begun to be characterized. Identifying a genetic basis for type 1 VWD, the most common variant, has proven to be particularly challenging with 3 large cohort studies identifying a putative mutation in only 65% of the tested subjects.[74–76] Inherited in an autosomal dominant manner, type 1 VWD has incomplete penetrance and expression, and as such, genetic testing, outside of a research study, is not recommended for diagnosing type 1 VWD. Type 2 VWD is inherited largely in an autosomal dominant manner (with the exception of type 2N, which is autosomal recessive) and usually occurs secondary to missense mutations.[69] The rare, type 3 VWD is autosomal recessive, with both parents carrying mutations in the VWF gene. Details of mutations identified in the VWF gene may be found through the International Society on Thrombosis and Haemostasis (ISTH)-sponsored database: http://www.vwf.group.shef.ac.uk/.

Classification and Laboratory Diagnosis

The current classification of VWD was established in 2006.[77] VWD is classified into 3 main categories: type 1 includes partial quantitative deficiency, type 2 includes qualitative defects, and type 3 VWD is associated with a complete deficiency of VWF (**Table 2**). Type 2 VWD is further subclassified into 4 secondary categories (A, B, M, and N), Laboratory evaluation of VWD includes the use of nonspecific tests such as the complete blood cell count (CBC), APTT, and FVIII activity, as well as tests specific for VWF. The platelet function analyzer (PFA-100) provides an *in vitro* measure of primary hemostasis under conditions of high shear using disposable cartridges containing collagen/epinephrine or collagen/adenosine diphosphate.[78] In a prospective study of 53 children with VWD, the sensitivity of PFA-100 for detecting VWD was 90%,[79] potentially allowing PFA-100 to be used as a screening test for VWD. Tests specific for VWF include measurement of the amount of circulating von Willebrand antigen (VWF:Ag) and measurement of von Willebrand function through either a ristocetin-based platelet aggregation study, known as von Willebrand ristocetin cofactor assay (VWF:RCo), or through a von Willebrand collagen binding assay.[70] The VWF:RCo to VWF:Ag ratio helps differentiate type 1 from type 2 A, B, and M VWD. In type 1 VWD, there is a proportionate decrease in the antigen and activity, and therefore the VWF:RCo/VWF:Ag is greater than or equal to 0.6. Conversely, in type 2 (A, B, and M) VWD, there is a disproportionate decrease in the VWF activity such that the VWF:RCo/VWF:Ag is less than 0.6. Other tests that aid in identification of the type 2 VWD subtypes include the ristocetin-induced platelet aggregation (RIPA; distinguishes type 2B from the others) and VWF multimer analysis (mainly used to differentiate type 2A from type 2M).

Type 1 VWD

Type 1 VWD accounts for 75% to 80% of all cases of VWD. Clinical diagnosis of type 1 VWD remains challenging because there are multiple factors such as patient age and blood group that contribute significantly to plasma VWF levels.[69] Plasma VWF levels increase by 1% to 2% per year of age and are 25% higher in individuals with non–blood group O than in those with blood group O.[80,81] VWF is also an acute-phase reactant, and plasma levels may be high in conditions of stress, inflammation, exercise, and pregnancy and in women using oral contraceptives. To make matters even more complicated, the plasma level of VWF, used as a cutoff to make the

Table 2
Laboratory findings in von Willebrand disease

Disease Subtype	VWF:Ag	VWF:RCo	VWF:RCo/ VWF:Ag Ratio	FVIII Level	Multimer Pattern	RIPA
1	↓	↓	>0.60	↓ or ↔	Normal	↔
2A	↓	↓↓	<0.60	↓ or ↔	Abnormal	↓
2B	↓	↓↓	<0.60	↓ or ↔	Abnormal	↑
2M	↓	↓↓	<0.60	↓ or ↔	Normal	↓
2N	↓ or ↔	↓ or ↔	>0.60	0.10–0.40 IU/dL	Normal	↔
3	<0.05 IU/dL	<0.05 IU/dL	NA	<0.10 IU/dL	Absent	Absent

↑, elevated/raised; ↓, mild reduction; ↓↓, severe reduction; ↔, normal.
Abbreviations: NA, not applicable; RIPA, ristocetin-induced platelet aggregation; VWF:Ag, von Willebrand antigen; VWF:RCo, von Willebrand ristocetin cofactor assay.

diagnosis of type 1 VWD, remains a matter of debate.[82] Different cutoffs ranging from 0.15 to 0.50 IU/dL have been suggested in the literature but with no consensus.[70,77,79] Using a cutoff of 0.40 IU/dL for both VWF:Ag and VWF:RCo seems to be practical and avoids both overdiagnosing and underdiagnosing VWD. CBC and PT/INR usually have normal values in type 1 VWD. The FVIII activity and consequently the APTT may have abnormal values when the VWF:Ag is <0.35 IU/dL, although a normal value of APTT by no means rules out VWD.[70]

Type 2 VWD

Type 2 VWD accounts for 20% to 25% of all VWD cases and is characterized by a VWF:RCo/VWF:Ag less than 0.6. Clinical presentation of type 2 VWD is similar to that of type 1 VWD.

Type 2A VWD Type 2A VWD is characterized by the selective loss of high- and medium-molecular-weight multimers either secondary to a defect in the synthesis of these multimers or due to increased cleavage of the multimers by ADAMTS13.[70] VWF multimer analysis can aid in the diagnosis (**Fig. 6**).

Type 2B VWD Type 2B VWD is caused by gain-of-function mutations in the GPIb/IX/V binding site of the von Willebrand gene, causing spontaneous binding of VWF to platelets and the subsequent removal of the HMW-VWF multimers together with platelets from the circulation.[6] Patients may have thrombocytopenia, which can be aggravated by conditions associated with increased VWF secretion. Type 2B VWD is also associated with loss of high-molecular-weight multimers (see **Fig. 6**). This condition may be differentiated from type 2A VWD by performing an RIPA assay. Type 2B VWD typically shows hyperresponsiveness with low-dose ristocetin, whereas the RIPA is reduced in type 2A.

Type 2M VWD Type 2M VWD occurs secondary to decreased interaction between VWF and platelets. VWF multimer analysis distinguishes type 2A from type 2M; in the former, multimer distribution is abnormal, whereas in the latter, it is typically normal.

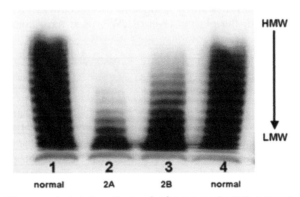

Fig. 6. VWF multimer analysis in 2 patients who have type 2 VWD. Lanes 1 and 4 represent normal plasma multimer patterns. Lane 2 shows the plasma VWF multimers for a patient who has type 2A, and lane 3 shows the plasma multimers for a patient who has type 2B VWD. HMW, high molecular weight; LMW, low molecular weight. (*From* Robertson J, Lillicrap D, James PD. Von Willebrand disease. Pediatr Clin North Am 2008;55(2):382. viii–ix; with permission.)

Type 2N (Normandy) VWD Type 2N VWD, an autosomal recessive variant of VWD, occurs secondary to mutations in the FVIII binding site in the von Willebrand gene and may be misdiagnosed as mild or moderate hemophilia.[83] The values of VWF:Ag and VWF:RCo may be borderline low or normal, with a disproportionate decrease in the FVIII activity (FVIII activity: 0.05–0.4 IU/dL). RIPA and VWF multimer pattern are normal. The diagnosis is made either using an enzyme-linked immunosorbent assay-based VWF:FVIII binding assay or by genetic analysis of the VWF gene.

Type 3 VWD

Type 3 VWD is a rare autosomal recessive variant of VWD. Patients present with severe mucocutaneous and hemophilia-like bleeding (hemarthrosis and muscle bleeds) early in life. The VWF:Ag and VWF:RCo are less than 0.05 IU/dL, with an FVIII activity less than 0.1 IU/dL.

Clinical Management

Anticipatory guidance, education of patients and parents, and use of local measures and antifibrinolytics is similar to hemophilia (please see preceding section on "clinical management of hemophilia"). Additional therapeutic interventions specific for VWD are elaborated.

Estrogens

Estrogen-containing oral contraceptive pills may be used for females with menorrhagia. Estrogen ointment (Premarin) has been used intranasally on a prophylactic basis for pediatric patients with recurrent epistaxis with some success.[84]

Desmopressin

Over 80% of patients with type 1 VWD will show a response to DDAVP,[85] although response in type 2 VWD is less predictable. DDVAP is not beneficial in type 3 VWD, and given the risk of exacerbating the thrombocytopenia, it is usually contraindicated in type 2B VWD. Similar to hemophilia, it is important to perform a DDAVP challenge test before using it in a clinical setting. Dose and side effects of DDAVP are elaborated in the hemophilia section of this article.

VWF/FVIII concentrate

For life-threatening bleeds, major surgery, and for patients in whom DDAVP is either contraindicated (type 2B VWD) or not beneficial (all patients with type 3 and those with type 2 or 1 VWD shown to be inadequate responders to DDAVP), viral-inactivated, plasma-derived, VWF/FVIII concentrates are the treatment of choice. There are several products available that are differentiated based on the ratio of VWF to FVIII. Infusions are usually given every 12 to 24 hours. For patients requiring repeated infusions of VWF/FVIII concentrates, it is recommended that trough FVIII and VWF levels be measured to ensure that the patient does not have supra-physiological levels of FVIII, which may be associated with an increased risk of thrombosis.[70] A recent retrospective study showed that prophylaxis with VWF/FVIII concentrates is safe and efficacious in patients with severe VWD.[86] For details about VWD management, readers are referred to the following excellent reviews.[82,87]

RARE INHERITED COAGULATION DISORDERS

RICD account for 3% to 5% of all coagulation disorders and include qualitative and quantitative deficiencies of fibrinogen (afibrinogenemia, hypofibrinogenemia, and dysfibrinogenemia), prothrombin (FII), FV, combined FV and FVIII, FVII, FX, FXI, and FXIII.[88–90] These conditions are inherited in an autosomal recessive manner with affected

Table 3
Prevalence, molecular basis, and clinical characteristics of rare inherited coagulation disorders

Deficient Factor	Prevalence	Gene Involved	Clinical Features	Coagulation Assays	Factor Replacement	Half-life of Factor
Afibrinogenemia	1 in 1 million	FGA (4q31.3) FGB (4q31.3) FGG (4q32.1)	Umbilical stump bleeding, CNS bleeds, hemarthrosis and recurrent first-trimester pregnancy loss; splenic rupture and rarely thrombosis	PT↑ APTT↑ TT↑	pd Fibrinogen, cryoprecipitate, FFP	2–4 d
Prothrombin (FII)	1 in 2 million	F2 (11p11.2)	Complete deficiency not compatible with life; mucosal bleeds, hemarthrosis, and muscle hematomas	PT↑ APTT↑ TT↔	FFP, PCCs	3–4 d
FV	1 in 1 million	F5 (1q24.2)	Mucosal bleeds, hemarthrosis, and muscle hematomas	PT↑ APTT↑ TT↔	FFP	36 h
Combined FV + FVIII	1 in 1 million	LMAN1 (18q21.32) MCFD2 (2p21)	Mucosal bleeds	PT↑ APTT↑ TT↔	FFP + pdFVIII/rFVIII	As for individual factors
FVII	1 in 500,000	F7 (13q34)	Mucosal bleeds, hemarthrosis, and muscle hematomas	PT↑ APTT↔ TT↔	pdFVII, rFVIIa, PCCs, FFP	4–6 h
FX	1 in 1 million	F10 (13q34)	Umbilical stump bleeding, CNS bleeds, hemarthrosis, and muscle hematomas	PT↑ APTT↑ TT↔	PCC, FFP	40–60 h
FXI	1 in 1 million	F11 (4q35.2)	Postsurgical hemorrhage	PT↔ APTT↑ TT↔	pdFXI, FFP	40–70 h
FXIII	1 in 2 million	F13B (1q31.3) F13A (6p25.1)	Umbilical stump bleeding, CNS bleeds, hemarthrosis, and muscle hematomas	PT↔ APTT↔ TT↔[a]	pdFXIII, rFXIII, cryoprecipitate, FFP	11–14 d

↑ Indicates prolonged; ↔ indicates normal.
Abbreviations: CNS, central nervous system; FGA, fibrinogen α-chain gene; FGB, fibrinogen β-chain gene; FGG, fibrinogen γ-chain gene; PCCs, prothrombin complex concentrate; pd, plasma-derived viral inactivated; rFVIII, recombinant FVIII; rFVIIa, recombinant activated factor VII; rFXIII, recombinant factor XIII.
[a] Note that the global coagulation assays, APTT, PT, and TT, yield completely normal results in patients with FXIII deficiency.

individuals being homozygous or compound heterozygous for disease-causing mutations. Data collected from international registries show a variable prevalence for homozygous forms, with FVII (1 in 500,000) deficiency being the most prevalent and prothrombin and FXIII (1 in 1–2 million) deficiencies being the least prevalent.[91–93] Given the rarity of these conditions, their molecular basis, phenotypic manifestations, and therapeutic modalities are less well understood as compared to hemophilia and VWD.

Bleeding risk in patients with RICD is less predictable as compared to HA and HB, and definitions of severity used for patients with hemophilia cannot be applied to patients with RICD.[88] The scientific and standardization committee of the ISTH concluded that while there was a strong association between clinical severity and coagulation factor activity for fibrinogen, FII, FX, and FXIII deficiencies; there was poor to no association for FV, FVII, and FXI deficiencies.[94] Typical bleeding symptoms in patients with RICD include epistaxis, menorrhagia, and bleeding after dental and surgical interventions. Severe life-threatening hemorrhage, including bleeding from the umbilical cord, recurrent hemoperitoneum with ovulation, and hemarthrosis are reported in patients with FII, FX, and FXIII deficiencies. Recurrent first-trimester pregnancy loss is typically seen with afibrinogenemia, and ICH is associated with both afibrinogenemia and FXIII deficiency.[94] Attention must be paid to women affected by RICD, as they may experience significant menorrhagia and postpartum hemorrhage.

Standard coagulation assays (APTT, PT, and thrombin time [TT]) may be used to screen patients suspected of having an RICD (**Table 3**). Based on the results, specific assays of factor coagulant activity can be performed to confirm the diagnosis. Standard laboratory screening assays (APTT, PT/INR, and TT) are however, completely normal in patients with FXIII deficiency. The ISTH recommends using a quantitative functional FXIII assay for screening for FXIII deficiency followed by measurement of FXIII-A2B2 antigen concentration to confirm the diagnosis.[95] Once a diagnosis of RICD is made, patients should be referred to a specialty center for further evaluation and management. Similar to hemophilia, replacement of the deficient coagulation factor forms the mainstay of therapy for RICD.[89] Plasma-derived, viral-inactivated factor concentrates are available for fibrinogen, FVII, FXI, and FXIII,[91,92,96,97] whereas recombinant factor concentrates are available only for FVII (NovoSeven), and more recently for FXIII (NovoThirteen).[98] There are no purified factor concentrates currently available for FII, FV, and FX, and bleeding in these conditions can be treated with FFP or prothrombin complex concentrates (for FII and FX deficiencies).[99–101] In patients with RICD, factor concentrates are usually used on-demand, although prophylactic replacement is recommended for patients with FXIII deficiency[97] and for select patients with severe deficiencies of FVII and fibrinogen who have sustained life-threatening bleeds. Antifibrinolytic agents such as ε-aminocaproic acid and tranexamic acid may be used for mucosal bleeds. Hormonal therapy with estrogen-containing oral contraceptive pills may be used in patients with menorrhagia.[89] Characteristic clinical findings, molecular basis, laboratory abnormalities, and factor concentrates available for the RICD are summarized in **Table 3**. For more advanced reading on the laboratory diagnosis and clinical management of RICD, the reader is referred to recommendations made by the United Kingdom Haemophilia Centre Doctors' Association (UKHC-DO).[102]

REFERENCES

1. Israels SJ, Kahr WH, Blanchette VS, et al. Platelet disorders in children: a diagnostic approach. Pediatr Blood Cancer 2011;56(6):975–83.
2. Israels SJ, Rand ML. What we have learned from inherited platelet disorders. Pediatr Blood Cancer 2013;60(Suppl 1):S2–7.

3. Revel-Vilk SR, Rand ML, Israles SJ. Primary and secondary hemostasis, regulators of coagulation, and fibrinolysis: understanding the basics. SickKids handbook of pediatric thrombosis and hemostasis. 1st edition. Basel (Switzerland): Karger; 2013.

4. Lippi G, Franchini M, Montagnana M, et al. Inherited disorders of blood coagulation. An Med 2012;44(5):405–18.

5. Lippi G, Favaloro EJ, Franchini M, et al. Milestones and perspectives in coagulation and hemostasis. Semin Thromb Hemost 2009;35(1):9–22.

6. Goodnight SH, Hathaway WE. Mechanisms of Hemostasis and Thrombosis. Disorders of Haemostasis and Thrombosis. 2nd edition. Lancester (PA): McGraw-Hill; 2001.

7. Kamal AH, Tefferi A, Pruthi RK. How to interpret and pursue an abnormal prothrombin time, activated partial thromboplastin time, and bleeding time in adults. Mayo Clin Proc 2007;82(7):864–73.

8. Mann KG. Biochemistry and physiology of blood coagulation. Thromb Haemost 1999;82(2):165–74.

9. Stonebraker JS, Bolton-Maggs PH, Michael Soucie J, et al. A study of variations in the reported haemophilia B prevalence around the world. Haemophilia 2012; 18(3):e91–4.

10. Stonebraker JS, Bolton-Maggs PH, Soucie JM, et al. A study of variations in the reported haemophilia A prevalence around the world. Haemophilia 2010;16(1): 20–32.

11. Soucie JM, Evatt B, Jackson D. Occurrence of hemophilia in the United States. The Hemophilia Surveillance System Project Investigators. Am J Hematol 1998; 59(4):288–94.

12. White GC 2nd, Rosendaal F, Aledort LM, et al. Definitions in hemophilia. Recommendation of the scientific subcommittee on factor VIII and factor IX of the scientific and standardization committee of the International Society on Thrombosis and Haemostasis. Thromb Haemost 2001;85(3):560.

13. Bowen DJ. Haemophilia A and haemophilia B: molecular insights. Mol Pathol 2002;55(2):127–44.

14. Gitschier J, Wood WI, Goralka TM, et al. Characterization of the human factor VIII gene. Nature 1984;312(5992):326–30.

15. Yoshitake S, Schach BG, Foster DC, et al. Nucleotide sequence of the gene for human factor IX (antihemophilic factor B). Biochemistry 1985;24(14):3736–50.

16. Carcao MD. The diagnosis and management of congenital hemophilia. Semin Thromb Hemost 2012;38(7):727–34.

17. Graw J, Brackmann HH, Oldenburg J, et al. Haemophilia A: from mutation analysis to new therapies. Nat Rev Genet 2005;6(6):488–501.

18. Lillicrap D. The molecular basis of haemophilia B. Haemophilia 1998;4(4):350–7.

19. Antonarakis SE, Rossiter JP, Young M, et al. Factor VIII gene inversions in severe hemophilia A: results of an international consortium study. Blood 1995;86(6): 2206–12.

20. Rossiter JP, Young M, Kimberland ML, et al. Factor VIII gene inversions causing severe hemophilia A originate almost exclusively in male germ cells. Hum Mol Genet 1994;3(7):1035–9.

21. Picketts DJ, Mueller CR, Lillicrap D. Transcriptional control of the factor IX gene: analysis of five cis-acting elements and the deleterious effects of naturally occurring hemophilia B Leyden mutations. Blood 1994;84(9):2992–3000.

22. Carcao MD, van den Berg HM, Ljung R, et al. Correlation between phenotype and genotype in a large unselected cohort of children with severe hemophilia A. Blood 2013;121(19):3946–52.

23. Mannucci PM, Franchini M. Is haemophilia B less severe than haemophilia A? Haemophilia 2013;19(4):499–502.
24. Kulkarni R, Soucie JM. Pediatric hemophilia: a review. Semin Thromb Hemost 2011;37(7):737–44.
25. Kulkarni R, Soucie JM, Lusher J, et al. Sites of initial bleeding episodes, mode of delivery and age of diagnosis in babies with haemophilia diagnosed before the age of 2 years: a report from The Centers for Disease Control and Prevention's (CDC) Universal Data Collection (UDC) project. Haemophilia 2009;15(6): 1281–90.
26. Richards M, Lavigne Lissalde G, Combescure C, et al. Neonatal bleeding in haemophilia: a European cohort study. Br J Haematol 2012;156(3):374–82.
27. Kulkarni R, Lusher JM. Intracranial and extracranial hemorrhages in newborns with hemophilia: a review of the literature. J Pediatr Hematol Oncol 1999; 21(4):289–95.
28. James AH, Hoots K. The optimal mode of delivery for the haemophilia carrier expecting an affected infant is caesarean delivery. Haemophilia 2010;16(3): 420–4.
29. Ljung R. The optimal mode of delivery for the haemophilia carrier expecting an affected infant is vaginal delivery. Haemophilia 2010;16(3):415–9.
30. Chalmers E, Williams M, Brennand J, et al. Guideline on the management of haemophilia in the fetus and neonate. Br J Haematol 2011;154(2):208–15.
31. Witmer C, Presley R, Kulkarni R, et al. Associations between intracranial hae-morrhage and prescribed prophylaxis in a large cohort of haemophilia patients in the United States. Br J Haematol 2011;152(2):211–6.
32. van Dijk K, Fischer K, van der Bom JG, et al. Variability in clinical phenotype of severe haemophilia: the role of the first joint bleed. Haemophilia 2005;11(5): 438–43.
33. Franchini M, Montagnana M, Targher G, et al. Interpatient phenotypic inconsis-tency in severe congenital hemophilia: a systematic review of the role of in-herited thrombophilia. Semin Thromb Hemost 2009;35(3):307–12.
34. van Dijk K, van der Bom JG, Fischer K, et al. Do prothrombotic factors influence clinical phenotype of severe haemophilia? A review of the literature. Thromb Haemost 2004;92(2):305–10.
35. Valentino LA. Blood-induced joint disease: the pathophysiology of hemophilic arthropathy. J Thromb Haemost 2010;8(9):1895–902.
36. Sorensen B, Benson GM, Bladen M, et al. Management of muscle haematomas in patients with severe haemophilia in an evidence-poor world. Haemophilia 2012;18(4):598–606.
37. Kumar R, Pruthi RK, Kobrinsky N, et al. Pelvic pseudotumor and pseudoaneur-ysm in a pediatric patient with moderate hemophilia B: successful management with arterial embolization and surgical excision. Pediatr Blood Cancer 2011; 56(3):484–7.
38. Berntorp E, Halimeh S, Gringeri A, et al. Management of bleeding disorders in children. Haemophilia 2012;18(Suppl 2):15–23.
39. de Moerloose P, Fischer K, Lambert T, et al. Recommendations for assessment, monitoring and follow-up of patients with haemophilia. Haemophilia 2012;18(3): 319–25.
40. Barnes C. Importance of pharmacokinetics in the management of hemophilia. Pediatr Blood Cancer 2013;60(Suppl 1):S27–9.
41. Collins PW, Bjorkman S, Fischer K, et al. Factor VIII requirement to maintain a target plasma level in the prophylactic treatment of severe hemophilia A: influences of

variance in pharmacokinetics and treatment regimens. J Thromb Haemost 2010; 8(2):269–75.

42. Batorova A, Holme P, Gringeri A, et al. Continuous infusion in haemophilia: current practice in Europe. Haemophilia 2012;18(5):753–9.

43. Batorova A, Martinowitz U. Continuous infusion of coagulation factors: current opinion. Curr Opin Hematol 2006;13(5):308–15.

44. Srivastava A, Brewer AK, Mauser-Bunschoten EP, et al. Guidelines for the management of hemophilia. Haemophilia 2013;19(1):e1–47.

45. Robertson JD, Curtin JA, Blanchette VS. Managing Hemophilia in Children and Adolescents. Sick Kids Handbook of pediatric thrombosis and hemostasis. 1st edition. Basel (Switzerland) Karger; 2013.

46. Mannucci PM, Ghirardini A. Desmopressin: twenty years after. Thromb Haemost 1997;78(2):958.

47. Seary ME, Feldman D, Carcao MD. DDAVP responsiveness in children with mild or moderate haemophilia A correlates with age, endogenous FVIII: C level and with haemophilic genotype. Haemophilia 2012;18(1):50–5.

48. Nilsson IM, Hedner U, Ahlberg A. Haemophilia prophylaxis in Sweden. Acta Paediatr Scand 1976;65(2):129–35.

49. Ahlberg A. Haemophilia in Sweden. VII. Incidence, treatment and prophylaxis of arthropathy and other musculo-skeletal manifestations of haemophilia A and B. Acta Orthop Scand Suppl 1965;(Suppl 77):73–132.

50. Nilsson IM, Berntorp E, Lofqvist T, et al. Twenty-five years' experience of prophylactic treatment in severe haemophilia A and B. J Intern Med 1992;232(1): 25–32.

51. Manco-Johnson MJ, Abshire TC, Shapiro AD, et al. Prophylaxis versus episodic treatment to prevent joint disease in boys with severe hemophilia. N Engl J Med 2007;357(6):535–44.

52. Valentino LA, Kawji M, Grygotis M. Venous access in the management of hemophilia. Blood Rev 2011;25(1):11–5.

53. Feldman BM, Pai M, Rivard GE, et al. Tailored prophylaxis in severe hemophilia A: interim results from the first 5 years of the Canadian Hemophilia Primary Prophylaxis Study. J Thromb Haemost 2006;4(6):1228–36.

54. Fogarty PF. Biological rationale for new drugs in the bleeding disorders pipeline. Hematology Am Soc Hematol Educ Program 2011;2011:397–404.

55. Nathwani AC, Tuddenham EG, Rangarajan S, et al. Adenovirus-associated virus vector-mediated gene transfer in hemophilia B. N Engl J Med 2011;365(25): 2357–65.

56. Santagostino E, Morfini M, Auerswald GK, et al. Paediatric haemophilia with inhibitors: existing management options, treatment gaps and unmet needs. Haemophilia 2009;15(5):983–9.

57. Gouw SC, van den Berg HM, Oldenburg J, et al. F8 gene mutation type and inhibitor development in patients with severe hemophilia A: systematic review and meta-analysis. Blood 2012;119(12):2922–34.

58. Pavlova A, Delev D, Lacroix-Desmazes S, et al. Impact of polymorphisms of the major histocompatibility complex class II, interleukin-10, tumor necrosis factor-alpha and cytotoxic T-lymphocyte antigen-4 genes on inhibitor development in severe hemophilia A. J Thromb Haemost 2009;7(12):2006–15.

59. Gouw SC, van der Bom JG, Auerswald G, et al. Recombinant versus plasma-derived factor VIII products and the development of inhibitors in previously untreated patients with severe hemophilia A: the CANAL cohort study. Blood 2007;109(11):4693–7.

60. Gouw SC, van der Bom JG, Ljung R, et al. Factor VIII products and inhibitor development in severe hemophilia A. N Engl J Med 2013;368(3):231–9.
61. Iorio A, Halimeh S, Holzhauer S, et al. Rate of inhibitor development in previously untreated hemophilia A patients treated with plasma-derived or recombinant factor VIII concentrates: a systematic review. J Thromb Haemost 2010;8(6): 1256–65.
62. Astermark J, Donfield SM, DiMichele DM, et al. A randomized comparison of bypassing agents in hemophilia complicated by an inhibitor: the FEIBA NovoSeven Comparative (FENOC) Study. Blood 2007;109(2):546–51.
63. Hay CR, DiMichele DM. The principal results of the International Immune Tolerance Study: a randomized dose comparison. Blood 2012;119(6):1335–44.
64. Berntorp E, Shapiro A, Astermark J, et al. Inhibitor treatment in haemophilias A and B: summary statement for the 2006 international consensus conference. Haemophilia 2006;12(Suppl 6):1–7.
65. Hay CR, Brown S, Collins PW, et al. The diagnosis and management of factor VIII and IX inhibitors: a guideline from the United Kingdom Haemophilia Centre Doctors Organisation. Br J Haematol 2006;133(6):591–605.
66. Rodeghiero F, Castaman G, Dini E. Epidemiological investigation of the prevalence of von Willebrand's disease. Blood 1987;69(2):454–9.
67. Werner EJ, Broxson EH, Tucker EL, et al. Prevalence of von Willebrand disease in children: a multiethnic study. J Pediatr 1993;123(6):893–8.
68. Bowman M, Hopman WM, Rapson D, et al. The prevalence of symptomatic von Willebrand disease in primary care practice. J Thromb Haemost 2010;8(1):213–6.
69. James PD, Lillicrap D. The molecular characterization of von Willebrand disease: good in parts. Br J Haematol 2013;161(2):166–76.
70. Robertson J, Lillicrap D, James PD. Von Willebrand disease. Pediatr Clin North Am 2008;55(2):377–92, viii–ix.
71. Mancuso DJ, Tuley EA, Westfield LA, et al. Structure of the gene for human von Willebrand factor. J Biol Chem 1989;264(33):19514–27.
72. Fowler WE, Fretto LJ, Hamilton KK, et al. Substructure of human von Willebrand factor. J Clin Invest 1985;76(4):1491–500.
73. Dong JF, Moake JL, Nolasco L, et al. ADAMTS-13 rapidly cleaves newly secreted ultralarge von Willebrand factor multimers on the endothelial surface under flowing conditions. Blood 2002;100(12):4033–9.
74. Cumming A, Grundy P, Keeney S, et al. An investigation of the von Willebrand factor genotype in UK patients diagnosed to have type 1 von Willebrand disease. Thromb Haemost 2006;96(5):630–41.
75. Goodeve A, Eikenboom J, Castaman G, et al. Phenotype and genotype of a cohort of families historically diagnosed with type 1 von Willebrand disease in the European study, Molecular and Clinical Markers for the Diagnosis and Management of Type 1 von Willebrand Disease (MCMDM-1VWD). Blood 2007; 109(1):112–21.
76. James PD, Notley C, Hegadorn C, et al. The mutational spectrum of type 1 von Willebrand disease: results from a Canadian cohort study. Blood 2007;109(1): 145–54.
77. Sadler JE, Budde U, Eikenboom JC, et al. Update on the pathophysiology and classification of von Willebrand disease: a report of the Subcommittee on von Willebrand Factor. J Thromb Haemost 2006;4(10):2103–14.
78. Carcao MD, Blanchette VS, Dean JA, et al. The Platelet Function Analyzer (PFA-100): a novel in-vitro system for evaluation of primary haemostasis in children. Br J Haematol 1998;101(1):70–3.

79. Dean JA, Blanchette VS, Carcao MD, et al. von Willebrand disease in a pediatric-based population–comparison of type 1 diagnostic criteria and use of the PFA-100 and a von Willebrand factor/collagen-binding assay. Thromb Haemost 2000;84(3):401–9.

80. Conlan MG, Folsom AR, Finch A, et al. Associations of factor VIII and von Willebrand factor with age, race, sex, and risk factors for atherosclerosis. The Atherosclerosis Risk in Communities (ARIC) Study. Thromb Haemost 1993;70(3):380–5.

81. Jenkins PV, O'Donnell JS. ABO blood group determines plasma von Willebrand factor levels: a biologic function after all? Transfusion 2006;46(10):1836–44.

82. Nichols WL, Hultin MB, James AH, et al. von Willebrand disease (VWD): evidence-based diagnosis and management guidelines, the National Heart, Lung, and Blood Institute (NHLBI) Expert Panel report (USA). Haemophilia 2008;14(2):171–232.

83. Gupta M, Lillicrap D, Stain AM, et al. Therapeutic consequences for misdiagnosis of type 2N von Willebrand disease. Pediatr Blood Cancer 2011;57(6):1081–3.

84. Ross CS, Pruthi RK, Schmidt KA, et al. Intranasal oestrogen cream for the prevention of epistaxis in patients with bleeding disorders. Haemophilia 2011;17(1):164.

85. Ben-Ami T, Revel-Vilk S. The use of DDAVP in children with bleeding disorders. Pediatr Blood Cancer 2013;60(Suppl 1):S41–3.

86. Abshire TC, Federici AB, Alvarez MT, et al. Prophylaxis in severe forms of von Willebrand's disease: results from the von Willebrand Disease Prophylaxis Network (VWD PN). Haemophilia 2013;19(1):76–81.

87. Rodeghiero F, Castaman G, Tosetto A. How I treat von Willebrand disease. Blood 2009;114(6):1158–65.

88. Bolton-Maggs PH. The rare inherited coagulation disorders. Pediatr Blood Cancer 2013;60(Suppl 1):S37–40.

89. Mannucci PM, Duga S, Peyvandi F. Recessively inherited coagulation disorders. Blood 2004;104(5):1243–52.

90. Peyvandi F, Bolton-Maggs PH, Batorova A, et al. Rare bleeding disorders. Haemophilia 2012;18(Suppl 4):148–53.

91. Gomez K, Bolton-Maggs P. Factor XI deficiency. Haemophilia 2008;14(6):1183–9.

92. Lapecorella M, Mariani G. Factor VII deficiency: defining the clinical picture and optimizing therapeutic options. Haemophilia 2008;14(6):1170–5.

93. Peyvandi F, Spreafico M. National and international registries of rare bleeding disorders. Blood Transfus 2008;6(Suppl 2):s45–8.

94. Peyvandi F, Di Michele D, Bolton-Maggs PH, et al. Classification of rare bleeding disorders (RBDs) based on the association between coagulant factor activity and clinical bleeding severity. J Thromb Haemost 2012;10(9):1938–43.

95. Kohler HP, Ichinose A, Seitz R, et al. Diagnosis and classification of factor XIII deficiencies. J Thromb Haemost 2011;9(7):1404–6.

96. Acharya SS, Dimichele DM. Rare inherited disorders of fibrinogen. Haemophilia 2008;14(6):1151–8.

97. Hsieh L, Nugent D. Factor XIII deficiency. Haemophilia 2008;14(6):1190–200.

98. Inbal A, Oldenburg J, Carcao M, et al. Recombinant factor XIII: a safe and novel treatment for congenital factor XIII deficiency. Blood 2012;119(22):5111–7.

99. Brown DL, Kouides PA. Diagnosis and treatment of inherited factor X deficiency. Haemophilia 2008;14(6):1176–82.

100. Huang JN, Koerper MA. Factor V deficiency: a concise review. Haemophilia 2008;14(6):1164–9.

101. Meeks SL, Abshire TC. Abnormalities of prothrombin: a review of the pathophysiology, diagnosis, and treatment. Haemophilia 2008;14(6):1159–63.
102. Bolton-Maggs PH, Perry DJ, Chalmers EA, et al. The rare coagulation disorders–review with guidelines for management from the United Kingdom Haemophilia Centre Doctors' Organisation. Haemophilia 2004;10(5):593–628.

Pediatric Thrombophilia

Janet Y.K. Yang, MBBS, MRCPCH, FHKAM (Pediatrics), FHKC.Paed,
Anthony K.C. Chan, MBBS, FRCPC, FRCPCH, FRCPI, FRCP (Glas), FRCPath*

KEYWORDS

- Pediatric thrombosis • Venous thromboembolic event • Arterial ischemic stroke
- Cerebral sinus venous thrombosis • Thrombophilia

KEY POINTS

- Venous thromboembolic events (VTE), arterial thrombosis, and stroke (arterial ischemic stroke [AIS] or cerebral sinus venous thrombosis [CSVT]) are increasingly recognized in the pediatric population, and occur during 2 peak times during childhood, in the neonatal and adolescent age groups.
- In comparison with adults, acquired medical risk factors play a larger role than inherited thrombophilia in the mechanism of disease in children.
- Inherited thrombophilias have a stronger influence than VTE on pediatric stroke.
- Thrombophilia testing is indicated in adolescents with spontaneous thrombosis, and in neonates/children with non–catheter-related thrombosis and stroke.
- There are insufficient data to recommend routine thrombophilia testing in neonates/children with catheter-related thrombosis; the need for thrombophilia testing should be determined by individual institutions and on a case-by-case basis.

INTRODUCTION

Venous thromboembolic events (VTE), arterial thromboses, and stroke (arterial ischemic stroke [AIS] or cerebral sinus venous thrombosis [CSVT]) are uncommon in children but are increasingly recognized, with serious morbidity and mortality. A Canadian registry estimated an incidence of 2.4 per 1000 admissions to the neonatal intensive care units for neonatal thrombosis, whereas for older children (>1 month old), the incidence is about 5.3 per 100,000 hospital admissions.[1,2] For CSVT, the Canadian Pediatric Ischemic Stroke Registry reported an incidence of 0.67 cases per 100,000 children per year,[3] with neonates in this age group most commonly affected. The estimated incidence of neonatal CSVT is 40.7 per 100,000 live births per year.[4] With the advance of radiologic imaging such as diffusion-weighted magnetic resonance imaging, and the increased awareness of the syndrome, the reported incidence for neonatal AIS

The authors declare no conflicts of interest.
Division of Hematology and Oncology, Department of Pediatrics, McMaster University, 1280 Main Street West, Hamilton, Ontario L8S 4K1, Canada
* Corresponding author. McMaster University, 1280 Main Street West, Room 3N27, Hamilton, Ontario L8S 4K1, Canada.
E-mail address: akchan@mcmaster.ca

Pediatr Clin N Am 60 (2013) 1443–1462
http://dx.doi.org/10.1016/j.pcl.2013.09.004 **pediatric.theclinics.com**

continues to increase, with current estimates of approximately 1 in 2300 live births.[5–7] In the National Hospital Discharge Survey (NHDS) from 1980 through 1998, the rate of ischemic stroke for infants (mostly term) less than 30 days of age was 17.8 per 100,000 live births per year. The Canadian Pediatric Ischemic Stroke Registry reported ischemic stroke in 2.7 per 100,000 children younger than 18 years per year.[8]

Thrombophilia is the term used to describe the tendency to develop thrombosis because of certain acquired clinical conditions or hereditary risk factors. The inherited and acquired thrombophilias can be categorized using the classic elements of Virchow's triad: stasis, hypercoagulable state, and vascular injury. To have a better understanding of each, this article addresses thrombophilia in neonates and children, and the risk factors for inherited and acquired thrombophilia.

THROMBOPHILIA IN THE NEONATAL PERIOD
Inherited Thrombophilia Disorders: Hypercoagulable States

Protein C and protein S deficiencies
Mechanism Both protein C and protein S are vitamin K–dependent plasma proteins, which play important roles in the human protein C anticoagulation pathway. Protein C is activated on the endothelial cell surface by the thrombin-thrombomodulin complex, generated during vessel injury to form the serine protease activated protein C (APC). On the other hand, protein S functions as a cofactor for protein C, so that the APC activity is increased 10-fold in the presence of protein S. Once APC is generated, it binds as a complex with its cofactor protein S, which can inactivate clotting factors (F) Va and FVIIIa. As a result the pathway can effectively regulate further thrombin formation and thrombosis.

Classification Protein C deficiency or protein S deficiency may be acquired or hereditary. The hereditary form can be categorized as heterozygous, homozygous, and compound heterozygous. Phenotypically, 2 types of protein C deficiency have been described: type 1 whereby both the antigenic levels and functional activities are reduced, and type 2 whereby protein C activity levels are reduced to a greater extent than antigenic levels.

Homozygous (or compound heterozygous) deficiencies of protein C and protein S are rare conditions, and usually present as life-threatening disorders on the first few days of life. Homozygous protein C deficiency affects approximately 1 in 400,000 to 1 in 1 million live births.[9,10] The first clinical manifestation is usually purpura fulminans, associated with laboratory evidence of disseminated intravascular coagulation (DIC). In some cases, massive major vessel thrombosis (renal vein, vena cava) can be the presenting features. By contrast, heterozygous protein C and protein S deficiencies rarely present in the neonatal period.

Epidemiology In a Canadian registry of 171 children (including neonates) with VTE, the prevalence of protein C deficiency and protein S deficiency was 0.6% and 1.2%, respectively, which was considered to be low, not considerably different from the general population.[11] The most significant etiologic factors for neonatal thrombosis are the presence of an intravascular catheter and/or other medical conditions.[1,12] By contrast, the pathophysiology of neonatal CSVT and perinatal AIS are considered more complex and multifactorial, and include maternal disorders, placental problems, and perinatal and neonatal risk factors. However, meta-analysis of studies on CSVT and AIS in neonates and children indicates that genetic thrombophilia serves as an important risk factor for stroke. The calculated odds ratio (OR) for protein C deficiency and protein S deficiency were 8.76 (95% confidence interval [CI] 4.53–16.96) and 3.20 (95% CI 1.22–8.40), respectively.[13]

Diagnosis The diagnosis of homozygous (or compound heterozygous) deficiency can be confirmed by the findings of undetectable activity (<1% or <0.01 U/mL) on measuring the functional protein C (or protein S) activity, with heterozygous activity levels demonstrated in both parents. Heterozygous anticoagulant protein-deficiency states are difficult to diagnose in the acute stage of neonatal thrombosis, for 2 reasons. First, because of developmental hemostasis, all anticoagulant protein levels are physiologically lower (mean value for all <50%) in normal healthy term or preterm infants, in comparison with adult levels, until 6 months of age. Second, acquired deficiency states are common because of underlying medical conditions or consumption of coagulation proteins at the time of an acute thrombotic event. Therefore, for neonates suspected of having heterozygous protein C or protein S deficiencies, functional protein C (or protein S) assays must be repeated at 6 months of age or later to accurately confirm the diagnosis.

Acute treatment For patients with neonatal purpura fulminans, assays of protein C and protein S levels must be drawn before the initiation of treatment. However, treatment should not be delayed while awaiting the results. Exogenous replacement of the deficient naturally occurring anticoagulant proteins forms the basis of treatment for this condition. Heparin and fibrinolytic agents are not effective treatments for this complex situation.

Fresh frozen plasma (FFP), given at a dose of 10 to 20 mL/kg every 12 hours, has proved to be successful for the management of patients with homozygous protein C deficiency or protein S deficiency. More frequent dosing may be required for protein C deficiency because protein C has a short plasma half-life, approximately 6 to 16 hours. However, the frequency of dosing is limited by the risk of hypervolemia and hypertension, and limited venous access. Protein C concentrate (Ceprotin; Baxter Healthcare Corp, Deerfield, IL) is another option. A starting dose of 100 U/kg, followed by 50 U/kg every 6 hours, is usually sufficient. Subsequent dosing with FFP or protein C concentrate depends on the patient's response. The dose is titrated to achieve a trough level of protein C activity of 50 IU/dL. For homozygous protein S deficiency there is no currently available protein S concentrate; however, the same dose of FFP can be started at the acute stage. As protein S has a longer half-life of approximately 36 hours, the frequency of treatment can be titrated to achieve a trough level of free protein S of 30 IU/dL. The replacement therapy should be continued until purpuric lesions have resolved (typically 6–8 weeks) and the neonate has transitioned to anticoagulation therapy.[14]

Long-term management Neonates with homozygous/compound heterozygous protein C or protein S deficiency require life-long anticoagulation therapy to prevent thrombosis. Options for long-term treatment include low molecular weight heparin (target anti-FXa concentration of 0.5–1.0 U/mL), protein C supplementation, oral warfarin therapy, or a combination of all these therapies. Recent studies reported subcutaneous administration of protein C concentrate with a dose of 250 U/kg every third day provides protective levels of protein C (>25 IU/dL)[15,16] and can be considered as an alternative.

Antithrombin deficiency
Mechanism Antithrombin (AT) is a glycoprotein of the family of serine protease inhibitors, and is synthesized in the liver. AT circulates in the blood in a quiescent form, slowly reacts with and irreversibly inhibits its primary targets thrombin and FXa, as well as secondary targets including FIXa, FXIa, FXIIa, and FVIIa. At the site of injury, thrombin is bound to thrombomodulin on the endothelial surface. The neutralization

of thrombin is enhanced by the interaction with the thrombin-thrombomodulin complex. The inactive thrombin and AT then dissociates from thrombomodulin and is cleared rapidly in the liver. The removal of thrombin also prevents further activation of protein C.

Classification Similarly to protein C/S deficiencies, AT deficiency can be acquired or inherited. Type I AT deficiency is characterized by parallel reductions of both antigen and activity levels, whereas type II deficiency covers all types of inherited dysfunctional AT variants, resulting in decreased functional activity. Among the group of dysfunctional AT, AT deficiencies may involve the reactive site (type II RS), the heparin-binding site (type II HBS), or both ("pleiotropic effect"; type II PE).[17] Homozygous AT deficiency type I is most likely not compatible with life, and only patients with homozygous type II deficiency have been reported, of whom the majority are type II HBS.[17-20] This AT variant was identified as a result of G2759T mutation, a Leu-Phe change at codon 99 (Antithrombin Budapest 3). Several other mutations of AT with heparin-binding defects were also reported, including 47 Arg-Cys,[21-24] 47 Arg-His,[25] and 41 Pro-Leu.[26] Acquired low AT levels and dysfunctional AT have been reported in neonates with respiratory distress syndrome and in other sick premature infants.[27,28]

Epidemiology From the Canadian registry[1] of VTE in children and neonates, none of the patients (out of 171) were found to have AT deficiency. This fact is in keeping with the notion that the most significant etiologic factor for neonatal thrombosis is still the presence of an intravascular catheter and/or other medical conditions.[12,13] By contrast, for stroke, including both AIS and CSVT, meta-analysis indicated that inherited thrombophilia contributed significantly as risk factors, and the OR for AT deficiency was 7.06 (95% CI 2.44–22.42).[6]

Diagnosis As a result of developmental hemostasis,[29-31] functional AT levels are normally reduced in healthy term neonates, and more so in premature infants. Therefore, establishing the diagnosis of AT deficiency in the neonatal period is especially challenging. The diagnosis of homozygous AT type II HBS deficiency in the neonatal period may require even more attention and suspicion. The presentation of heparin resistance and thrombosis suggests a type II HBS AT deficiency.[19] The routine chromogenic AT assays may miss the diagnosis of AT type II HBS variant. These assays commonly recommend a preincubation time varying from 90 seconds to 5 minutes with the heparin-containing buffer and the patient's plasma. The AT type II HBS variant binds to heparin slowly and, therefore, their anti-FIIa and anti-FXa activity will be low in the assay with a short incubation time, but significantly higher (or close to the normal range) in the assay with a longer incubation time.[32,33] Thus, in patients suspected of inherited thrombophilia based on family history, or in the presence of heparin resistance, a 2-step AT assay measuring anti-FIIa activity with a short incubation time (10–30 seconds) and normal incubation time (>90 seconds) is recommended.[33] Nevertheless, because AT activity is normally low in neonates, the 2-step assays could still yield nearly normal results in suspected cases in this age group. Molecular analysis of the AT gene will be particularly helpful in making the diagnosis of homozygous AT type II HBS deficiency in these situations.[19,34]

Treatment Neonates with suspected homozygous AT deficiency may present with arterial or venous thrombosis, as well as stroke. In the absence of medical risk factors and family history of thrombosis, thrombophilia screening (including AT assay) should be performed before the commencement of anticoagulation therapy. Cases with AT type II HBS deficiency typically also present with heparin resistance, in which case, despite increasing the heparin doses, the activated partial thromboplastin time (aPTT) will remain subtherapeutic.[19] Again, this should alert the physician to the possibility of a type II HBS AT deficiency. The AT anti-FIIa activity (with short incubation time) will typically be less than 50% of normal. Formerly, human plasma-derived AT concentrate was used for patients with acquired or hereditary AT deficiency. Recombinant AT concentrate is now licensed in the United States, approved by Food and Drug Administration in 2009. Calculation of initial loading dose should be individualized, based on the actual level of AT activity, using the formula: IU/infused intravenously over 24 hours = (100 − baseline AT activity level (in % of normal)/2.3) × body weight (kg). The target level should be 80% to 120% of normal (30 minutes postinfusion), and the dose should be increased or decreased if the AT level is below 80% or above 120% of normal, respectively. Repeated AT level should be measured at 30 minutes and 4 hours after any rate change to confirm AT level is within the target range. As there are not currently any pediatric safety and efficacy studies published, this dosing recommendation is based on adult studies.[35,36] Hence, clinicians should take extra precautions if considering the usage of recombinant AT concentrate. Frequent monitoring of bleeding symptoms, as well as close monitoring of AT activity, aPTT, and adjustment of the heparin dosage are required. For all patients with confirmed homozygous AT deficiency, long-term anticoagulation therapy is indicated. The advice of a pediatric hematologist should be sought to help manage these patients.

Homozygous/heterozygous factor V Leiden mutation

Mechanisms Factor V Leiden (FVL) is characterized by a point mutation in the FV gene with a single amino-acid substitution (arginine 506 to glutamine at the APC cleavage site). The thrombin activation of FVL to Va is normal, whereas APC is not able to cleave FVa Leiden variant, leading to an excess of activated FVL and, hence, a hypercoagulable state.

Genetics and epidemiology Inheritance of FVL is autosomal dominant. Approximately 4% of Caucasians are heterozygous for the gene defect. Meta-analysis of studies on inherited thrombophilia and pediatric VTE have shown that FVL is significantly associated with first VTE in all pediatric age groups (neonates/infants/older children), with the summary OR of 3.56 (95% CI 2.57–4.93).[34] This figure is concordant with data from adult studies, in which FV mutation increases the risk of a first episode of VTE by 3- to 7-fold.[37] Regarding the risk of pediatric AIS and CSVT, a meta-analysis demonstrated that the calculated OR for FVL is 3.26 (95% CI 2.59–4.1).

Prothrombin 20210A (factor II) mutation

Mechanisms Prothrombin (FII G20210A) variant is characterized by a single G to A nucleotide substitution at position 20,210 in the prothrombin gene. FVa bound in the prothrombin-FVa complex is normally resistant to APC inactivation. This prothrombin mutation is associated with an increase in production of plasma prothrombin. An elevated plasma prothrombin level increases the half-life of FVa in the circulation by protecting it from APC cleavage, leading to a hypercoagulable state.

Genetics and epidemiology Inheritance of prothrombin mutation is autosomal dominant. The prevalence of this mutation in Caucasians is approximately 2%. Meta-analysis demonstrated that the OR for FII G20210A and onset of VTE in pediatric age group is 2.63 (95% CI 1.61–4.29), and the OR for recurrent VTE in children is 2.15 (95% CI 1.12–4.1).[34] These data concur with those from adult studies in which FII mutation increases the risk of first VTE by 2- to 3-fold.

MTHFR C677T genotype

Mechanisms Hyperhomocysteinemia has been identified as an independent risk factor for VTE, CSVT, and AIS. The mechanisms appear to be related to the effect of high levels of homocysteine on vessel walls by inducing endothelial injury and dysfunction, with associated decreased thrombomodulin activity. The thermolabile homozygous methylenetetrahydrofolate reductase (MTHFR) C677T (alanine 677 to valine) genotype has half of the catalytic activity of the normal MTHFR enzyme, and can result in mild hyperhomocysteinemia. However, in individuals with adequate folate levels, the effect of the genetic defect will be canceled out and plasma homocysteine levels will remain normal. Therefore, not everyone with the MTHFR C677T genotype will develop high homocysteine levels and be prone to develop VTE or stroke.

Epidemiology The MTHFR C677T genotype is present in up to 10% of the healthy population. In children with a first-episode stroke, homozygosity of MTHFR C677T mutation has been shown to be an independent risk factor.[38–41] However, because homocysteine levels were not always studied, the potential associated risk could not be accurately determined.

Lipoprotein(a)

Mechanisms A plasma lipoprotein(a) (Lp(a)) level higher than 30 mg/mL is considered to be elevated. The plasminogen gene on chromosome 6 is linked closely to the structurally similar apolipoprotein(a) gene. The gene product associates with a low-density lipoprotein to form Lp(a). Owing to molecular mimicry, Lp(a) competes with plasminogen for the binding domain on the endothelial cell surface. A hypercoagulable state results from the decreased activity of plasminogen on the endothelial cell surface.

Epidemiology Elevated Lp(a) was found to be present in 7% to 10.3% of the normal population.[35,42] The OR of elevated Lp(a) associated with a first VTE onset in children was 4.49 (95% CI 3.26–6.18); however, no significant association with recurrent VTE was found for elevated Lp(a).[34] From another meta-analysis, the calculated OR associated with first AIS/CSVT onset in children was 6.27 (95% CI 4.52–8.69).[13]

Acquired Thrombophilia States: Disturbance of Blood Flow/Stasis

Central venous lines

In view of the small caliber of blood vessels in neonates, the use of central venous lines (CVL) is logically associated with significant disruption of blood flow, which can lead to increased blood stasis and a higher risk of thrombosis. In the Canadian registry of neonatal thrombosis, 89% of all cases were associated with an intravascular catheter.[1]

Congenital heart disease

Neonates with congenital heart disease (CHD), such as transposition of great arteries, tricuspid atresia, and tetralogy of Fallot, are at risk of developing VTE, arterial thrombosis, or stroke. Disturbance of blood flow can occur because of the underlying cardiac pathology, or the presence of prosthetic material, stent, or conduit used in the palliative/corrective surgery.[43] In the Canadian Childhood Thrombophilia Registry, CHD was the underlying disease in 19% (75 of 405) of children with VTE.[44]

Acquired Thrombophilia States: Vascular Injury

Central venous lines

A recent study has also shown that the insertion technique of CVL is associated with VTE because of the relative trauma to the venous wall at the insertion site.[45]

Acquired Thrombophilia States: Blood Components/Hypercoagulable State

Central venous lines
The presence of an intravascular foreign material and associated endothelial irritation by the CVL can be considered a procoagulant state.

Cyanotic heart disease
Polycythemia is commonly present in neonates with uncorrected cyanotic heart disease, increasing the hematocrit and related blood viscosity, and leading to a hypercoagulable state.

Septicemia
In the Canadian registry, systemic infection is the second most common risk factor associated with neonatal thrombosis. Nearly one-third of cases were associated with systemic infection.[1] In another study, 67% of neonates with catheter-related thrombosis have associated bloodstream infection.[46] Although the acquired deficiency state of protein C and AT III functional activity have been well reported for meningococcemia and associated purpura fulminans,[47,48] further studies are warranted to determine the pathophysiology of the association between septicemia and normal VTE.

Dehydration
Dehydration commonly occurs in preterm and sick neonates because of iatrogenic causes such as fluid restriction, excessive insensible water loss, or diarrhea. The increase in hematocrit predisposes the neonate to a higher risk of VTE.

Total parenteral nutrition
Parenteral nutrition (PN) is commonly administered to preterm or sick neonates. Studies have demonstrated that PN is another important acquired factor associated with thrombosis. Dextrose in the PN mixture may favor the procoagulant state of monocytes.[49] The high concentration of calcium in the PN solution, an important activator of the coagulation cascade, may promote thrombus propagation.[49]

Maternal antiphospholipid antibodies
Antiphospholipid syndrome (APS) in adults is characterized by persistent presence of antiphospholipid antibodies (APLA) and clinical manifestations such as thrombosis, recurrent fetal loss, thrombocytopenia, livedo reticularis, and neurologic manifestations. APLA include anticardiolipin antibodies (aCL), anti–β2-glycoprotein I antibodies (anti–β2GPI), and lupus anticoagulant.

Neonatal APS is a rare clinical entity characterized by neonatal thrombosis resulting from transplacental passage of maternal APLA from a mother with APS/systemic lupus. In a recent meta-analysis of 16 infants with perinatal thrombosis and positive APLA,[50] 80% had arterial thrombosis and one-half (8) had arterial ischemic stroke. Nine of 14 evaluable infants had additional perinatal prothrombotic risk factors or inherited thrombophilia. A recent study of 60 mother-infant pairs with neonatal AIS established the contribution of APLA to perinatal stroke.[51] In a recent large meta-analysis, the OR of first stroke onset in a pediatric age group (neonate/children) for APLA was 6.95 (95% CI 3.67–13.14).[13]

THROMBOPHILIA IN OLDER CHILDREN
Inherited Thrombophilia Disorders: Hypercoagulable State

Protein C and protein S deficiencies
Adult studies have shown a strong association between inherited thrombophilia disorders and an increased risk of thrombosis. Overall, 50% of adult VTE are associated

with inherited thrombophilia. By contrast, in the pediatric age group various studies have demonstrated that compared with acquired medical risk factors, inherited thrombophilic disorders are uncommon in the totality of pediatric VTE. From the prospective cohort study by Albisetti and colleagues,[52] none of the 48 patients (mean age 3.4 years) had protein C/protein S deficiency. In the Canadian prospective cohort, only 1 (0.6%) and 2 (1.2%) of 171 consecutive children had protein C and protein S deficiency, respectively.[11] This result confirmed that the prevalence of inherited thrombophilia disorders in children with VTE is low, and not considerably different from that in the general population. These data suggested that the yield of thrombophilia screening in children with VTE is low.

Nevertheless, keeping in mind that not all children with the same acquired medical risk factors develop VTE, it is apparent that genetic factors do contribute to which children will develop thrombosis. From a recent meta-analysis, the summary ORs for protein C deficiency and protein S deficiency associated with a first VTE onset in children was 7.72 (95% CI 4.44–13.42) and 5.77 (95% CI 3.03–10.97), respectively.[34]

Antithrombin deficiency

Similarly to protein C and protein S deficiencies, AT deficiency is uncommon in pediatric patients with VTE. In the same Canadian prospective cohort, none of the 171 pediatric patients with VTE was found to have AT deficiency.[11] Calculated OR for AT deficiency associated with a first VTE onset in children was 9.44 (95% CI 3.34–26.66).[34]

Homozygous/heterozygous factor V Leiden mutation, prothrombin 20210A (factor II) mutation

MTHFR C677T genotype and lipoprotein(a) Similar to data from studies on neonates, FVL, prothrombin G20210A, MTHFR mutation, and elevated Lp(a) are also not commonly present in pediatric VTE, as the majority have associated underlying acquired or medical risk factors. All these inherited thrombophilia disorders have significant ORs associated with first VTE onset in the pediatric age group[34] (**Table 1**), but without associated acquired precipitating prothrombotic conditions it is apparent that most patients with these genetic defects will not develop thrombosis in childhood.

Table 1
Summary of the odds ratio for inherited thrombophilia associated with a first VTE onset in children

Genetic Traits (No. of Studies)	Patients/Controls, n	OR (95% CI), Fixed Model	OR (95% CI), Random Model
Protein C deficiency (16)	1079/1979	7.72 (4.44–13.42)	7.75 (4.48–13.38)
Protein S deficiency (16)	1075/1979	5.77 (3.03–10.97)	5.77 (3.07–10.85)
Antithrombin deficiency (16)	1072/1979	9.44 (3.34–26.66)	8.73 (3.12–24.42)
Factor V Leiden (23)	1430/2623	3.77 (2.98–4.77)	3.56 (2.57–4.93)
Prothrombin G20210A (14)	916/1673	2.64 (1.6–4.41)	2.63 (1.61–4.29)
Lipoprotein(a) (8)	599/1441	4.49 (3.26–6.18)	4.50 (3.19–6.35)
≥2 Genetic traits (12)	965/1625	9.5 (4.92–18.39)	8.89 (3.43–23.06)

Abbreviations: CI, confidence interval; OR, odds ratio (95% CI; meta-analysis); VTE, venous thromboembolism.

Data from Young G, Albisetti M, Bonduel M, et al. Impact of inherited thrombophilia on venous thromboembolism in children: a systematic review and meta-analysis of observational studies. Circulation 2008;118:1373–82.

Familial elevated FVIII

Several recent adult studies have demonstrated that elevated FVIII levels are associated with increased risk of first episode of VTE in young and elderly adults.[53,54] A recent study reported that familial elevated FVIII levels (>90th percentiles) increase the risk of first VTE in children, with OR of 6.7 (95% CI 2.7–16.7).[55]

Combined genetic defects

Combination of 2 or more inherited thrombophilia disorders is associated with higher OR of 9.5 (95% CI 4.92–18.39) with a first VTE onset in children.[34] The OR of combined defect is even higher in children, with OR of a first AIS/CSVT at 11.86 (95% CI 5.93–23.73).[13]

Spontaneous/idiopathic VTE in children

Recent evidence suggested a higher prevalence rate of inherited thrombophilia disorders in children with spontaneous VTE when compared with other pediatric VTE patients. In the Canadian cohort, of the 5 older children with spontaneous VTE, 3 (60%) were found to have inherited prothrombotic conditions, compared with 6 (10%) of 58 older children with a VTE secondary to an underlying medical condition (P = .02; OR 13, 95% CI 1.8–94).[11] Recurrent VTE was also much more common, occurring in 21.3% of children with spontaneous VTE,[56] compared with an average of 8% in all children with or without an underlying medical condition.[34]

Recurrent VTE

Significant association with recurrent VTE was found for all inherited thrombophilia disorders except for FVL and elevated Lp(a). The OR ranged from 1.88 (95% CI 1.01–3.29) for prothrombin G20210A to 3.12 (95% CI 1.50–6.45) for protein S deficiency. A combination of 2 or more gene defects have the highest OR of 4.46 (95% CI 2.89–6.89) for recurrent VTE.[34]

VTE versus AIS and CSVT Recent evidence also suggested that children with AIS/CSVT have a much higher prevalence rate of inherited thrombophilia disorders compared to children with VTE only (**Table 2**).[11,57,58] This finding supports the concept of having a different perspective, and separating children with AIS/CSVT from all pediatric thrombosis when considering thrombophilia screening.

Acquired Thrombophilia States: Disturbance of Blood Flow/Stasis

Anatomic cause

Congenital inferior vena cava anomalies Congenital inferior vena cava (IVC) anomalies include the congenital absence, interruption, or hypoplasia of IVC, which are

Table 2
Summary of the odds ratio (95% CI, meta-analysis) for inherited thrombophilia associated with a first AIS/CSVT onset in neonates/children

Genetic Traits (No. of Studies)	Patients/Controls, n	OR (95% CI), Fixed Model
Protein C deficiency (10)	1031/1468	9.31 (4.81–18.02)
Protein S deficiency (6)	761/941	3.20 (1.22–8.40)
Antithrombin deficiency (6)	826/1153	7.06 (2.44–22.42)
Factor V Leiden (21)	1625/2842	3.26 (2.59–4.10)
Prothrombin G20210A (17)	1409/2613	2.43 (1.67–3.51)
Lipoprotein(a) (5)	722/727	6.27 (4.51–8.69)
≥2 Genetic traits (12)	926/1720	11.86 (5.93–23.73)

Abbreviations: AIS, arterial ischemic stroke; CSVT, cerebral sinovenous thrombosis.

usually associated with other cardiovascular anomalies, such as hypoplastic right iliac veins.[59] Absent IVC is found in 0.3% of healthy individuals, but in 5% of adults with deep venous thrombosis (DVT).[60–62] Of note, patients with VTE associated with absent IVC are usually much younger than those with normal venous anatomy, and more commonly have bilateral VTE involvement.[59,62]

May-Thurner syndrome May-Thurner syndrome (iliac vein compression syndrome) occurs when the left iliac vein is compressed by the overlying right common iliac artery, thus increasing the risk of thrombosis in the iliac vein and femoral vein. DVT caused by May-Thurner syndrome always occurs in the left lower extremity.[63] If the thrombus propagates into the distal IVC, swelling of bilateral lower extremities can occur. Although May-Thurner syndrome is infrequently described in the pediatric literature, it was found in 19% to 49% of adults with left lower extremity VTE.[64,65] Stenting of the left iliac vein can be performed to correct the anatomic abnormalities after confirmation of the diagnosis.

Paget-Schroetter syndrome Upper extremity VTE can occur as a result of Paget-Schroetter syndrome (thoracic outlet syndrome), whereby the subclavian vein is impinged on by the overlying cervical ribs, long transverse processes of the cervical spine, musculofascial bands, and clavicular or first rib abnormalities. Paget-Schroetter syndrome predominantly affects the right side, which may be secondary to the more common right-hand dominance in adolescents. In most circumstances, the extrinsic compression can be relieved by surgery such as resection of the first rib.

Recommendation Most pediatric VTE attributable to anatomic causes were diagnosed in teenagers who were otherwise healthy, without other clinical risk factors. Ultrasonography is rarely adequate to image the IVC, the proximal iliac vein, or the subclavian vein in adolescent patients. Magnetic resonance venography (MRV) and/or venography must be routinely performed with the diagnosis of proximal DVT in adolescents, to detect any underlying congenital vascular or anatomic abnormalities that can predispose them to recurrence. Diagnosing an underlying vascular malformation is important, as corrective surgical procedures such as stenting or rib resection can be undertaken to modify this important risk factor.

Central venous lines
CVLs are commonly inserted in sick pediatric patients receiving intensive care, PN, or chemotherapy. Similarly to neonates, the use of CVLs disrupts the blood flow, leading to stasis and an increased risk of thrombosis. According to the Canadian registry, DVT was associated with the presence of CVLs in 33% of children[2]; similarly, in the Netherlands registry[12] 37% in children with DVT have CVLs.

Congenital heart disease
From the neonatal period to early childhood, several complex forms of CHD require stepwise corrective surgical approaches and the insertion of prosthetic stents or conduits. These procedures lead to disturbance of blood flow and persistently predispose the children to the risk of thrombosis.[43] From the Canadian and Netherlands registry, 14.6% (20 of 137) and 19% (10 of 52), respectively, of children with VTE were found to have associated CHD.

Acquired Thrombophilia States: Vascular Injury

Central venous lines
As described in the neonatal section, the insertion technique of CVL is associated with VTE because of the relative trauma to the venous wall at the insertion site.[45]

Acquired Thrombophilia States: Blood Components/Hypercoagulable States

Pediatric antiphospholipid syndrome

The diagnosis of pediatric APS is usually established by the presence of thrombosis in a child, together with persistently positive APLA on at least 2 occasions between the minimum intervals of 12 weeks. Primary APS and APS associated with autoimmune disease occur with similar frequency in children. According to the most recent data from the international registry of pediatric APS, DVT of upper/lower extremities occurred in 42% (52 of 121) of patients, CSVT in 7% (8 of 121), and AIS in 26% (31 of 121).[66] The percentage of stroke (CSVT and AIS) is higher than that reported in adults (16%–21%).[67,68] It was also noted that children with primary APS were significantly younger and had a higher frequency of arterial thrombotic events, in particular cerebrovascular events, than children with secondary APS with an autoimmune disease. The etiology is still unclear.[66] Overall, 19% (23 of 121) of pediatric patients with APS developed recurrent thrombotic events.

Infection-induced antiphospholipid syndrome

Many childhood viral or bacterial infections can induce the production of APLA, which tend to be transient and are usually not associated with thrombosis or the manifestation of APS.[69,70] However, recent evidence suggested that there are several infectious agents that can trigger APS, which include parvovirus B19, cytomegalovirus, varicella zoster virus, human immunodeficiency virus, streptococcal and staphylococcal infections, and gram-negative and *Mycoplasma* pneumonia.[70]

Malignancy

The reported incidence of thromboembolic events (TE) ranged from 7% to 10% in children with cancer,[71,72] which is much higher than the incidence of 0.07 events per 10,000 children in the general population.[2] The risk is highest in patients with acute lymphoblastic leukemia (ALL) (OR 4.6), followed by sarcoma and lymphoma, and the lowest risk is seen in children with brain tumors.[73] CVL dysfunction (difficulty of blood draw, infusion or documented CVL infection) and intrathoracic disease are significantly associated with thrombosis.

The etiology of VTE in ALL is particularly multifactorial, and includes increased thrombin generation related to leukemia at diagnosis, the procoagulant effects of high-dose corticosteroids, and asparaginase-induced profound and prolonged deficiency of AT and other natural anticoagulants, as well as the presence of CVLs.[72,73] Inherited thrombophilia disorders may also increase the risk of thrombosis in children with cancer. However, currently available studies vary widely in the ethnicity of the study populations and in the extent of thrombophilia testing, so it is difficult to interpret the data and determine the impact of inherited thrombophilia on the development of VTE in children with cancer.[73]

Nephrotic syndrome

TE is one of the common complications of nephrotic syndrome. The pathophysiologic mechanism is multifactorial, owing to the imbalance of the inhibitor and procoagulant system. Such factors include urinary loss of anticoagulants (AT, protein C, total and free protein S), increased procoagulatory activity (fibrinogen, FV, and FVIII), urinary loss of fibrinolytic proteins, thrombocytosis, and platelet hyperaggregability.[74] Hyperviscosity and hyperlipidemia secondary to nephrotic syndrome, as well as medications including steroids and diuretics, exaggerate the risk of thrombosis in children with nephrotic syndrome.[75]

The reported incidence of TE in children with idiopathic nephrotic syndrome was 1.8% to 5%, although a recent retrospective cohort that included both primary and secondary nephrotic syndrome reported the incidence of TE as 9.2%.[75]

Total parenteral nutrition

PN is commonly used in sick children with protein-losing enteropathy or severe mucositis secondary to chemotherapy or radiotherapy, to maintain or enhance their nutritional status. Studies have demonstrated that PN is another important acquired thrombophilia factor for thrombosis. As previously mentioned in the section on neonates, older children who require PN may experience hypercoagulability, as the high concentration of dextrose in the PN mixture may favor the procoagulatory state of monocytes[49]; in addition, the high concentration of calcium in the PN solution may promote thrombus propagation.[49]

Dehydration

Dehydration can occur in children secondary to severe diarrhea, ketoacidosis in type I diabetes mellitus, polyuria secondary to diabetes insipidus, extremely poor oral intake during sickness, or excessive insensible water loss resulting from high fever or burn injury. The constriction of blood volume increases the risk of thrombosis in these children.

Septicemia

Sepsis induces activation of coagulation through the extrinsic pathway. At the same time, sepsis interferes with many of the natural anticoagulant mechanisms, leading to a net imbalance of hemostasis. Various coagulation proteins, including AT, protein C, protein S, tissue factor, and thrombin, act as important mediators of sepsis that induce inflammatory reactions.[76,77] Gram-positive organisms can release mucopolysaccharides, leading to activation of platelets and serine proteases in the clotting cascade. Similarly, gram-negative organisms release endotoxin, which can also activate the proinflammatory cytokines, leading to endothelial damage and a state similar to vasculitis.[78]

Varicella infection

Varicella infection is well known to be associated with neurologic complications such as encephalitis, cerebellar ataxia, aseptic meningitis, and transverse myelitis. The estimated risk is about 0.01% to 0.03%.[79] In recent years, varicella zoster infection has been recognized as a cause of pediatric AIS. The absolute risk of varicella-associated AIS was reported as 1 in 15,000 children.[80] The mean interval from varicella infection to AIS was 2.6 months (range 0.2–12 months).[80] The underlying mechanism is not well established. It was thought that varicella infection may cause vasculopathy from damage to the vessel-wall media by direct viral invasion. It is further proposed that varicella-autoantibody syndrome,[81] through the production of lupus anticoagulant, and acquired protein C/protein S deficiency resulting from autoantibody production, also play an important role in the pathogenesis of AIS.[82–84]

Another clinical entity called postinfectious purpura fulminans, which is clinically nondistinguishable from neonatal purpura fulminans attributable to homozygous protein C/protein S deficiency, has been reported after varicella zoster infection.[85] The disease usually begins 7 to 10 days after the onset of the precipitating infection, with rapidly progressive purpura leading to extensive areas of skin necrosis and peripheral gangrene.[85] Multiorgan failure with pulmonary embolism and TE in other organs usually will subsequently develop. The disease is mediated by autoantibodies (immunoglobulins M and G) against protein S, which persists in the circulation for less than 3 months. The initial level of total protein S is always markedly reduced, and the level of free protein S is virtually undetectable. Prompt recognition of the clinical entity, immediate heparinization, infusion of FFP, and, in organ-threatening situations, the use of tissue plasminogen activator may limit the progression of TEs.[85,86]

THROMBOPHILIA SCREENING
Who and Why to Test?

In 2002, the Subcommittee for Perinatal and Pediatric Thrombosis of the Scientific and Standardization Committee (SSC) of the International Society of Thrombosis and Hemostasis (ISTH) recommended that all pediatric patients with thrombosis should to be tested on a full panel of inherited thrombophilia disorders.[87] The rationale for this recommendation was that it was common for pediatric patients to have a combination of both inherited and acquired risk factors, and therefore, even if several acquired risk factors were present, evaluation for inherited thrombophilia should also be performed.[87]

Nevertheless, the clinical situation of every patient is diverse, and no single recommendation to be applied to all patients is optimal. Most physicians would agree that thrombophilia screening should not be performed if the likelihood of an abnormal result and outcome is not increased in the population of interest.[88] With the current available evidence, 3 groups of patients are strongly recommended to have thrombophilia screening: (1) adolescents with spontaneous thrombosis, (2) neonates with non–catheter-related VTE/stroke (CSVT/AIS), and (3) neonates/children participating in thrombosis research (**Table 3**).

Testing asymptomatic children with a family history of thrombosis

Comprehensive thrombophilia testing in asymptomatic children should be avoided. The family member with thrombosis, if still alive, should undergo thrombophilia testing initially; if an inherited thrombophilia is identified, the child's appropriate parent should be tested before deciding whether to pursue testing in the child. The decision to perform thrombophilia testing in this circumstance should be made on an individual basis, and only after proper counseling of the family regarding the benefits and limitations of thrombophilia screening. The physician should be experienced in the management of children with thrombosis.[88]

Screening asymptomatic children without a family history in high-risk situations

At present there are no data to support screening asymptomatic children who encounter high-risk situations, such as those with ALL before starting chemotherapy, or prior to CVL insertion.[88] Universal thrombophilia screening of adolescent girls and young women before initiating oral contraceptive pills (OCPs) is also not recommended.[89]

What Laboratory Tests Should be Performed?

The most common laboratory thrombophilia tests are listed in **Table 4**. It is noteworthy that, as described earlier, MTHFR mutation by itself may or may not be prothrombotic because with adequate folate intake, patients can have normal homocysteine levels. Hence, only fasting homocysteine levels are recommended to be included in the screening panel, and not the MTFHR mutation.

Level I testing, including thrombophilia conditions, is the most prevalent in pediatrics. If level I testing is normal and thrombophilia disorders are strongly suspected, level II testing can be performed.

When Should Testing be Performed?

Physicians must be aware that the levels of protein C, protein S, and AT may be transiently decreased because of consumption in the setting of acute thrombosis. Similarly, FVIII and Lp(a) can be elevated in inflammatory conditions. Therefore, any of the aforementioned that is abnormal during the acute stage should be repeated later, usually after the patient has recovered and is off anticoagulation medication. For children with low

Table 3
Recommendations for thrombophilia testing in children

Who, Indication	Recommendation	Why, Rationale	Comments
Adolescents with spontaneous thrombosis (ie, no identifiable acquired risk factors)	Testing strongly recommended	Identify combined defects Counsel risk of recurrence Counsel/test family members	This group has the highest prevalence of inherited thrombophilia
Neonates/children with non–catheter-related VTE or stroke	Testing strongly recommended	Identify combined defects Counsel risk of recurrence Counsel/test family members	—
Neonates/children with symptomatic catheter-related thrombosis	Not enough evidence to support recommendation	Variation in study results regarding role of thrombophilia in catheter-related thrombosis	—
Asymptomatic children with a positive family history	Decision should be made on an individual basis and only after counseling	Counseling adolescent females on risk of OCPs Thromboprophylaxis in high-risk situations	Caution about false reassurance Test parents first Encourage testing until child is older
Asymptomatic children prior to high-risk setting (leukemia chemotherapy, CVL insertion, OCPs)	Testing not recommended	Not cost-effective Most patients with risk factor will not have thrombosis No effective prophylaxis	—
Neonates/children participating in thrombosis research	Testing recommended	More data needed on long-term outcome to determine the role of inherited thrombophilia and optimal management	—

Abbreviations: CVL, central venous line; OCP, oral contraceptive pills.

levels of protein C, protein S, or AT, testing of both parents should be performed before committing to a diagnosis of hereditary deficiency. Molecular analysis such as polymerase chain reaction testing of genetic mutations can be performed during the acute setting. This analysis is reliable and its repetition is not necessary.[88]

Contraceptive Advice for an Asymptomatic Adolescent Female with Family History of Thrombosis

All young women should be informed about the increased risk of thrombosis with OCPs. The risk of VTE in all women of reproductive age is about 1 per 12,500, which increases to 1 per 3500 for those on OCPs.[90]

In circumstances when an adolescent female with a family history of thrombosis is considering OCPs, thrombophilia testing may be justified, as the patient can be counseled on how her risk of VTE is influenced by the presence or absence of an inherited thrombophilia. For women who are heterozygous for FVL, their risk of VTE while on

Table 4
Common thrombophilia testing

	Thrombophilia	Laboratory Tests
Level I testing	Protein C deficiency	Chromogenic or clotting assay
	Protein S deficiency	Clotting assay or immunologic assay of free and total protein S antigen
	Antithrombin deficiency	Chromogenic or clotting assay
	Factor V Leiden mutation	PCR or screening with clotting assay
	Prothrombin G20210A mutation	PCR
	Hyperhomocysteinemia	Fasting homocysteine level
	Elevated lipoprotein(a)	ELISA
	Antiphospholipid antibodies	Phospholipid-based clotting assays (PTT, DRVVT, Staclot LA) with confirmatory assay using exogenous phospholipid ELISA assays for IgM and IgG anticardiolipin and β2-glycoprotein antibodies
	Elevated factor VIII	One-stage clotting assay, chromogenic assay
Level II testing	Dysfibrinogenemia	Thrombin time, clotting assay Immunologic assay
	Elevated factor IX, factor XI	One-stage clotting assay

Abbreviations: DRVVT, dilute Russell viper venom test; ELISA, enzyme-linked immunosorbent assay; IgG, immunoglobulin G; IgM, immunoglobulin M; PCR, polymerase chain reaction; PTT, partial thromboplastin time.

OCPs increases to approximately 1 per 500 compared with 1 per 3500 for the general female population on OCPs.[90] These women can then be counseled regarding their risk, choices, and alternatives such as progesterone-only preparations that may be a safer but equivalently effective choice.

SUMMARY

Pediatric thrombosis is often a multifactorial disease, with acquired risk factors such as the presence of CVLs and the underlying medical condition playing a more important role than inherited thrombophilia. The acute management is seldom affected by the identification of inherited thrombophilia except in neonates or older children suspected of having severe (homozygous/compound heterozygous) protein C/protein S or AT deficiencies, as replacement with FFP/factor concentrate is crucial in acute management. Understanding the rationale and the limitations of thrombophilia screening is important. More future prospective studies are required to help determine the long-term outcomes and management in patients with thrombosis and inherited thrombophilia disorders.

REFERENCES

1. Schmidt B, Andrew M. Neonatal thrombosis: report of a prospective Canadian and international registry. Pediatrics 1995;96:939–43.
2. Andrew M, David M, Adams M, et al. Venous thromboembolic complications (VTE) in children: first analyses of the Canadian Registry of VTE. Blood 1994; 83:1251–7.
3. deVeber G, Andrew M, Adams C, et al. Cerebral sinovenous thrombosis in children. N Engl J Med 2001;345(6):417–23.

4. Shroff M, deVeber G. Sinovenous thrombosis in children. Neuroimaging Clin N Am 2003;13:115–38.

5. Lynch JK, Nelson KB. Epidemiology of perinatal stroke. Curr Opin Pediatr 2001; 13:499–505.

6. Nelson KB, Lynch JK. Stroke in newborn infants. Lancet Neurol 2004;3:150–8.

7. Schulzke S, Weber P, Luetschg J, et al. Incidence and diagnosis of unilateral arterial cerebral infarction in newborn infants. J Perinat Med 2005;33:170–5.

8. Lynch JK, Hirtz DG, deVeber G, et al. Report of the National Institute of Neurological Disorders and Stroke workshop on perinatal and childhood stroke. Pediatrics 2002;109:116–23.

9. Nizzi FA, Kaplan HS. Protein C and S deficiency. Semin Thromb Hemost 1999; 25:265–72.

10. Manco-Johnson MJ, Knapp-Clevenger R. Activated protein C concentrate reverses purpura fulminans in severe genetic protein C deficiency. J Pediatr Hematol Oncol 2004;26:25–7.

11. Revel-Vilk S, Chan A, Bauman M, et al. Prothrombotic conditions in an unselected cohort of children with venous thromboembolic disease. J Thromb Haemost 2003; 1:915–21.

12. van Ommen CH, Heijboer H, Buller HR, et al. Venous thromboembolism in childhood: a prospective two-year registry in the Netherlands. J Pediatr 2001;139: 676–81.

13. Kenet G, Lütkhoff LK, Albisetti M, et al. Impact of thrombophilia on risk of arterial ischemic stroke or cerebral sinovenous in neonates and children. A systematic review and meta-analysis of observational studies. Circulation 2010;121: 1838–47.

14. Monagle P, Chan AK, Goldenberg NA, et al. Antithrombotic therapy in neonates and children: antithrombotic therapy and prevention of thrombosis, 9th ed: American College of Chest Physicians Evidence-Based Clinical Practice Guidelines. Chest 2012;141:e737S–801S.

15. Sanz-Rodriguez C, Gil-Fernández JJ, Zapater P, et al. Long-term management of homozygous protein C deficiency: replacement therapy with subcutaneous purified protein C concentrate. Thromb Haemost 1999;81:887–90.

16. Minford AM, Parapia LA, Stainforth C, et al. Treatment of homozygous protein C deficiency with subcutaneous protein C concentrate. Br J Haematol 1996;93:215–6.

17. Kuhle S, Lane DA, Jochmanns K, et al. Homozygous antithrombin deficiency type II (99 Leu to Phe mutation) and childhood thromboembolism. Thromb Haemost 2001;86:1007–11.

18. Chowdhury V, Lane DA, Mille B, et al. Homozygous antithrombin deficiency: report of two new cases (99 Leu toPhe) associated with arterial and venous thrombosis. Thromb Haemost 1994;72:198–202.

19. Brown SA, Mitchell M, Cutler JA, et al. Rapid genetic diagnosis in neonatal pulmonary artery thrombosis caused by homozygous antithrombin Budapest 3. Clin Appl Thromb Hemost 2000;6:181–3.

20. Olds RJ, Lane DA, Caso R, et al. Antithrombin III Budapest: a single amino acid substitution (429Pro to Leu) in a region highly conserved in the serpin family. Blood 1992;79:1206–12.

21. Sakuragawa N, Takahashi K, Kondo S, et al. Antithrombin III Toyama: a hereditary abnormal antithrombin III of a patient with recurrent thrombophlebitis. Thromb Res 1983;31:305–17.

22. Fischer AM, Cornu P, Sternberg C, et al. Antithrombin III Alger: a new homozygous AT III variant. Thromb Haemost 1986;55:218–21.

23. Okajima K, Ueyama H, Hashimoto Y, et al. Homozygous variant of antithrombin III that lacks affinity for heparin, AT III Kumamoto. Thromb Haemost 1989;61: 20–4.
24. Bauters A, Zawadzki C, Bura A, et al. Homozygous variant of antithrombin with lack of affinity for heparin: management of severe thrombotic complications associated with intrauterine fetal demise. Blood Coagul Fibrinolysis 1996;7:705–10.
25. Owen MC, Borg JY, Soria C, et al. Heparin binding defects in a new antithrombin III variant: Rouen, 47 Arg to His. Blood 1987;69:1275–9.
26. Chang JY, Tran TH. Antithrombin III basel. Identification of a Pro-Leu substitution in a hereditary abnormal antithrombin with impaired heparin cofactor activity. J Biol Chem 1986;261:1174–6.
27. Peters M, Ten Cate JW, Breederveld C, et al. Low antithrombin III levels in neonates with idiopathic respiratory distress syndrome: poor prognosis. Pediatr Res 1984;18:273–6.
28. Andrew M, Massicotte-Nolan P, Mitchell L, et al. Dysfunctional antithrombin III in sick premature infants. Pediatr Res 1985;19:237–9.
29. Andrew M, Paes B, Milner R, et al. Development of the human coagulation system in the healthy premature infant. Blood 1988;72:1651–7.
30. Andrew M, Paes B, Milner R, et al. Development of the human coagulation system in the full-term infant. Blood 1987;70:165–72.
31. Monagle P, Barnes C, Ignjatovic V, et al. Developmental haemostasis: impact for clinical haemostasis laboratories. Thromb Haemost 2006;95:362–72.
32. Harper PL, Daly M, Price J, et al. Screening for heparin binding variants of antithrombin. J Clin Pathol 1991;44:477–9.
33. Kristensen SR, Basmussen B, Pedersen S, et al. Detecting antithrombin deficiency may be a difficult task-more than one test is necessary. J Thromb Haemost 2007;5: 617–8.
34. Young G, Albisetti M, Bonduel M, et al. Impact of inherited thrombophilia on venous thromboembolism in children: a systematic review and meta-analysis of observational studies. Circulation 2008;118:1373–82.
35. Fyfe A, Tait RC. Antithrombin-α for the prophylaxis of venous thrombosis in congenital antithrombin deficiency. Expert Rev Hematol 2009;2:499–507.
36. Tiede A, Tait RC, Shaffer DW, et al. Antithrombin alfa in hereditary antithrombin deficient patients: a Phase III study of prophylactic intravenous administration in high-risk situations. Thromb Haemost 2008;99:616–22.
37. De Stefano V, Rossi E, Paciaroni K, et al. Screening for inherited thrombophilia: indication and therapeutic implications. Haematologica 2002;87:1095–108.
38. Prengler M, Sturt N, Krywawych S, et al. Homozygous thermolabile variant of the methylenetetrahydrofolate reductase gene: a potential risk factor for hyperhomocysteinaemia, CVD, and stroke in childhood. Dev Med Child Neurol 2001; 43:220–5.
39. van Beynum IM, Smeitink JA, den Heijer M, et al. Hyperhomocysteinemia: a risk factor for ischemic stroke in children. Circulation 1992;99:2070–2.
40. von Depka M, Nowak-Göttl U, Eisert R, et al. Increased lipoprotein (a) levels as an independent risk factor for venous thromboembolism. Blood 2000;96:3363–8.
41. Nowak-Göttl U, Junker R, Hartmeier M, et al. Increased lipoprotein (a) is an important risk factor for venous thromboembolism in childhood. Circulation 1999;100:743–8.
42. Kristensen SR, Käehne M, Petersen NE. Hemizygous antithrombin-deficiency (Budapest III) in a newborn presenting with a thrombosis at birth. Br J Haematol 2007;138:397–8.

43. McCrindle BW, Manlhiot C, Cochrane A, et al. Factors associated with thrombotic complications after the Fontan procedure: a secondary analysis of a multicenter, randomized trial of primary thromboprophylaxis for 2 years after the Fontan procedure. J Am Coll Cardiol 2013;61:346–53.

44. Monagle P, Adams M, Mahoney M, et al. Outcome of pediatric thromboembolic disease: a report from the Canadian Childhood Thrombophilia Registry. Pediatr Res 2000;47:763–6.

45. Male C, Chait P, Andrew M, et al. Central venous line-related thrombosis in children: associated with central venous line location and insertion technique. Blood 2003;101:4273–8.

46. Thornburg CD, Smith PB, Smithwick ML, et al. Association between thrombosis and bloodstream infection in neonates with peripherally inserted catheters. Thromb Res 2008;122:782–5.

47. Rivard GE, David M, Farrell C, et al. Treatment of purpura fulminans in meningococcemia with protein C concentrate. J Pediatr 1995;126:646–52.

48. Clarke RC, Johnston JR, Mayne EE. Meningococcal septicaemia: treatment with protein C concentrate. Intensive Care Med 2000;26:471–3.

49. Kakzanov V, Monagle P, Chan AK. Thromboembolism in infants and children with gastrointestinal failure receiving long term parenteral nutrition. JPEN J Parenter Enteral Nutr 2008;32:88–93.

50. Boffa MC, Lachassine E. Infant perinatal thrombosis and antiphospholipid antibodies: a review. Lupus 2007;16:634–41.

51. Curry CJ, Bhullar S, Holmes J, et al. Risk factors for perinatal arterial stroke: a study of 60 mother-child pairs. Pediatr Neurol 2007;37:99–107.

52. Albisetti M, Moeller A, Waldvogel K, et al. Congenital prothrombotic disorders in children with peripheral venous and arterial thromboses. Acta Haematol 2007; 117:149–55.

53. Kamphuisen PW, Eikenboom JCJ, Vos HL, et al. Increased levels of factor VIII and fibrinogen in patients with venous thrombosis are not caused by acute phase reactions. Thromb Haemost 1999;81:680–3.

54. O'Donnell J, Mumford AD, Manning RA, et al. Elevation of FVIII: C in venous thromboembolism is persistent and independent of the acute phase response. Thromb Haemost 2000;83:10–3.

55. Kreuz W, Stoll M, Junker R, et al. Familial elevated factor VIII in children with symptomatic venous thrombosis and post-thrombotic syndrome: results of a multicenter study. Arterioscler Thromb Vasc Biol 2006;26:1901–6.

56. Nowak-Göttl U, Junker R, Kreuz W, et al. Risk of recurrent venous thrombosis in children with combined prothrombotic risk factors. Blood 2001;97:858–62.

57. deVeber G, Monagle P, Chan A, et al. Prothrombotic disorders in infants and children with cerebral thromboembolism. Arch Neurol 1998;55:1539–43.

58. Kenet G, Sadetzki S, Murad H, et al. Factor V Leiden and antiphospholipid antibodies are significant risk factors of ischemic stroke in children. Stroke 2000;31:1283–8.

59. Bruins B, Masterson M, Drachtman RA, et al. Deep venous thrombosis in adolescents due to anatomic causes. Pediatr Blood Cancer 2008;51:125–8.

60. Ruggeri M, Tosetto A, Castaman G, et al. Congenital absence of the inferior vena cava: a rare risk factor for idiopathic deep-vein thrombosis. Lancet 2001;357:441.

61. Timmers GJ, Falke TH, Rauwerda JA, et al. Deep vein thrombosis as a presenting symptoms of congenital interruption of the inferior vena cava. Int J Clin Pract 1999;53:75–6.

62. Obernosterer A, Aschauer M, Schnedl W, et al. Anomalies of the inferior vena cava in patients with iliac venous thrombosis. Ann Intern Med 2002;136:37–41.
63. Raffini L, Raybagkar D, Cahill AM, et al. May-Thurner syndrome (iliac vein compression) and thrombosis in adolescents. Pediatr Blood Cancer 2006;47: 834–8.
64. Oguzkurt L, Tercan F, Pourbagher MA, et al. Computed tomography findings in 10 cases of iliac vein compression (May-Thurner) syndrome. Eur J Radiol 2005; 55:421–5.
65. Chung JW, Yoon CJ, Jung SI, et al. Acute iliofemoral deep vein thrombosis: evaluation of underlying anatomic abnormalities by spiral CT venography. J Vasc Interv Radiol 2004;15:249–56.
66. Avcin T, Cimaz R, Silverman ED, et al. Pediatric antiphospholipid syndrome: clinical and immunologic features of 121 patients in an international registry. Pediatrics 2008;122:e1100–7.
67. Cervera R, Piette JC, Font J, et al. Antiphospholipid syndrome: clinical and immunologic manifestations and patterns of disease expression in a cohort of 1000 patients. Arthritis Rheum 2002;46:1019–27.
68. García-Carrasco M, Galarza C, Gómez-Ponce M, et al. Antiphospholipid syndrome in Latin American patients: clinical and immunological characteristics and comparison with European patients. Lupus 2007;16:366–73.
69. Shoenfeld Y, Blank M, Cervera R, et al. Infectious origin of the antiphospholipid syndrome. Ann Rheum Dis 2006;65:2–6.
70. Avcin T, Toplak N. Antiphospholipid antibodies in response to infection. Curr Rheumatol Rep 2007;9:212–8.
71. Journeycake JM, Buchanan GR. Catheter-related deep vein thrombosis and other catheter complications in children with cancer. J Clin Oncol 2006;24: 4575–80.
72. Athale U, Siciliano S, Thabane L, et al. Epidemiology and clinical risk factors predisposing to thromboembolism in children with cancer. Pediatr Blood Cancer 2008;51:792–7.
73. Athale U, Chan AK. Thromboembolic complications in pediatric hematologic malignancies. Semin Thromb Hemost 2007;33:416–26.
74. Schlegel N. Thromboembolic risks and complications in nephrotic children. Semin Thromb Hemost 1997;23:271–80.
75. Kerlin BA, Blatt NB, Fuh B, et al. Epidemiology and risk factors for thromboembolic complications of childhood nephrotic syndrome: a Midwest Pediatric Nephrology Consortium (MWPNC) study. J Pediatr 2009;155:105–10.
76. Hack CE. Tissue factor pathway of coagulation in sepsis. Crit Care Med 2000; 28:S25–30.
77. Esmon C. The protein C pathway. Crit Care Med 2000;28:S44–8.
78. Aird WC. Vascular bed-specific hemostasis: role of endothelium in sepsis pathogenesis. Crit Care Med 2001;29:S28–34.
79. Yaramis A, Herguner S, Kara B, et al. Cerebral vasculitis and obsessive-compulsive disorder following varicella infection in childhood. Turk J Pediatr 2009;51:72–5.
80. Askalan R, Laughlin S, Mayank S, et al. Chickenpox and stroke in childhood: a study of frequency and causation. Stroke 2001;32:1257–62.
81. Josephson C, Nuss R, Jacobson L, et al. The varicella autoantibody syndrome. Pediatr Res 2001;50:345–52.
82. Ganesan V, Kirkham FJ. Mechanisms of ischemic stroke after chickenpox. Arch Dis Child 1997;76:522–5.

83. Alehan FK, Boyvat F, Baskin E, et al. Focal cerebral vasculitis and stroke after chickenpox. Eur J Paediatr Neurol 2002;6:331–3.

84. Massano J, Ferreira D, Toledo T, et al. Stroke and multiple peripheral thrombotic events in an adult with varicella. Eur J Neurol 2008;15:e90–1.

85. Levin M, Eley BS, Louis J, et al. Postinfectious purpura fulminans caused by an autoantibody directed against protein S. J Pediatr 1995;127:355–63.

86. D'Angelo A, Della Valle P, Crippa L, et al. Brief report: autoimmune protein S deficiency in a boy with severe thromboembolic disease. N Engl J Med 1993; 328:1753–7.

87. Manco-Johnson MJ, Grabowski EF, Hellgreen M, et al. Laboratory testing for thrombophilia in pediatric patients. On behalf of the Subcommittee for Perinatal and Pediatric Thrombosis of the Scientific and Standardization Committee of the International Society of Thrombosis and Haemostasis (ISTH). Thromb Haemost 2002;88:155–6.

88. Raffini L. Thrombophilia in children: who to test, how, when and why? Hematology Am Soc Hematol Educ Program 2008;228–35.

89. Wu O, Robertson L, Twaddle S, et al. Screening for thrombophilia in high-risk situations: systematic review and cost-effectiveness analysis. The Thrombosis: Risk and Economic Assessment of Thrombophilia Screening (TREATS) study. Health Technol Assess 2006;10:1–110.

90. Rosendaal FR, Helmerhorst FM, Vandenbroucke JP. Oral contraceptives, hormone replacement therapy and thrombosis. Thromb Haemost 2001;86:112–23.

Antithrombotic Therapies
Anticoagulation and Thrombolysis

Ruchika Goel, MD[a], Suresh Vedantham, MD[b], Neil A. Goldenberg, MD, PhD[c,d,e,*]

KEYWORDS

- Deep vein thrombosis • Venous thromboembolism • Pediatrics • Anticoagulant
- Thrombolysis

KEY POINTS

- Pediatric deep vein thrombosis (DVT) is an increasingly recognized phenomenon, especially with advances in treatment and supportive care of critically ill children and with better diagnostic capabilities.
- High-quality evidence and uniform management guidelines for antithrombotic treatment, particularly thrombolytic therapy, remain limited.
- Use of a thrombolytic approach is considered when rapid clot lysis could ameliorate limb/organ/life-threatening sequelae, reverse the inability to ambulate due to pain from occlusive DVT of the lower limb, or reduce the risk of clinically significant post-thrombotic syndrome in patients deemed to be at high risk for this adverse outcome.
- Optimal dosing, intensity and duration strategies for anticoagulation as well as thrombolytic regimens that maximize efficacy and safety need to be determined through well-designed clinical trials using use of a risk-stratified approach.

OBJECTIVES

This article aims to summarize the available evidence, guidelines, and practice considerations regarding conventional anticoagulation as well as less-conventional antithrombotic strategies in the treatment of venous thromboembolism (VTE) in children. Conventional agents are briefly overviewed to provide context (and are extensively reviewed elsewhere), whereas the latter approaches are discussed in detail, with

Funding Sources: None.
Conflict of Interest: None.
[a] Division of Hematology and Oncology, Department of Pediatrics, Johns Hopkins School of Medicine, Baltimore, MD, USA; [b] Mallinckrodt Institute of Radiology, Washington University School of Medicine, St. Louis, MO, USA; [c] Division of Hematology, Department of Pediatrics, Johns Hopkins School of Medicine, Baltimore, MD, USA; [d] Division of Hematology, Department of Medicine, Johns Hopkins School of Medicine, Baltimore, MD, USA; [e] Pediatric Thrombosis and Stroke Programs, All Children's Hospital Johns Hopkins Medicine, St. Petersburg, FL, USA
* Corresponding author. 501 Sixth Avenue South, St. Petersburg, FL 33701.
E-mail address: Neil.Goldenberg@allkids.org

Pediatr Clin N Am 60 (2013) 1463–1474
http://dx.doi.org/10.1016/j.pcl.2013.09.005
0031-3955/13/$ – see front matter © 2013 Elsevier Inc. All rights reserved.

pediatric.theclinics.com

main emphasis on thrombolysis and the new oral anticoagulants coming under study in pediatric trials.

EPIDEMIOLOGY OF VTE

Although still rare in comparison with adults, pediatric VTE is being recognized with increasing frequency particularly in the tertiary care setting.[1–3] In 2001, data from a prospective 2-year registry of children in Netherlands showed that in 85% of cases, thrombosis occurred in hospitalized patients. Although neonatal VTE was almost exclusively catheter related and located in the upper venous system, VTE was catheter related in only one-third of older children, more often located in the lower extremity.[4] The Canadian Childhood Thrombophilia Registry reported significant long-term morbidity in pediatric DVT with 33/405 children (8.1%) having recurrent thrombosis, and 50/405 children (12.4%) having post-thrombotic syndrome (PTS) at about 3 years follow-up. Mortality directly attributable to DVT/pulmonary embolism (PE) occurred in 9/405 children (2.2%), all of whom had central venous line–associated thrombosis.[5]

Data from the National Hospital Discharge Survey in 2004 identified an overall in-hospital incidence rate of 4.9 VTE/100,000 children/year in the United States, with bimodal distribution in which incidence peaked in neonates and adolescents.[6] In a retrospective study, using the Pediatric Health Information System administrative database during the period from 2001 to 2007, Raffini and colleagues[7] demonstrated that the annual rate of VTE in pediatric hospitals in the United States showed a dramatic increase of 70%, from 34 to 58 cases per 10,000 hospital admissions. The US Surgeon General's Call-to-Action in 2008 on DVT and PE Prevention highlighted the growing incidence of VTE and the need to identify risk predictors and risk-stratified preventative and therapeutic strategies for this growing problem in adults as well as children.[8]

CONVENTIONAL ANTICOAGULANTS

Conventional anticoagulants attenuate hypercoagulability, thus reducing the risk for thrombus progression and embolism. Nearly 50% of the VTE events treated with anticoagulant agents resolve over weeks to months.[9] However, the evidence basis for the indication of anticoagulation in VTE (derived from early adult studies) is the reduction of life-threatening pulmonary embolism.[10]

Conventional anticoagulants in pediatric VTE include unfractionated heparin (UFH), low molecular weight heparins (LMWHs, enoxaparin and dalteparin in the United States), and vitamin K antagonists (warfarin in the United States).[5]

UFH has a shorter half-life than LMWH and is typically preferred in clinical situations with higher bleeding risk and/or higher acuity, due to rapid extinction of anticoagulant activity on discontinuing the drug.[11] UFH is also preferred for acute VTE therapy in the setting of diminished renal function because of the relatively greater renal elimination of LMWH.

LMWH is increasingly being used as a first-line agent for anticoagulation in children[7] due to (1) ease of subcutaneous over intravenous administration; (2) less frequent need for monitoring when compared with warfarin or UFH; and (3) decreased risk for the development of heparin-induced thrombocytopenia when compared with UFH.[12] Raffini and colleagues[7] reported that the proportion of children with VTE treated with enoxaparin increased from 29% to 49% during the time period from 2001 to 2007. Despite the widespread use of LMWH, the therapeutic and prophylactic guidelines for these agents in children are extrapolated from adult guidelines. The REVIVE trial aimed to assess the efficacy of another LMWH, reviparin sodium, compared with UFH and warfarin for the treatment of VTE in children. However, the trial was closed prematurely and thus not adequately powered to assess comparative efficacy.[13] Hence, at present, the considerations for specific agents/regimens are largely guided by the considerations listed earlier, including the patient's clinical status, bleeding risk, and renal function. Anticoagulant choices can also strongly be guided by patient preferences, particularly to achieve optimal adherence to a prescribed regimen in the outpatient settings.

Available studies regarding the pharmacokinetics, effectiveness, side effects profile, and optimum dosing for LMWH therapy in children[14–17] suggest that a bolus (loading) dose is not necessary. The starting dose of enoxaparin in children (except neonates) should be 1.0 to 1.25 mg/kg subcutaneously Q12-hour. In term neonates, a higher dose of enoxaparin (1.5 mg/kg Q12 h) typically is necessary with even higher requirements in preterm infants.[15,18–20] Bauman and colleagues[17] also recently reported that age-based enoxaparin doses are required to achieve therapeutic levels in infants and children, observing an inverse relationship between dose/kg and age. These investigators found that increasing the starting dose of enoxaparin might result in faster acquisition of the therapeutic range with fewer venipunctures or dose adjustments and without an appreciable increase in bleeding events.

The FondaKIDS study recently reported prospective data on pharmacokinetics and safety of fondaparinux (a synthetic and specific inhibitor of activated Factor X) in children, with 0.1 mg/kg once daily dosing in children resulting in pharmacokinetic profiles comparable to adults, suggesting fondaparinux as a potential alternative to LMWH.[21,22] Comparative efficacy studies are warranted.

THROMBOLYSIS
Settings

Although conventional anticoagulation therapy continues to be the mainstay of VTE management,[5] thrombolytic therapy represents a key treatment choice in select circumstances of pediatric DVT, with the aim of improving short-term outcomes and decreasing long-term morbidity and mortality.[11] However, the current limited understanding of the risks and benefits results in limited use of thrombolysis in pediatric DVT.[2,23,24] A recent survey among active and trainee members of ASPHO reveals a wide variability in the clinical practice and decision making pertaining to the use of thrombolytic agents in childhood VTE.[25]

The latest evidence-based practice guidelines for antithrombotic therapy for VTE in the pediatric population vary with respect to recommendations for the use of thrombolytic therapy. Although American Heart Association guidelines suggest considering thrombolytic therapy in children in whom the "benefit may outweigh risk", American College Chest Physicians (ACCP) guidelines discourage the "routine" use of thrombolytic therapy for pediatric DVT and recommend that thrombolysis be reserved for patients with life- or limb-threatening events.[11,26]

Those VTE that have strong consensus for thrombolysis based on ACCP pediatric antithrombotic therapy guidelines include (1) massive PE with cardiovascular instability; (2) obstructive superior vena cava syndrome; (3) bilateral renal vein thrombosis; (4) cerebral sinus venous thrombosis with deteriorating neurologic status; (5) large atrial thrombi; and (6) VTE causing life-threatening shunt obstructions in patients with complex congenital heart disease status-post staged surgical repairs.[2] Relatively weaker "indications" by consensus (which nevertheless remain important clinical considerations) include acute iliofemoral or inferior vena cava thrombosis and anatomic compressive syndromes, including May-Thurner (**Fig. 1**) and Paget-Schroetter syndromes.[24]

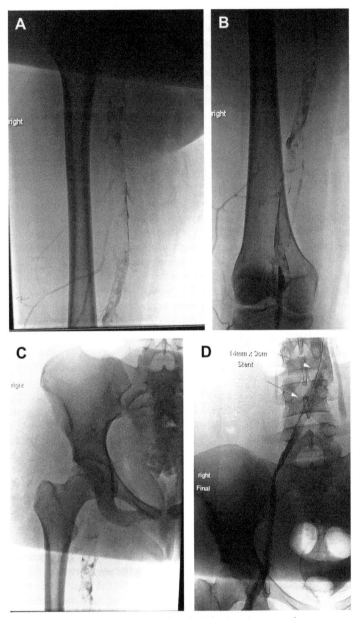

Fig. 1. Catheter venogram in a 15-year-old girl with situs inversus demonstrates globular filling defects in (*A*) the right popliteal and (*B*) right femoral veins, with (*C*) no contrast entry into the iliac vein, consistent with occlusion. (*D*) After thrombolysis and stent placement in the right common iliac vein, there is restoration of inline flow in the iliac vein with mild residual narrowing but without significant residual thrombus. This patient has right-sided May-Thurner syndrome.

In adult patients, management guidelines from the American Heart Association recommended thrombolysis as a therapeutic modality in "young patients" with extensive and/or occlusive thrombus of recent onset and an anticipated long lifespan as well as low bleeding risk.[27] Prospective studies and clinical trials aimed at reducing the risk of PTS are particularly important in children, given the sustained burden that PTS could have throughout a patient's lifespan.

It has been suggested, and some evidence supports the notion, that prompt administration of thrombolysis can reduce venous obstruction and the risks of venous valvular insufficiency and PTS when compared with conventional anticoagulation alone.[28,29] In a small cohort study in pediatric patients with complete veno-occlusive proximal lower-limb DVT who had up to an 80% risk of PTS at 1 year if managed by conventional anticoagulation alone, the use of acute thrombolysis (low-dose systemic tPA, followed by catheter-directed thrombolysis for any residual occlusion) significantly reduced the risk of PTS to 22% (odds ratio [OR], 0.02; 95% confidence interval [CI], <0.001–0.48).[30] The findings of this study are preliminary, and the question would best be answered by a definitive prospective randomized clinical trial (RCT).

Agents

Major thrombolytic agents include streptokinase, urokinase, recombinant tPA (rt-tPA), tenecteplase, and reteplase; published use of the latter two agents in pediatric VTE is limited to case reports/series. These thrombolytic agents are plasminogen activators, which promote fibrinolysis by converting plasminogen to plasmin. The thrombolytic agent used most frequently in children over more than the past 10 years is rt-tPA.[11,25] This agent is produced in Chinese hamster cell lines using recombinant DNA technology. It is rapidly cleared through the liver, with an intravascular half-life of approximately 5 minutes.

Modalities

Systemic thrombolysis

In a pooled analysis of adult RCT's of systemic thrombolysis using streptokinase compared with heparin, greater than 50% clot lysis was seen more often in proximal DVT patients treated with streptokinase (62% vs 17%, $P<.0001$), albeit at the cost of substantively increased bleeding risk.[31] In small RCTs with substantial methodological limitations, the use of thrombolytic therapy with streptokinase showed a trend toward PTS prevention.[32,33] RCTs in adults comparing dosing regimens of systemic intravenous rt-PA plus heparin compared with heparin alone in the treatment of acute proximal DVT have provided evidence that rt-PA and rt-PA plus heparin result in more clot lysis than heparin alone. The addition of heparin to rt-PA does not improve the lysis rate. This study also found a trend toward PTS reduction with rt-tPA use.[28,34] A recent Cochrane database systematic review of RCTs of thrombolysis (systemic thrombolysis or catheter-directed thrombolytic infusion) versus standard anticoagulation alone in adult VTE concluded that the acute rate of achieving complete patency is significantly increased (RR = 4.14, 95% CI = 1.22–14.01) with thrombolysis, and the risk of PTS is correspondingly decreased (RR = 0.66, 95% CI = 0.47–0.94). However, mortality and the risk of recurrent VTE were not reduced by thrombolysis and a slight increase in acute major bleeding risk was attributed to thrombolysis as compared with standard anticoagulation (RR, 1.73; 95% CI, 1.04–2.88).[35]

There are several reports available citing the use of tPA in infancy and childhood in various clinical settings.[36–39] Systemic thrombolytic therapy in children typically follows one of two dose-based regimens: (1) so-called "standard-dose" tPA (0.1–0.5 mg/kg per hour) and (2) low-dose tPA with a dose of 0.03 mg/kg to 0.06 mg/kg per hour.[2,40] Wang and colleagues[40] reported on 35 pediatric subjects of which 29 had acute thrombi and 6 had chronic thrombi. In this analysis, low-dose tPA was used at 0.01 to 0.06 mg/kg per hour (a higher dose of 0.06 mg/kg/hr was used in neonates) in 17 subjects and standard dose tPA at 0.1 to 0.5 mg/kg per hour in 12 subjects. In approximately half of the study population, tPA dosing regimens used concomitant antithrombotic therapy with UFH (5–10 U/kg per hour) or LMWH (enoxaparin 0.5 mg/kg twice daily). Systemic therapy was used in 25 of 35 cases, whereas catheter-directed infusion of tPA was administered in the remaining patients. Major bleeding occurred in only 1 subject (a preterm infant). Complete thrombolysis was observed in 28 of 29 (97%) cases of acute thrombi. Partial clot resolution was seen in each of 6 chronic thrombi. Low-dose systemic tPA has since been used effectively, with seemingly lower bleeding risk than with standard/high-dose regimens.[41] In 2007, Goldenberg and colleagues[30] also reported favorable by the responses and safety for low-dose systemic tPA, albeit requiring salvage local lytic therapy in some cases.

Catheter-directed thrombolysis/thrombolytic infusion

In the CaVenT multicenter RCT, adults with proximal lower extremity DVT and symptoms less than 21 days were randomized to receive additional CDT or standard treatment alone. The trial showed that the use of additional CDT was associated with a 26% relative reduction in the risk of PTS at 2 years follow-up and a major bleeding rate of 3.3%.[42] There were no intracranial bleeds or fatal bleeds. Other reported bleeds were time-limited events that did not ultimately affect the patients' long-term health.

In 2000, Manco-Johnson and colleagues[43] reported retrospective data in 32 children with VTE using urokinase for CDTI with concurrent low-dose UFH at 10 U/kg/h. At 48 hours, 50% of the children showed substantial clot lysis, and at 1-year follow-up, these children had continued complete resolution. There was one thrombotic death, one thrombus progression, and one pulmonary embolism. Three children with poor early clot lysis had recurrent VTE.

Two pediatric studies have reported on experience with CDTI using tPA. In the retrospective study by Wang and colleagues,[40] of the 35 subjects, 10 received tPA through a local catheter; no difference in outcome was detected when systemic administration was compared with local tPA administration. Major bleeding occurred in only one premature infant, and minor bleeds (mostly oozing at IV sites) occurred in 27% of infants during TPA infusion. In 2007, Goldenberg and colleagues[30] reported the use of tPA in a dose of 0.5 to 1.0 mg/h using CDTI, as part of a thrombolytic regimen that directly followed pharmacomechanical thrombectomy (PMT, see later discussion) as salvage therapy for suboptimal response to initial systemic tPA. No major bleeds were attributed to CDTI.

Percutaneous mechanical/pharmaco-mechanical thrombectomy

PMT refers to the use of a catheter-based device that contributes to mechanical clot lysis by causing clot fragmentation, maceration, and/or subsequent aspiration. Pharmacomechanical CDT or percutaneous pharmacomechanical thrombectomy (PPMT) are used interchangeably and refer to clot dissolution using a combined approach with CDT and PMT. In adults, there are retrospective data providing evidence of equivalent outcomes with clot lysis with PMT/PMMT than CDT alone but with (1) significant reductions in the thrombolytic agent dose and (2) drug infusion time, thus being more resource efficient. However, there are very limited prospective data supporting the evidence, and the data were generated in the setting of few reported cases of PMT/PMMT in the context of studies essentially focused on CDT.[44,45] In the retrospective adult data, although the initial results have been very promising with rapid response,[46,47] data on PTS risk are as yet lacking, and data on long-term vessel patency are limited.

In small neonates and children, the needed technical expertise and limited manufacturing of age-adapted devices limit the wide availability for mechanical thrombectomy.[48] Goldenberg and colleagues[49] recently provided prospective evidence of efficacy as well as safety of PMT/PPMT in a cohort of adolescents with VTE (*a priori* judged to be at high risk for PTS because of complete vaso-occlusion and dual elevation of factor VIII and D-dimer) who underwent PMT/PPMT, with adjunctive catheter-directed thrombolytic infusion of tPA post-procedure. The investigators reported a technical initial success rate of 94% with no periprocedural major hemorrhage events and one symptomatic pulmonary embolism. They further reported an early local DVT recurrence of 40% with successful clot relysis in 83% cases and a late DVT recurrence rate at median follow-up of 14 months (range: 1–42 months) of 27% with a cumulative PTS incidence of 13%.[50] Previously, Goldenberg and colleagues[30] had reported that thrombolysis with systemic tPA by low-dose continuous intravenous infusion with salvage PMT/PPMT intervention (for persistent thrombi) led to a significant reduction in the risk of PTS (OR, 0.02; 95% CI, <0.001–0.48). Interestingly, ASPHO physician members and trainees identified PMT/PPMT as the most common preferred approach to thrombolysis in DVT.[25]

Contraindications/Safety Issues

Standards of safety and efficacy in treatment of pediatric and neonatal DVT with thrombolytic therapy are evolving. Recently, standards for safety and efficacy endpoint reporting and definitions in pediatric VTE studies were published from the Scientific and Standardization Committee of the International Society on Thrombosis and Hemostasis.[51] Bleeding definitions were standardized.

The main complication of thrombolytic therapy, much like for other antithrombotic therapies such as conventional anticoagulation, is bleeding. "Major bleeding" complications include CNS hemorrhage, retroperitoneal hemorrhage, any bleeding significant enough to require a surgical intervention and/or cause a decline in hemoglobin by greater than or equal to 2 g/dL in a 24 hour period. Reported bleeding complications following thrombolysis in the pediatric population range from 0% to up to 40%.[2,24,53,54] Zenz and colleagues[54] reported on a review of 30 years of reported literature that the risk of intracerebral hemorrhage (ICH) from thrombolytic therapy in the pediatric age group was lower in children than in neonates, and lower in term infants than in preterm infants.

Contraindications to systemic and local tPA use are largely modeled after those used in adult studies, but have been suggested and used in several pediatric studies.[30,50] Some of the well-recognized contraindications for thrombolytic therapy adapted from adult literature include (1) active bleeding, (2) recent major surgery or invasive procedure (in past 7–14 days), (3) central nervous system (CNS) surgery, trauma, or hemorrhage with in the last 30 days, (4) seizures in the last 48 hours, (5) uncontrolled hypertension, (6) severe and uncontrolled coagulopathy with inability to maintain platelet count greater than 75,000/μL and/or fibrinogen greater than 100 mg/dL, (7) sepsis, and (8) serum creatinine greater than 2mg/dL.[2,24,50,52]

NEW ORAL ANTICOAGULANTS: DIRECT FACTOR XA AND IIA (THROMBIN) INHIBITORS

Although LMWH and warfarin are the most established subacute/extended anticoagulants used in children, there are many practical limitations to their use. Twice-daily subcutaneous administration is a barrier for adherence to a therapeutic LMWH regimen. Challenges to warfarin use include the need for frequent monitoring using venipuncture, absence of commercially-supplied liquid formulations, and the pharmacodynamic influences of dietary vitamin K intake and concomitant medications (such as CYP2C9 inhibitors and inducers). These limitations necessitate the study of alternative anticoagulants in children, particularly alternative nonparenteral agents.[20,55]

Several novel oral direct thrombin (eg, dabigatran) and factor Xa (eg, apixaban and rivaroxaban) inhibitors are currently in clinical development for a variety of antithrombotic indications in adults. As a result of newer and stricter regulations in Europe and the United States, manufacturers of these agents are required to have a drug development program for pediatrics. Dabigatran, apixaban, and rivaroxaban are all FDA and/or EMA approved for VTE prevention following elective knee or hip replacement surgery in adults and prevention of stroke in adult patients with nonvalvular atrial fibrillation. Pediatric VTE prevention and treatment studies registered on clinicaltrials.gov (ie, completed, ongoing, or planned) are summarized below.

A Canadian open-label safety and tolerability trial of dabigatran given for 3 days at the end of standard anticoagulant therapy in adolescents was recently completed (NCT00844415; results not yet published), and a similar study of children aged 1 to 12 years is underway outside the United States (NCT01083732). Because of once daily administration, absence of significant drug interactions, and high predictability of the anticoagulant action, laboratory monitoring is deemed not necessary,[56] which would be a particular advantage in the pediatric age group.

In November 2012, the FDA expanded the approval of rivaroxaban to include treating DVT or PE, to reduce the risk of recurrent DVT and PE following initial treatment, in adults only. A single-dose, pharmacokinetic/pharmacodynamic study of rivaroxaban is ongoing in pediatric subjects (6 mo–18 y of age) who have completed treatment of VTE but are considered to have increased risk for recurrence of VTE (NCT01145859), and a second study is planned for subjects treated for at least 60 days with conventional anticoagulants, to complete a 3-month total course of therapy for VTE in children aged 6 to 18 years (NCT01684423).

In addition, an international single-dose phase 1 study is evaluating the pharmacokinetics, pharmacodynamics, safety, and tolerability of apixaban in children (neonate, 18 y of age) at risk for a venous or arterial thrombosis, including patients with central venous catheters (NCT01707394). Planning for additional pediatric studies is underway.

SUMMARY

Pediatric VTE is an increasingly recognized phenomenon especially with advances in treatment and supportive care of critically ill children and with better diagnostic capabilities. Yet, high-quality evidence and uniform management guidelines for antithrombotic treatment, particularly thrombolytic therapy, remain limited. Although conventional anticoagulation remains at the mainstay of initial management, thrombolytic therapy represents a key treatment choice in select circumstances of pediatric VTE, with the aim of improving short-term outcomes and decreasing long-term morbidity and mortality. Compared to conventional anticoagulation, the use of a thrombolytic agent to provide prompt clot lysis has shown potential to decrease the risk of venous obstruction, venous valvular insufficiency, and PTS. Optimal dosing strategies for anticoagulation and thrombolytic regimens that maximize efficacy and safety need to be determined through well-designed clinical trials using a risk stratified approach.

REFERENCES

1. Goldenberg NA, Bernard TJ. Venous thromboembolism in children. Hematol Oncol Clin North Am 2010;24:151–66.
2. Raffini L. Thrombolysis for intravascular thrombosis in neonates and children. Curr Opin Pediatr 2009;21:9–14.
3. Setty BA, O'Brien SH, Kerlin BA. Pediatric venous thromboembolism in the United States: a tertiary care complication of chronic diseases. Pediatr Blood Cancer 2012;59:258–64.
4. van Ommen CH, Heijboer H, Buller HR, et al. Venous thromboembolism in childhood: a prospective two-year registry in The Netherlands. J Pediatr 2001;139: 676–81.
5. Monagle P, Adams M, Mahoney M, et al. Outcome of pediatric thromboembolic disease: a report from the Canadian Childhood Thrombophilia Registry. Pediatr Res 2000;47:763–6.
6. Stein PD, Kayali F, Olson RE. Incidence of venous thromboembolism in infants and children: data from the National Hospital Discharge Survey. J Pediatr 2004;145:563–5.
7. Raffini L, Huang YS, Witmer C, et al. Dramatic increase in venous thromboembolism in children's hospitals in the United States from 2001 to 2007. Pediatrics 2009;124:1001–8.
8. The Surgeon General's Call to Action to prevent deep vein thrombosis and pulmonary embolism. 2008. Available at: www.surgeongeneral.gov/library/calls/deepvein/call-to-action-on-dvt-2008.pdf.
9. Goldenberg NA. Long-term outcomes of venous thrombosis in children. Curr Opin Hematol 2005;12:370–6.
10. Barritt DW, Jordan SC. Anticoagulant drugs in the treatment of pulmonary embolism. A controlled trial. Lancet 1960;1:1309–12.
11. Monagle P, Chan AK, Goldenberg NA, et al. Antithrombotic therapy in neonates and children: antithrombotic therapy and prevention of thrombosis, 9th ed: American College Of Chest Physicians evidence-based clinical practice guidelines. Chest 2012;141(Suppl 2):e737S–801S.
12. Linkins LA, Dans AL, Moores LK, et al. Treatment and prevention of heparin-induced thrombocytopenia: antithrombotic therapy and prevention of thrombosis, 9th ed: American College of Chest Physicians evidence-based clinical practice guidelines. Chest 2012;141(Suppl 2):e495S–530S.
13. Massicotte P, Julian JA, Gent M, et al. An open-label randomized controlled trial of low molecular weight heparin compared to heparin and coumadin for the treatment of venous thromboembolic events in children: the REVIVE trial. Thromb Res 2003;109:85–92.
14. Michaels LA, Gurian M, Hegyi T, et al. Low molecular weight heparin in the treatment of venous and arterial thromboses in the premature infant. Pediatrics 2004; 114:703–7.
15. Andrade-Campos MM, Montes-Limon AE, Fernandez-Mosteirin N, et al. Dosing and monitoring of enoxaparin therapy in children: experience in a tertiary care hospital. Blood Coagul Fibrinolysis 2013;24:194–8.
16. Lewis TV, Johnson PN, Nebbia AM, et al. Increased enoxaparin dosing is required for obese children. Pediatrics 2011;127:e787–90.
17. Bauman ME, Belletrutti MJ, Bajzar L, et al. Evaluation of enoxaparin dosing requirements in infants and children. Better dosing to achieve therapeutic levels. Thromb Haemost 2009;101:86–92.

18. Hicks JK, Shelton CM, Sahni JK, et al. Retrospective evaluation of enoxaparin dosing in patients 48 weeks' postmenstrual age or younger in a neonatal intensive care unit. Ann Pharmacother 2012;46:943–51.

19. Malowany JI, Knoppert DC, Chan AK, et al. Enoxaparin use in the neonatal intensive care unit: experience over 8 years. Pharmacotherapy 2007;27:1263–71.

20. Chan VH, Monagle P, Massicotte P, et al. Novel paediatric anticoagulants: a review of the current literature. Blood Coagul Fibrinolysis 2010;21:144–51.

21. Young G, Yee DL, O'Brien SH, et al. FondaKIDS: a prospective pharmacokinetic and safety study of fondaparinux in children between 1 and 18 years of age. Pediatr Blood Cancer 2011;57:1049–54.

22. Young G. Old and new antithrombotic drugs in neonates and infants. Semin Fetal Neonatal Med 2011;16:349–54.

23. Albisetti M. Thrombolytic therapy in children. Thromb Res 2006;118:95–105.

24. Greene LA, Goldenberg NA. Deep vein thrombosis: thrombolysis in the pediatric population. Semin Intervent Radiol 2012;29:36–43.

25. Yee DL, Chan AK, Williams S, et al. Varied opinions on thrombolysis for venous thromboembolism in infants and children: findings from a survey of pediatric hematology-oncology specialists. Pediatr Blood Cancer 2009;53:960–6.

26. Jaff MR, McMurtry MS, Archer SL, et al. Management of massive and submassive pulmonary embolism, iliofemoral deep vein thrombosis, and chronic thromboembolic pulmonary hypertension: a scientific statement from the American Heart Association. Circulation 2011;123:1788–830.

27. Kearon C, Kahn SR, Agnelli G, et al. Antithrombotic therapy for venous thromboembolic disease: American College of Chest Physicians evidence-based clinical practice guidelines (8th Edition). Chest 2008;133(Suppl 6):454S–545S.

28. Turpie AG, Levine MN, Hirsh J, et al. Tissue plasminogen activator (rt-PA) vs heparin in deep vein thrombosis. Results of a randomized trial. Chest 1990; 97(Suppl 4):172S–5S.

29. Enden T, Klow NE, Sandvik L, et al. Catheter-directed thrombolysis vs. anticoagulant therapy alone in deep vein thrombosis: results of an open randomized, controlled trial reporting on short-term patency. J Thromb Haemost 2009;7:1268–75.

30. Goldenberg NA, Durham JD, Knapp-Clevenger R, et al. A thrombolytic regimen for high-risk deep venous thrombosis may substantially reduce the risk of post-thrombotic syndrome in children. Blood 2007;110:45–53.

31. Goldhaber SZ, Buring JE, Lipnick RJ, et al. Pooled analyses of randomized trials of streptokinase and heparin in phlebographically documented acute deep venous thrombosis. Am J Med 1984;76:393–7.

32. Arnesen H, Hoiseth A, Ly B. Streptokinase of heparin in the treatment of deep vein thrombosis. Follow-up results of a prospective study. Acta Med Scand 1982;211:65–8.

33. Elliot M, Immelman E, Jeffery P, et al. A comparative randomized trial of heparin versus streptokinase in the treatment of acute proximal venous thrombosis: an interim report of a prospective trial. Br J Surg 1979;66:838–43.

34. Goldhaber SZ, Meyerovitz MF, Green D, et al. Randomized controlled trial of tissue plasminogen activator in proximal deep venous thrombosis. Am J Med 1990;88:235–40.

35. Watson LI, Armon MP. Thrombolysis for acute deep vein thrombosis. Cochrane Database Syst Rev 2004;(18):CD002783.

36. Dillon PW, Fox PS, Berg CJ, et al. Recombinant tissue plasminogen activator for neonatal and pediatric vascular thrombolytic therapy. J Pediatr Surg 1993;28:1264–8 [discussion: 8–9].

37. Farnoux C, Camard O, Pinquier D, et al. Recombinant tissue-type plasminogen activator therapy of thrombosis in 16 neonates. J Pediatr 1998;133:137–40.

38. Leaker M, Massicotte MP, Brooker LA, et al. Thrombolytic therapy in pediatric patients: a comprehensive review of the literature. Thromb Haemost 1996;76:132–4.

39. Nowak-Gottl U, Schwabe D, Schneider W, et al. Thrombolysis with recombinant tissue-type plasminogen activator in renal venous thrombosis in infancy. Lancet 1992;340:1105.

40. Wang M, Hays T, Balasa V, et al. Low-dose tissue plasminogen activator thrombolysis in children. J Pediatr Hematol Oncol 2003;25:379–86.

41. Leary SE, Harrod VL, de Alarcon PA, et al. Low-dose systemic thrombolytic therapy for deep vein thrombosis in pediatric patients. J Pediatr Hematol Oncol 2010;32:97–102.

42. Enden T, Haig Y, Kløw NE, et al. Long-term outcome after additional catheter-directed thrombolysis versus standard treatment for acute iliofemoral deep vein thrombosis (the CaVenT study): a randomised controlled trial. Lancet 2012;379:31–8.

43. Manco-Johnson MJ, Nuss R, Hays T, et al. Combined thrombolytic and anticoagulant therapy for venous thrombosis in children. J Pediatr 2000;136:446–53.

44. Bjarnason H, Kruse JR, Asinger DA, et al. Iliofemoral deep venous thrombosis: safety and efficacy outcome during 5 years of catheter-directed thrombolytic therapy. J Vasc Interv Radiol 1997;8:405–18.

45. Verhaeghe R, Stockx L, Lacroix H, et al. Catheter-directed lysis of iliofemoral vein thrombosis with use of rt-PA. Eur Radiol 1997;7:996–1001.

46. Bush RL, Lin PH, Bates JT, et al. Pharmacomechanical thrombectomy for treatment of symptomatic lower extremity deep venous thrombosis: safety and feasibility study. J Vasc Surg 2004;40:965–70.

47. Jackson LS, Wang XJ, Dudrick SJ, et al. Catheter-directed thrombolysis and/or thrombectomy with selective endovascular stenting as alternatives to systemic anticoagulation for treatment of acute deep vein thrombosis. Am J Surg 2005; 190:864–8.

48. Kukreja K, Vaidya S. Venous interventions in children. Tech Vasc Interv Radiol 2011;14:16–21.

49. Goldenberg NA, Knapp-Clevenger R, Manco-Johnson MJ, et al. Elevated plasma factor VIII and D-dimer levels as predictors of poor outcomes of thrombosis in children. N Engl J Med 2004;351:1081–8.

50. Goldenberg NA, Branchford B, Wang M, et al. Percutaneous mechanical and pharmacomechanical thrombolysis for occlusive deep vein thrombosis of the proximal limb in adolescent subjects: findings from an institution-based prospective inception cohort study of pediatric venous thromboembolism. J Vasc Interv Radiol 2011;22:121–32.

51. Mitchell LG, Goldenberg NA, Male C, et al. Definition of clinical efficacy and safety outcomes for clinical trials in deep venous thrombosis and pulmonary embolism in children. J Thromb Haemost 2011;9:1856–8.

52. Manco-Johnson MJ, Grabowski EF, Hellgreen M, et al. Recommendations for tPA thrombolysis in children. On behalf of the Scientific Subcommittee on Perinatal and Pediatric Thrombosis of the Scientific and Standardization Committee of the International Society of Thrombosis and Haemostasis. Thromb Haemost 2002;88:157–8.

53. Zenz W, Zoehrer B, Levin M, et al. Use of recombinant tissue plasminogen activator in children with meningococcal purpura fulminans: a retrospective study. Crit Care Med 2004;32:1777–80.

54. Zenz W, Arlt F, Sodia S, et al. Intracerebral hemorrhage during fibrinolytic therapy in children: a review of the literature of the last thirty years. Semin Thromb Hemost 1997;23:321–32.

55. Bruce A, Bauman ME, Massicotte MP. Establishing safe and effective antithrombotic therapy use in children...finally. Thromb Res 2012;130:693–4.

56. Eikelboom JE, Weitz JI. Dabigatran etexilate for prevention of venous thromboembolism. Thromb Haemost 2009;101:2–4.

Inherited Disorders of Platelet Function

Dana C. Matthews, MD[a,b,*]

KEYWORDS

• Platelets • Bruising • Epistaxis • Menorrhagia • Platelet aggregation

KEY POINTS

- Patients with platelet function disorders (PFD) have abnormal primary hemostasis and typically present with bruising, epistaxis, and especially menorrhagia.
- PFD are more common than previously recognized and may be more common than von Willebrand disease, especially in adolescents with menorrhagia.
- Severe PFD such as Bernard-Soulier syndrome and Glanzmann thrombasthenia are rare but fairly straightforward to diagnose.
- Milder PFD are more common but may be more difficult to diagnose and may not be identified with the readily available platelet function screen tests.
- Advanced testing for PFD includes platelet light transmission aggregometry, electron microscopy, and biochemical analysis; such testing is less widely available and should be overseen by a pediatric hematologist.
- Supportive care measures such as oral contraceptives, antifibrinolytic agents, and iron replacement are the mainstay of management for patients with symptomatic PFD.
- Desmopressin, platelet transfusions, and recombinant activated factor VII may be indicated in certain clinical settings.

INTRODUCTION: NATURE OF THE PROBLEM

Previously thought to be a rare disorder, primary abnormalities of platelet function are increasingly recognized in pediatrics and can result in bleeding symptoms of varying severity (reviewed in Refs.[1–3]). In fact, recent studies have suggested that platelet function disorders (PFD) are at least as common as von Willebrand disease (VWD) in specific patient populations, such as adolescents with menorrhagia.[4] However, the diagnosis of PFD is challenging, especially for the less severe abnormalities.[5,6]

Platelets are critical for the process of primary hemostasis. At the time of vessel injury, the subendothelium is exposed, leading to the binding of von Willebrand factor

[a] Division of Hematology/Oncology, Department of Pediatrics, University of Washington School of Medicine, Seattle, WA, USA; [b] Cancer and Blood Disorders Center, Seattle Children's Hospital MS MB.8.501, 4800 Sand Point Way Northeast, Seattle, WA 98105, USA
* Cancer and Blood Disorders Center, Seattle Children's Hospital MS MB.8.501, 4800 Sand Point Way Northeast, Seattle, WA 98105.
E-mail address: dana.matthews@seattlechildrens.org

Pediatr Clin N Am 60 (2013) 1475–1488
http://dx.doi.org/10.1016/j.pcl.2013.08.004
0031-3955/13/$ – see front matter © 2013 Elsevier Inc. All rights reserved.

(VWF) multimers to collagen (**Fig. 1**).[7] In the setting of shear forces from flowing blood, this large molecule stretches, exposing binding sites for platelets. Once bound to collagen through the bridging VWF protein (via the platelet surface glycoprotein [GP] Ib/IX/V complex), enhanced by the binding of platelet agonists such as thrombin, epinephrine, and ADP, to surface receptors, platelets are activated. Activation results in a rapid cytoskeletal rearrangement, which leads to a configurational change and then recruitment of and aggregation with other platelets, primarily via the surface GPIIb-IIIa (mediated by fibrinogen and VWF). The activation of intracellular signaling pathways leads to the secretion of thromboxane. Platelet granules release their contents (dense [δ] granules contain serotonin and ADP, and α granules contain growth factors and adhesive proteins). The release of these granules contributes to the "second wave" of platelet aggregation, which involves recruiting and activating of additional platelets, contributing to the strength of the platelet plug formed. Platelets also serve as an important "platform" on which the proteins of the coagulation cascade interact.

These surprisingly complex cell fragments are critical to the initiation and perpetuation of thrombus formation. Abnormalities of platelet surface GPs, agonist receptors, intracellular signaling pathways, cytoskeleton structure, and granule content or release can lead to mild or severe bleeding disorders (**Fig. 2**).[8] Although a detailed

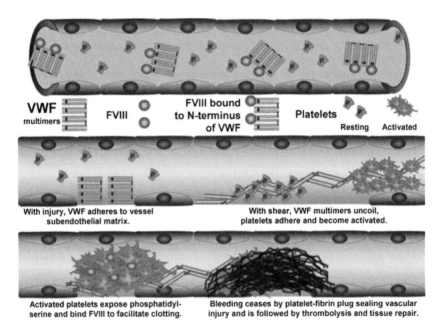

Fig. 1. Platelets and VWF in primary hemostasis. (*top*) Under normal conditions VWF does not interact with platelets or endothelial cells. (*middle left*) After vascular injury, VWF adheres to the exposed subendothelial matrix. (*middle right*) After VWF is uncoiled by local shear forces, platelets adhere to the altered VWF, undergo activation, and recruit other platelets to this injury site. (*bottom left*) The surface of activated and aggregated platelets binds clotting factors and initiates local deposition of fibrin. (*bottom right*) The combination of clotting and platelet aggregation and adhesion forms a platelet-fibrin plug. (*From* Nichols WL, Hultin MB, James AH, et al. von Willebrand disease (VWD): evidence-based diagnosis and management guidelines, the National Heart, Lung and Blood Institute (NHLBI) Expert Panel report (USA). Haemophilia 2008:14(2):177; with permission.)

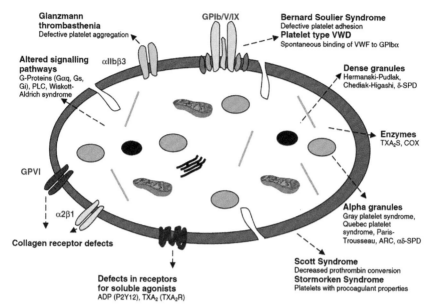

Fig. 2. Overview of the main inherited platelet disorders. (*From* Salles II, Feys HB, Iserbyt BF, et al. Inherited traits affecting platelet function. Blood Rev 2008;22(3):157; with permission.)

description of the specifics of each of these disorders is beyond the scope of this review, the most common and severe of these disorders are summarized in **Table 1**, along with clinical features and diagnostic results. More detailed discussions of specific PFD are available in several recent reviews.[1–3,5,6,8–11]

The classic textbook PFD, including Bernard-Soulier syndrome (BSS, absent GP1b/IX/V) or Glanzmann thrombasthenia (GT, absent GPIIb/IIIa), are associated with severe bleeding symptoms, are relatively straightforward to diagnose, and are fortunately, rare disorders. In contrast, milder PFD are more subtle in their presentation, and much more challenging to diagnose. There is increasing recognition that such mild disorders are far more common than previously recognized and may even be more common than VWD. For example, in a retrospective review of 105 patients with heavy menstrual bleeding referred to a pediatric hematology clinic for evaluation,[4] 62% were diagnosed with a bleeding disorder. Of these, platelet storage pool deficiency (36%) was 4 times as common as VWD (9%), and an additional 8% had other platelet function defects. In contrast, other studies have found different proportions of bleeding disorders in such patients. A study by Mikhail and colleagues[12] of 61 adolescents with menorrhagia referred to a different hematology center demonstrated that 36% had VWD and only 7% had platelet aggregation abnormalities. Such differences reflect, in part, referral differences as well as varying definitions of both menorrhagia and bleeding disorders, and even more importantly, differences in diagnostic testing. Nevertheless, these recent studies reinforce the importance of considering a PFD when evaluating a patient with excessive bleeding, particularly an adolescent with menorrhagia.

PATIENT HISTORY

The classic manifestations of a PFD are those of abnormal primary hemostasis and thus are generally mucocutaneous bleeding, particularly bruising, epistaxis, and

Table 1
Summary of most common PFD

Class of Abnormality	Defect	Severity and Inheritance	Clinical Features	Laboratory Diagnosis	Special Comments[a]
Platelet surface GP					
BSS	Absent GP1b/IX/V expression	• Severe • AR (usually)	• Mild-moderate thrombocytopenia, large platelets • Heterozygosity for BSS common cause of macrothrombocytopenia without bleeding	Platelet aggregation: no agglutination with ristocetin	Confirm with flow cytometry or immunoblot for GP1b expression
GT	Absent GPIIb/IIIa expression	• Severe • AR	• Normal platelet count and size • High risk of platelet alloimmunization and refractoriness	Platelet aggregation: severe impairment to all agonists except ristocetin	Confirm with flow cytometry or immunoblot for GP IIb/IIIa expression
Platelet-type ("pseudo") VWD	GPIbα mutation → increased avidity for VWF	• Mild to moderate • AD	• Mild macrothrombocytopenia • Platelet clumping may be present • Resembles VWD type 2B	Platelet aggregation: increased agglutination to low-dose ristocetin Decreased high-molecular weight VW multimers	Platelet-mixing studies and genetics required to distinguish from VWD type 2B
Platelet receptors for soluble agonists					
• ADP receptor P2Y12 • Thromboxane receptor A2 • Collagen receptor GPVI	Absent or abnormal receptor for platelet agonists	• Variable severity • Variable inheritance	Variable	Platelet aggregation: impaired aggregation to specific agonist	—

Platelet granules

Disorder	Defect	Inheritance/severity	Clinical features	Laboratory findings	Confirmation
δ-storage pool deficiency	Deficiency of dense granules	• Variable severity • AR or AD • Hermansky-Pudlak and Chediak-Higashi are both AR	"Nonsyndromic" or "syndromic": • Hermansky-Pudlak syndrome—abnormalities of melanosomes and lysosomes • Chediak-Higashi syndrome—oculocutaneous albinism, peroxidase-positive cytoplasmic granules, neutropenia, immunologic deficiency	• Variable abnormalities of platelet aggregation in some, but not all • Absent or decreased "2nd wave" of platelet aggregation	• Confirm with biochemical analysis of platelet ATP/ADP ratio, serotonin • Confirm with platelet EM
Gray platelet syndrome	Deficiency of α granules	• Variable severity • Most AR (AD, XR reported)	"Gray, ghostly" platelets, may be abnormally large ± thrombocytopenia • Splenomegaly may be present	Platelet aggregation: may have impaired response to thrombin and collagen	Confirm with platelet EM
αδ-granule disorder	Deficiency of α and δ granules	• AD or AR	Normal platelet count	Platelet aggregation: impaired 2nd wave	Reduced secretion of ATP or serotonin Confirm with platelet EM
Quebec platelet disorder	Abnormal proteolysis of α granules from increased expression of urokinase plasminogen activator	• Severe • AD	± thrombocytopenia Excessive fibrinolysis, resembles defect of secondary hemostasis • Unresponsive to platelet transfusions • Responsive to anti-fibrinolytic agent	Platelet aggregation: impaired to epinephrine	Reduced α granules

Signal-transduction pathways

Disorder	Defect	Inheritance/severity	Clinical features	Laboratory findings	Confirmation
Cyclooxygenase deficiency	—	Mild-moderate	Aspirin-like defect	Platelet aggregation: absent to arachidonic acid, diminished to other agonists	Absent COX expression by immunoblot
Thromboxane synthase defects	—	Mild-moderate	—	—	—

Abbreviations: AD, autosomal dominant; AR, autosomal recessive.
[a] Gene sequencing may be indicated in some disorders.

menorrhagia. Additional sites of bleeding may include the oropharynx or gastrointestinal track as well as surgical sites (especially mucosal). Given that both VWD and PFD result in abnormalities of primary hemostasis, it is not possible to distinguish the 2 diagnostic categories by clinical symptoms. In contrast to hemophilia, an abnormality of secondary hemostasis, musculoskeletal bleeds (joints, muscles), are uncommon, and ecchymoses are more likely to be superficial and spreading rather than deep and palpable. Severe PFD such as BSS and GT may present with extensive ecchymoses at birth. However, most PFD are milder and do not result in notable symptoms until children begin to be mobile. In fact, for many patients, the extent of bruising and epistaxis is difficult to clearly distinguish from "normal."

Because challenges to hemostasis may be relatively few in the first several years of a child's life, a detailed and probing family history may provide critical clues to a PFD in a child. In a young patient with relatively few symptoms who will be undergoing a surgical procedure, particular a surgery involving mucous membranes with a high risk for bleeding (such as tonsillectomy), a positive family history may provide the only clue to a diagnosis that might put the patient at risk. A good family history involves more than asking if anyone in the family has bleeding symptoms and should include specific questions regarding parents, siblings, aunts, uncles, and grandparents (**Table 2** provides examples).

A semi-quantitative pediatric bleeding questionnaire has been developed for VWD, where a patient's bleeding score of ≥ 2 was correlated with VWD.[13] More recently, this instrument has been assessed in patients with a PFD.[14] Early evaluation suggests heterogeneity between diagnostic groups of patients with various platelet disorders, as well as variability within patients with the same diagnosis. The full pediatric bleeding questionnaire may take longer to administer than can be easily performed in a busy clinic and has more utility in a research setting. However, the examples of specific bleeding symptoms assigned a higher bleeding score (see **Table 2**) provide a sense of the relative weight that should be given to bleeding symptoms when considering the likelihood of a PFD. The bleeding score also recognizes that having had certain procedures (eg, tooth extractions, surgeries) without bleeding is clinically important and the presence of this history subtracts from the overall bleeding score.

Menorrhagia is one of the bleeding symptoms most likely to bring a patient to medical attention. In one study of 63 teens with documented PFD,[15] 68% had heavy menstrual bleeding, the most common manifestation, with 86% of these diagnosed based on menorrhagia at or after menarche. Although many affected patients present primarily with heavy menses on a relatively regular schedule, in the study by Vo and colleagues,[4] more patients with bleeding disorders reported irregular menses than did girls with menorrhagia who did not have bleeding disorders.

PHYSICAL EXAMINATION

The physical examination of a child with a PFD is most likely to reveal ecchymoses. Although most ecchymoses will still be found on body areas that are at greatest risk for contact, especially the pretibial area, lateral thighs, and arms, they may also be present in areas such as the chest and trunk. Ecchymoses will be more prominent than "physiologic bruises," often more deeply colored, larger, multiple, and occasionally will be palpable, although these will rarely have the central hematoma common in patients with hemophilia. There may be fresh blood or a recent clot at the vascular plexus in the anterior nares. In rare cases of repetitive or persistent bleeding, pallor may be present. In addition, a few uncommon PFD are associated with clinical syndromes that have additional physical manifestations, such as the occulocutaneous

Table 2
Bleeding history: questions for patient and family

Additional Questions for Patient	Specific Queries
Has the patient taken medications in the last week?	Aspirin Nonsteroidal anti-inflammatory drug Valproic acid
What prior surgeries or significant injuries has the patient had?	Lacerations requiring sutures Tonsil surgery
Any bleeding with minor procedures?	Heel-stick blood sampling Venipuncture Injections
Additional questions for family members	Specific queries
Has anyone in the family been told they were a "bleeder"?	Specific treatment required Become anemic from bleeding Unexplained bleeding from their digestive tract
Has anyone in your family ever had unusual bleeding after procedures?	Tonsil surgery Childbirth Tooth extractions/wisdom teeth surgery Other surgeries
Specific bleeding symptoms	Details and examples of bleeding scores[a] (transfusion, replacement therapy, or desmopressin: +4 for any symptom)
Epistaxis	Duration? Associated with rhinitis or manipulation? >5/y or >10-min duration: +1 Packing, cauterization, antifibrinolytics: +3
Ecchymoses	Palpable/unusual locations >1 cm and no trauma: +1
Tooth extraction	No bleeding in at least 2 extractions: −1 No bleeding in 1 extraction: 0 Reported: +1 Resuturing, repacking, or antibrinolytics: +3
Mouth bleeding with injury	No bleeding in at least 2 injuries: −1 No bleeding in 1 injury: 0 Reported: +1 Suturing, packing or antifibrinolytics: +3
Surgery	No bleeding in at least 2 surgeries: −1 None done or no bleeding: 0 Reported: +1 Surgical hemostasis or antifibrinolytics: +3
Menorrhagia (patient if applicable, or close female relatives)	>80 mL/cycle; change pads/tampons more frequently than every 2 h, pads + tampons to avoid soiling clothes/bedding, flooding? Yes: +1 Oral contraceptives or antifibrinolytics: +2 D&C or iron therapy: +3
Postpartum bleeding (patient if applicable, or close female relatives)	No bleeding in >1 delivery: −1 No bleeding in 1, or no deliveries: 0 D&C or iron therapy: +2
Umbilical stump, circumcision, cephalohematoma, post venipuncture bleeding	Yes: +1 Surgical hemostasis, antifibrinolytics, or iron therapy: +3

[a] Bleeding score examples.
From Bowman M, Riddel J, Rand ML, et al. Evaluation of the diagnostic utility for von Willebrand disease of a pediatric bleeding questionnaire. J Thromb Haemost 2009;7(8):1418–21.

albinism seen in Hermansky-Pudlak and Chediak-Higashi syndromes, both dense granule disorders.

DIAGNOSTIC TESTING

The diagnosis of PFD remains a major clinical challenge and a matter of some controversy (summarized in Refs.[9,16]). In a patient with mucocutaneous bleeding and/or a suggestive family history of such bleeding, the initial evaluation should include a complete blood count including mean platelet volume with review of a blood smear, prothrombin time, and partial thromboplastin time. In addition, strong consideration should be given to testing for VWD, because it is relatively common and the relevant laboratory tests (VW activity and antigen, factor 8 activity, and in the proper context, VW multimers) can be readily performed at, or sent out by, most laboratories. See the article by Carcao and colleagues elsewhere in this issue for a full discussion of VWD. If VWD has been ruled out, then additional testing may be required. The direction of such a workup may be suggested by the complete blood count (eg, mild thrombocytopenia with high mean platelet volume in BSS, hypogranular platelets in gray platelet syndrome). For patients with a suspected PFD, referral to a pediatric hematologist will often be indicated. An overview of the evaluation of patients with suspected platelet disorders is shown in **Fig. 3**, as developed by the Rare Inherited Bleeding Disorders Subcommittee of the Association of Hemophilia Clinic Directors of Canada. Of note, this algorithm includes diagnoses not discussed in detail here, including some thrombocytopenic disorders.[2]

Historically, the template bleeding time was used as an in vivo test of platelet function. However, it has always been difficult to perform in small children, is poorly reproducible, and has poor sensitivity especially for disorders of mild to moderate severity. Many hospitals and laboratories no longer perform this test. Instead, the platelet function screen (PFS) is widely available, including at many community hospitals where the PFA-100 instrument (Dade-Behring, Deerfield, IL, USA) is used primarily to assess aspirin resistance in adults. This assay uses blood anticoagulated with citrate and pulled via capillary tube into a chamber coated with collagen and either epinephrine or ADP. In this condition of sheer, with dependence on VWF, platelets adhere to the collagen, become activated, and aggregate, ultimately plugging flow. The result is reported as "closure time" for each cartridge. However, in addition to the impact of a patient's VWF and platelet function, the closure times are also impacted by platelet count (especially if counts are <100,000/uL), and by hematocrit (especially when <30%). There is controversy about the utility of this screening test.[17–19] Advantages include its wide availability, reproducibility, the ability to perform it on all but the smallest infant, and its ability to identify the abnormal function in severe PFD, such as BSS and GT. However, the PFS is less sensitive in identifying the milder disorders. For example, in a study of 63 teens with documented PFD,[15] only 42% had an abnormal PFS.

The "gold standard" of testing for PFD has always been formal testing of platelet aggregation. This testing is most commonly performed by light transmission aggregometry (LTA), where platelets are carefully purified from anticoagulated blood from a fresh sample. Aliquots of suspended platelets are exposed to several platelet agonists at varying concentrations, and the transmission of light through the suspension is measured over time. The first wave of aggregation causes platelet clumps to settle out of solution, followed by even greater light transmission with the second wave of aggregation. Recent guidelines have been standardized for the performance of LTA, with moderate sensitivity and good specificity for the most common PFD.[6,20]

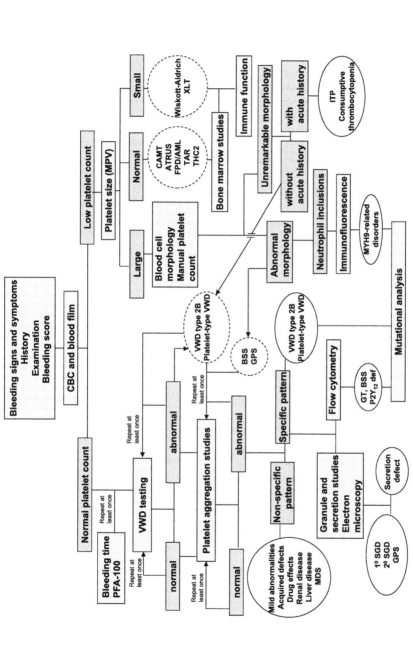

Fig. 3. Algorithm for evaluation of children with suspected platelet disorders. Suggested investigations are in gray boxes and potential results are in hatched boxes. The circles and dotted circles contain diagnoses and suspected diagnoses, respectively. ATRUS, amegakaryocytic thrombocytopenia with radio-ulnar synostosis; CAMT, congenital amegakaryocytic thrombocytopenia; FPD/AML, familial platelet disorder and predisposition to acute myelogenous leukemia; GPS, gray platelet syndrome; SGD, storage granule disorder; TAR, thrombocytopenia with absent radii; THC2, autosomal dominant thrombocytopenia; XLT, X-linked thrombocytopenia. (*From* Israels SJ, Kahr WH, Blanchette VS, et al. Platelet disorders in children: a diagnostic approach. Pediatr Blood Cancer 2011;56(6):978; with permission.)

However, platelet aggregation testing is available only at large centers, is not readily available at some children's hospitals, is complex to standardize, perform, and interpret, and is costly. Nevertheless, platelet aggregation testing is more sensitive than the more widely available PFS, with 60% of the teens reported by Amesse and colleagues[15] having abnormal platelet aggregation.

Platelet granule abnormalities often produce an impaired second wave of aggregation. Another way to assay for platelet granule abnormalities includes electron microscopy (EM) to determine the average number of each granule type per platelet, as well as biochemical analysis of platelet granule content. EM studies documented δ-granule deficiency in 26% of the adolescents studied by Amesse and colleagues[15] who had normal standard platelet studies including LTA. However, these studies are even less available than platelet aggregometry, and the clinical significance of abnormalities with EM or platelet granule content analysis is not always clear.

Additional diagnostic studies may include analysis for platelet GP (GP IIb/IIIa or GP Ib) using flow cytometry or immunoblotting assays.[1] Occasionally genotyping may be used to confirm a specific diagnosis like BSS or GT. In certain settings where a positive family history suggests the potential for autosomal-dominant inheritance, it may be preferred to refer the possibly affected parent for complete evaluation. If an abnormality of platelet function is identified in the parent, the child could then undergo focused laboratory testing to determine whether they have inherited this abnormality.

MUCOCUTANEOUS BLEEDING OF UNKNOWN CAUSE

There is increasing awareness that diagnostic testing for a subgroup of patients with significant and impressive mucocutaneous bleeding symptoms (bruising, epistaxis, and menorrhagia), consistent with an abnormality of primary hemostasis, may not identify a recognized, well-characterized disorder. Even in kindreds where multiple family members are affected in an apparently autosomal-dominant pattern, with every diagnostic test of coagulation and platelet function (including bleeding times) having been performed, 47% to 69% of such patients do not have a demonstrable laboratory abnormality.[5,21] In the past, such patients may have been told that they did not have a clotting problem or a bleeding disorder. Without a specific diagnosis, there is generally not a specific treatment for these patients. However, aggressive use of supportive measures described below may decrease bleeding with surgical or dental procedures or trauma. Thus the increasing recognition of this clinical entity of "mucocutaneous bleeding of unknown cause", and identification of patients and their family members as falling into this broad category, may help to reduce perioperative hemorrhage in such patients.

PHARMACOLOGIC TREATMENT OPTIONS

Treatment of PFD in children can be challenging and is often best overseen by a pediatric hematology center. Treatment options for patients with PFD are discussed in more detail elsewhere,[22,23] but the most important are reviewed here.

Desmopressin (DDAVP, Stimate, CSL Behring, King of Prussia, PA) is a synthetic analogue of L-arginine vasopressin that has been used in patients with PFD.[24–26] This analogue is an attractive therapeutic option because it does not involve exposure to blood products, and high-concentration desmopressin nasal spray (Stimate, CSL Behring, King of Prussia, PA) can be easily administered away from medical facilities. Although primarily used to increase the circulating levels of VWF and factor 8 transiently in patients with VWD or mild hemophilia A, its use has resulted in improved platelet function transiently in about two-thirds of patients with mild PFD. However, this has not been carefully or definitively studied. The challenges detailed above in laboratory assessment of platelet function make it difficult to prove the efficacy of desmopressin with a laboratory test and one must rely on clinical observation. Nevertheless, in patients with a PFS, the marked shortening of the closure times measured 60 to 90 minutes after a test dose suggests the potential for meaningful efficacy. Such a test dose should be considered before elective surgical or invasive procedures.

The mechanism for this temporary improvement in effective platelet function is not clear, but it is likely partly attributable to the release of high-molecular-weight VWF multimers. Most patients experience mild facial flushing and may have headache. Desmopressin also stimulates vasopressin V2 receptors and thus has an antidiuretic effect. It should generally not be used in young children (less than 2–3 years of age) and patients should be restricted to "maintenance" fluid intake for 24 hours after each dose to minimize the risk of excessive free water retention with potential hyponatremia and seizures. Consideration should be given to monitoring serum sodium, especially when repetitive doses are administered. There have been rare reports of thrombotic events following desmopressin, although not in pediatric patients.

Antifibrinolytic treatment options include epsilon-aminocaproic acid (Amicar, Clover Pharmaceuticals Corporation, Marietta, GA) and tranexamic acid (Lysteda, Ferring Pharmaceuticals, Parsippany, NJ). These options have most classically been used in the setting of oral mucosal injuries or dental extractions where the inhibition of salivary fibrinolytic enzymes helps to stabilize clots and prevent their degradation. Antifibrinolytic agents should be continued until the site of bleeding is completely healed, usually 5 to 10 days depending on the procedure. These agents may be adequate to facilitate hemostasis or may be used to stabilize clots after desmopressin or even a platelet transfusion. They may also be effective in the treatment of recurrent epistaxis, and menorrhagia.[27]

Hormonal management, including oral contraceptive agents, is a mainstay of treatment for women with recurrent menorrhagia from PFD. More recently, levonorgestrel-releasing intrauterine devices (Mirena; Bayer HealthCare Pharmaceuticals, Wayne, NJ) have gained acceptance as a way to minimize uterine lining buildup in older adolescents and young adults with bleeding disorders.[28]

Recombinant human activated FVII (NovoSeven RT, Novo Nordisk Inc, Plainsboro, NJ) has been used in patients with severe PFD, particularly GT, as a means of avoiding platelet transfusions or in patients who have become refractory to platelets.[29] However, its efficacy is variable, and many patients respond poorly if at all. Its use in this setting is not Food and Drug Administration–approved, although it has been approved by the European Medical Evaluation Agency.

NONPHARMACOLOGIC TREATMENT OPTIONS

Platelet transfusions are occasionally indicated for patients with PFD, but should be used sparingly. In addition to the usual risks associated with the transfusion of blood products such as allergic or febrile reactions, there is an important risk of alloimmunization with resultant platelet refractoriness. Not only can such patients form antibodies reactive with HLA antigens on donor platelets, patients whose PFD is the result of an absent platelet surface GP may quickly recognize the presence of this antigen on transfused platelets as "non-self" and make antibodies to the surface GP. This is a particular problem for patients with GT, who may become profoundly refractory to all transfused platelets, leaving them at risk of potentially fatal bleeding.[30] Because of this risk, platelet transfusions should be restricted to settings of severe or life-threatening bleeding in GT patients.

Patients with severe PFD who have become refractory to platelet transfusions have in a few cases been treated with hematopoietic stem cell transplant.[31]

SUPPORTIVE CARE AND OTHER ISSUES

Supportive care measures may be critical for patients with PFD, given that platelet transfusions should generally be reserved for significant bleeding or for injuries/surgeries. A detailed discussion about the management of epistaxis should include asking the family to describe, and even demonstrate, what they do when their child has epistaxis. In many cases, parents or the child themselves apply pressure to the bridge of the nose rather than the inferior aspect at the site of anterior plexus vascular bleeding. They should be instructed to hold the nose for at least 10 minutes before checking to see if bleeding has ceased, and for severe PFD, even longer. The regular, twice daily use of an ointment such as petroleum jelly or triple-antibiotic ointment to the anterior nasal plexus, applied by using the fifth finger of the child, if at all possible, may help to limit the clusters of epistaxis that are common in these patients by softening the drying eschar that forms, increasing the chance that it will not be pulled off before mucosal healing is complete, and by protecting the superficial vessels. In dry climates, the use of a humidifier for the child's bedroom may help. Saline nasal spray may also help. Discourage the use of packing or inserting items such as cotton-tipped swabs in the nares because that may further damage the fragile mucosa. Occasionally, nasal cautery may help decrease the frequency of epistaxis if resistant to other measures.

Children with frequent prolonged epistaxis or ongoing menorrhagia are at risk for iron deficiency. Determination of hemoglobin/hematocrit and iron studies may be appropriate, and some children need ongoing supplementation with oral iron.

As is true for all patients with bleeding disorders, affected patients should receive regular preventive dental care to minimize the need for more invasive dental procedures and extractions, and to optimize gingival health.

SUMMARY AND FUTURE DIRECTIONS

As described, PFD result in abnormal primary hemostasis and are most likely to manifest with menorrhagia, epistaxis, and bruising. The history and clinical course for patients with severe PFD are not subtle and can lead to a straightforward diagnosis, but nevertheless, confirmation of these rare diseases requires specialized laboratory testing. Mild PFD are much more common and may still cause significant menorrhagia, bothersome epistaxis, and problematic bleeding with procedures such as tonsillectomy. Their diagnosis, however, is much more challenging, and even though progress has been made toward standardization of assays such as LTA, there is still much to be learned about clinical and laboratory correlations. Thus, PFD are an area of great interest in pediatric hematology, and future studies may make their diagnosis more straightforward. Regardless of the diagnosis, for the most part supportive care measures, rather than specific therapies for a given subtype of PFD, are the mainstay of treatment.

REFERENCES

1. Podda G, Femia EA, Pugliano M, et al. Congenital defects of platelet function. Platelets 2012;23(7):552–63.

2. Israels SJ, Kahr WH, Blanchette VS, et al. Platelet disorders in children: a diagnostic approach. Pediatr Blood Cancer 2011;56(6):975–83.
3. Neunert CE, Journeycake JM. Congenital platelet disorders. Hematol Oncol Clin North Am 2007;21(4):663–84, vi.
4. Vo KT, Grooms L, Klima J, et al. Menstrual bleeding patterns and prevalence of bleeding disorders in a multidisciplinary adolescent haematology clinic. Haemophilia 2013;19(1):71–5.
5. Israels SJ, El-Ekiaby M, Quiroga T, et al. Inherited disorders of platelet function and challenges to diagnosis of mucocutaneous bleeding. Haemophilia 2010; 16(Suppl 5):152–9.
6. Hayward CP. Diagnostic evaluation of platelet function disorders. Blood Rev 2011;25(4):169–73.
7. Nichols WL, Hultin MB, James AH, et al. von Willebrand disease (VWD): evidence-based diagnosis and management guidelines, the National Heart, Lung, and Blood Institute (NHLBI) Expert Panel report (USA). Haemophilia 2008;14(2):171–232.
8. Salles II, Feys HB, Iserbyt BF, et al. Inherited traits affecting platelet function. Blood Rev 2008;22(3):155–72.
9. Hayward CP, Moffat KA, Liu Y. Laboratory investigations for bleeding disorders. Semin Thromb Hemost 2012;38(7):742–52.
10. Israels SJ, Rand ML. What we have learned from inherited platelet disorders. Pediatr Blood Cancer 2013;60(Suppl 1):S2–7.
11. Nurden AT, Freson K, Seligsohn U. Inherited platelet disorders. Haemophilia 2012;18(Suppl 4):154–60.
12. Mikhail S, Varadarajan R, Kouides P. The prevalence of disorders of haemostasis in adolescents with menorrhagia referred to a haemophilia treatment centre. Haemophilia 2007;13(5):627–32.
13. Bowman M, Riddel J, Rand ML, et al. Evaluation of the diagnostic utility for von Willebrand disease of a pediatric bleeding questionnaire. J Thromb Haemost 2009;7(8):1418–21.
14. Biss TT, Blanchette VS, Clark DS, et al. Use of a quantitative pediatric bleeding questionnaire to assess mucocutaneous bleeding symptoms in children with a platelet function disorder. J Thromb Haemost 2010;8(6):1416–9.
15. Amesse LS, Pfaff-Amesse T, Gunning WT, et al. Clinical and laboratory characteristics of adolescents with platelet function disorders and heavy menstrual bleeding. Exp Hematol Oncol 2013;2(1):3.
16. Mezzano D, Quiroga T, Pereira J. The level of laboratory testing required for diagnosis or exclusion of a platelet function disorder using platelet aggregation and secretion assays. Semin Thromb Hemost 2009;35(2):242–54.
17. Hayward CP, Harrison P, Cattaneo M, et al. Platelet function analyzer (PFA)-100 closure time in the evaluation of platelet disorders and platelet function. J Thromb Haemost 2006;4(2):312–9.
18. Favaloro EJ. Clinical utility of the PFA-100. Semin Thromb Hemost 2008;34(8): 709–33.
19. Karger R, Donner-Banzhoff N, Muller HH, et al. Diagnostic performance of the platelet function analyzer (PFA-100) for the detection of disorders of primary haemostasis in patients with a bleeding history-a systematic review and meta-analysis. Platelets 2007;18(4):249–60.
20. Dawood BB, Lowe GC, Lordkipanidze M, et al. Evaluation of participants with suspected heritable platelet function disorders including recommendation and validation of a streamlined agonist panel. Blood 2012;120(25):5041–9.

21. Pereira J, Quiroga T, Mezzano D. Laboratory assessment of familial, nonthrombo-cytopenic mucocutaneous bleeding: a definitive diagnosis is often not possible. Semin Thromb Hemost 2008;34(7):654–62.
22. Seligsohn U. Treatment of inherited platelet disorders. Haemophilia 2012; 18(Suppl 4):161–5.
23. O'Brien SH. Common management issues in pediatric patients with mild bleeding disorders. Semin Thromb Hemost 2012;38(7):720–6.
24. Coppola A, Di Minno G. Desmopressin in inherited disorders of platelet function. Haemophilia 2008;14(Suppl 1):31–9.
25. Ben-Ami T, Revel-Vilk S. The use of DDAVP in children with bleeding disorders. Pediatr Blood Cancer 2013;60(Suppl 1):S41–3.
26. Rose SS, Faiz A, Miller CH, et al. Laboratory response to intranasal desmopressin in women with menorrhagia and platelet dysfunction. Haemophilia 2008;14(3): 571–8.
27. James AH, Kouides PA, Abdul-Kadir R, et al. Evaluation and management of acute menorrhagia in women with and without underlying bleeding disorders: consensus from an international expert panel. Eur J Obstet Gynecol Reprod Biol 2011;158(2):124–34.
28. Kaunitz AM, Inki P. The levonorgestrel-releasing intrauterine system in heavy menstrual bleeding: a benefit-risk review. Drugs 2012;72(2):193–215.
29. Poon MC. The evidence for the use of recombinant human activated factor VII in the treatment of bleeding patients with quantitative and qualitative platelet dis-orders. Transfus Med Rev 2007;21(3):223–36.
30. Poon MC, D'Oiron R, Von Depka M, et al. Prophylactic and therapeutic recombi-nant factor VIIa administration to patients with Glanzmann's thrombasthenia: results of an international survey. J Thromb Haemost 2004;2(7):1096–103.
31. Kitko CL, Levine JE, Matthews DC, et al. Successful unrelated donor cord blood transplantation for Glanzmann's thrombasthenia. Pediatr Transplant 2011;15(3): e42–6.

Diagnosis and Management of Autoimmune Cytopenias in Childhood

David T. Teachey, MD*, Michele P. Lambert, MD

KEYWORDS

- Autoimmune hemolytic anemia • Immune thrombocytopenia
- Autoimmune neutropenia • Evans syndrome
- Autoimmune lymphoproliferative syndrome

KEY POINTS

- Most children with autoimmune cytopenias have idiopathic disease with no secondary cause and enter a spontaneous remission with time.
- Chronic or multi-lineage disease should prompt testing for secondary causes of autoimmune cytopenias, including human immunodeficiency virus, systemic lupus erythematosus, autoimmune lymphoproliferative syndrome (ALPS), and common variable immune deficiency.
- First-line treatments typically include corticosteroids and intravenous IgG. Second-line treatments vary depending on the cell lineage(s) affected and whether or not there is an underlying cause.
- Corticosteroids can cause significant long-term morbidity; therefore, their long-term use should be avoided, because numerous safe and effective alternatives exist.
- Recent advances have led to targeted therapies for select patients, including the use of thrombopoeitin (TPO) receptor agonists (TPO mimetics) for immune thrombocytopenia and sirolimus for ALPS.

INTRODUCTION

Autoimmune cytopenias are a group of heterogeneous but closely related conditions defined by immune-mediated destruction of hematologic cell lineages, including white blood cells (neutrophils), red blood cells (RBC), and platelets. This destruction can be

Conflict of Interest: M.P. Lambert has participated in clinical trials funded by GSK and Amgen. This work was supported by R56A1091791, R21A1099301, and the Cures within Reach (formerly Partnership for Cures) (D.T. Teachey).
Pediatric Hematology, Children's Hospital of Philadelphia, University of Pennsylvania School of Medicine, 3501 Civic Center Boulevard, Philadelphia, PA 19104, USA
* Corresponding author. Children's Hospital of Philadelphia, 3008 CTRB, 3501 Civic Center Boulevard, Philadelphia, PA 19104.
E-mail address: teacheyd@email.chop.edu

Pediatr Clin N Am 60 (2013) 1489–1511
http://dx.doi.org/10.1016/j.pcl.2013.08.009   **pediatric.theclinics.com**
0031-3955/13/$ – see front matter © 2013 Elsevier Inc. All rights reserved.

primary or secondary to other illnesses. Primary autoimmune cytopenias, formerly classified as idiopathic, consist of single-lineage destruction, including immune thrombocytopenia (ITP), autoimmune hemolytic anemia (AIHA), and autoimmune neutropenia (AIN), as well as multi-lineage destruction, known as Evans syndrome (ES). Secondary autoimmune cytopenias result from another cause, including medications, rheumatologic disorders, immunodeficiencies, lymphoproliferative disorders, malignancies, or as a complication of organ or hematopoietic stem cell transplant (HSCT). Despite their complex and heterogeneous nature, treatment is relatively straightforward, primarily using drugs that suppress or modulate the immune system. Many patients require no treatment; however, others need multi-agent therapy and occasionally autologous or allogeneic HSCT.

This review focuses on challenges encountered in the diagnosis and management of single-lineage and multi-lineage autoimmune cytopenias in children. New treatments for ITP and autoimmune lymphoproliferative syndrome (ALPS) are discussed as paradigms for the translation of basic science into clinic progress, as thrombopoietin (TPO) mimetics (TPO receptor agonists [TPO-RAs]) and mammalian target of rapamycin (mTOR) inhibitors have revolutionized therapy for these 2 conditions, respectively. With modern genomics, this paradigm will likely be used in the near future for other autoimmune cytopenia syndromes.

PRIMARY AUTOIMMUNE CYTOPENIA SYNDROMES

Most children with autoimmune cytopenias have idiopathic destruction of a single-cell lineage, most commonly idiopathic destruction of platelets (ITP). Primary autoimmune cytopenia syndromes are diagnoses of exclusion. However, in children, single-lineage primary autoimmune cytopenias are more common than secondary autoimmune cytopenias. Thus, the default is often to presume that a child who presents acutely with single-lineage destruction has a primary autoimmune cytopenia. Patients with chronic disease or multi-lineage cytopenias, in contrast, more commonly have a predisposing cause, necessitating a more extensive diagnostic evaluation. Patients with primary ITP frequently have a preceding viral syndrome or other immune trigger, such as vaccination. The key difference is that the triggering event is not a chronic illness or a medication. The distinction between primary and secondary autoimmune cytopenias is becoming blurred as genetic alterations and polymorphisms predisposing patients to autoimmune cytopenias are being identified.

ITP

Primary ITP is a rare, generally benign autoimmune bleeding disorder characterized by isolated thrombocytopenia, defined as a platelet count less than 100×10^9/L in the absence of other causes or diseases that may cause thrombocytopenia. The thrombocytopenia is often severe (with platelet counts $<10 \times 10^9$/L), but life-threatening bleeding is rare.[1] Antibodies are often directed against the 2 most prevalent receptors on the platelet surface, GPIb/IX complex (von Willebrand factor receptor) and the GPIIb/IIIa receptor (collagen/fibrinogen receptor) and are detectable in 60% of patients.[2] ITP is caused by a complex interplay of immune dysregulation involving a shift toward Th1 cells, a decrease in regulatory T-cell (Treg) function/number, and cytotoxic T-cell–mediated direct lysis of platelets and megakaryocytes.[3] Dysmegakaryopoiesis plays a critical role in the development of thrombocytopenia.[4]

In 2011, an international ITP working group recommended changing the terminology to immune thrombocytopenia to reflect that many patients may not have bleeding or purpura.[5] The phases of illness in ITP have also been redefined to allow for better uniformity (**Table 1**).[5]

Clinically, patients with ITP present most commonly with variable degrees of mucocutaneous bleeding. In a report from the International Consortium of ITP Study Group, most pediatric patients presenting with ITP (77%) had no or mild bleeding at diagnosis, despite the fact that 74% of children had platelet counts less than 20×10^9/L at the time of diagnosis.[1] Severe bleeding is rare in pediatric ITP, and in the same report, only 1 patient (of 863 evaluable patients) had central nervous system bleeding, whereas 3% of patients had severe bleeding (epistaxis, mouth, gastrointestinal [GI], urinary tract, menorrhagia, or multiple sites), and 20% of patients had moderate bleeding. Given the rare occurrence of significant bleeding in children with ITP, the recommendation is careful observation for children with newly diagnosed ITP and mild to no bleeding symptoms.[6]

In children requiring therapy to increase the platelet count, a single dose of intravenous IgG (IVIgG) or a short course of corticosteroids is recommended as first-line therapy, with a single dose of anti-Rho(D) immunoglobulin as an alternative first-line therapy in Rh(D)-positive patients. Second-line therapies addressed in the evidence-based practice guidelines include rituximab, high-dose dexamethasone, and splenectomy. Splenectomy is effective in 70% to 80% of children with ITP, and most of these responses are durable.[7] Twenty percent to 30% of children do not respond, and the permanent effects of splenectomy include an increased risk of infection with encapsulated organisms and the theoretic risks of venous thromboembolism and pulmonary hypertension. Because most children with ITP have spontaneous remissions, splenectomy should be reserved for children who have persistent disease (>12 months) or have serious treatment-refractory disease.

Rituximab has been studied extensively in both children and adults with ITP, although there have been no pediatric randomized placebo-controlled trials. Response rates to rituximab vary from 25% to 80% in different series.[6] Many of these responses are durable, but a significant percent of patients with chronic ITP relapse ~12 to 18 months after treatment.[8] A randomized trial comparing rituximab and high-dose dexamethasone versus dexamethasone alone in newly diagnosed childhood ITP reported improved responses with the addition of rituximab (63% vs 36% sustained response, $P = .004$).[9] More often, rituximab is used in patients with chronic ITP. Other immunosuppressive therapies, including mercaptopurine, danazol,

Table 1	
Revised classification of ITP	
Primary ITP	Isolated thrombocytopenia (platelet count <100 $\times$ 10⁹/L) occurring in the absence of other disease known to be associated with thrombocytopenia
Secondary ITP	All forms of immune-mediated thrombocytopenia other than primary ITP
Phases of the disease	Newly diagnosed ITP: <3 mo of diagnosis
	Persistent ITP: 3–12 mo from diagnosis; includes patients not reaching spontaneous remission or not maintaining complete response off therapy
	Chronic ITP: lasting >12 mo
	Severe ITP: presence of bleeding symptoms at presentation sufficient to mandate treatment or occurrence of new bleeding symptoms requiring additional therapeutic intervention with a different platelet-enhancing agent or an increased dose

Data from Rodeghiero F, Stasi R, Gernsheimer T, et al. Standardization of terminology, definitions and outcome criteria in immune thrombocytopenic purpura of adults and children: report from an international working group. Blood 2009;113:2386–93.

vincristine, mycophenolate mofetil (MMF), and sirolimus, have all been used in small series of patients with reported efficacy in ~60% of patients with ITP refractory to first-line and second-line therapies (see treatment section).

Recently, TPO-RAs have emerged as novel therapies for ITP. TPO was described in the 1950s but was not cloned and sequenced until 1994.[10] Shortly after that development, recombinant TPO was developed as an adjunct for chemotherapy-induced thrombocytopenia and to stimulate increased platelet counts in platelet donors.[11] Subsequently, however, several healthy volunteers developed neutralizing antibodies that cross-reacted with endogenous TPO, causing severe thrombocytopenia, and development of recombinant TPO was halted because of this safety concern.[12] More recently, TPO-RAs were developed that bind within the receptor pocket but do not share any sequence homology with the endogenous receptor. Since the development of these drugs, a few patients have developed antibodies against the TPO-RAs, but these have not been clinically significant. Several randomized clinical trials have reported durable response rates of 60% to 85% in adults with ITP.[13] Some of these patients are able to stop taking the drugs and remain in remission; however, others have rebound thrombocytopenia. Less is known about the safety and efficacy of TPO-RAs in children. Several case series and 1 randomized clinical trial have been published suggesting that TPO-RAs may be efficacious in pediatric patients with ITP.[14] Given the lack of significant data in pediatric patients, use of these medications should be limited to ongoing clinical trials to evaluate safety and efficacy of these agents.

AIHA

Immune-mediated hemolytic anemia can be autoimmune (AIHA) or isoimmune/alloimmune. Isoimmune hemolytic anemia arises from alloimmunization against RBC-specific antigens via placental exposure (hemolytic disease of the newborn) or RBC transfusion. In contrast, AIHA is caused by autoantibodies against RBC antigens. Isoimmune hemolytic anemia and hemolytic disease of the newborn are reviewed elsewhere.[15,16] Primary AIHA affects 1 in 80,000 adults and children. AIHA is classified as warm-reactive (W-AIHA), cold-agglutinin (C-AIHA), or paroxysmal cold hemoglobinuria (PCH).

W-AIHA is the most common form of AIHA in children (~90% of cases) and is usually caused by IgG antibodies against RBC antigens; however, rarely, antibodies can be IgM or IgA.[17] It is classified as a warm antibody, because the maximal activity of the antibody is at approximately 37°C. Children with W-AIHA can present with mild anemia or severe, sudden-onset life-threatening disease. W-AIHA is typically self-limiting in childhood. Clinical manifestations include pallor, fatigue, jaundice, dark-colored urine, and occasionally, splenomegaly. The best diagnostic test is the direct antiglobulin test (DAT, Coombs test), which is usually IgG+ (with or without C3 positivity) at 37°C. Other laboratory abnormalities include anemia, reticulocytosis, increased lactate dehydrogenase level, hyperbilirubinemia, and decreased haptoglobin. Peripheral blood smear most commonly reveals polychromasia, nucleated RBCs, spherocytes, and red cell agglutination.

Treatment of primary W-AIHA is usually immune suppression or modulation, most commonly with corticosteroids, IVIgG, or rituximab (see treatment section). Unlike patients with ITP, IVIgG is often not effective as a single-agent, and usually requires treatment with very high doses for benefit, although it may be a useful adjunctive therapy in severe cases.[18] Corticosteroids are the first line, especially in acutely presenting, very ill patients.[19] Most children with W-AIHA are corticosteroid responsive, with published response rates from 50% to 80% in larger series.[20] Splenectomy was previously the treatment of choice for patients who failed or become steroid refractory or intolerant, as well as those who developed chronic disease, with response rates as high as 60%.[21] Splenectomy is used less commonly because better therapies have been developed and the short-term and long-term risks of splenectomy are increasingly apparent, especially in children. Plasmapheresis can be used for acutely ill patients; however, benefits are usually short-lived, and it is not effective for IgG antibodies.[20]

Most published guidelines recommend rituximab as the agent of choice for corticosteroid-refractory patients or for children unable to wean off corticosteroids.[17] Many small series and case reports have described the benefit of rituximab for children and adults with refractory W-AIHA, with overall response rates ranging from 40% to 100% (median ~50%–60%).[17,20] Some patients require multiple courses. Other agents with activity against W-AIHA include antimetabolites (mercaptopurine, azathioprine, MMF, methotrexate), calcineurin inhibitors (cyclosporine), alkylating agents (cyclosphosphamide), mTOR inhibitors (sirolimus), mitotic inhibitors (vincristine or vinblastine), or other antibody-based therapy (alemtuzumab).[20] None of these has been formally studied in randomized controlled trials. Also, the published case series often group patients with primary and secondary W-AIHA or patients treated with combinations of medications. Danazol, a commonly used agent in adults, is generally not used in children with AIHA because of its masculinizing effects.[22]

Transfusions should be avoided if possible in W-AIHA. Identification of compatible units for transfusion is challenging, because warm antibodies are typically panreactive. Also, the panreactive autoantibodies may destroy the transfused cells in vivo, leading to increased hemolysis, hemoglobinuria, and renal failure. For patients who are very ill or not responding to immune suppression, safety of transfusions may be increased by using special absorption techniques to help distinguish alloantibodies versus autoantibodies in vitro and by transfusing the patient slowly to observe for clinical reactions as well as for free hemoglobin in the plasma and urine during transfusion.

C-AIHA is considerably less common in children than W-AIHA and is typically caused by anti-IgM antibodies that destroy erythrocytes when exposed to cold temperatures. A DAT is typically positive for complement only. In children, C-AIHA is usually triggered by infection, mostly commonly with *Mycoplasma pneumonia*. Patients tend to present with less severe anemia than in W-AIHA. Peripheral smear commonly shows agglutination, but spherocytes are rare. Treatment of C-AIHA differs significantly from W-AIHA, because corticosteroids are often ineffective. A primary goal is to treat the underlying infection, if possible. The patient should remain as warm as possible until the condition improves, and if transfused, the packed RBCs (pRBC) should be warmed. Plasmapheresis is often effective in C-AIHA and may be combined with rituximab. Recent reports, mostly in adults, have described the efficacy of rituximab in C-AIHA, with response rates more than 50%.[23]

Rarely, children can develop PCH, which is caused by a biphase hemolysin IgG antibody against the P-antigen on RBCs (Donath-Landsteiner antibody).[24] It can bind and fix complement at cold temperatures or warm temperatures, but only after cooling and rewarming the sample, leading to complement amplification and hemolysis. Similar to C-AIHA, pRBC for transfusion should be kept warm. PCH patients often respond to plasmapheresis, and several reports have described responses to rituximab.[24] Unlike C-AIHA, PCH is often corticosteroid responsive, because it is caused by an IgG-mediated antibody.

AIN

Similar to immune-mediated destruction of platelets and erythrocytes, immune neutropenia can be alloimmune or autoimmune. Neonatal alloimmune neutropenia, not discussed in detail here, is caused by alloimmunization against fetal neutrophil-specific antigens that are not present on maternal WBCs.[25] Neonates can also develop autoimmune neutropenia, secondary to placental transfer of maternal anti-neutrophil autoantibodies when the mother has AIN.

Primary single-lineage AIN is rare, most commonly presents in infancy or early childhood after viral infection, and is often self-limiting, with more than 95% of children having a complete resolution of AIN.[26] Neonatal AIN secondary to passive transfer of maternal antibodies typically resolves by 2 to 3 months of age.[27] Other forms of childhood AIN typically recover a few months after diagnosis, with only a small percentage of children developing chronic disease.[26] Similar to children with ITP or AIHA, chronic disease is more likely to be secondary to another disease process than is the acute self-resolving form.[28]

Patients with AIN rarely present with significant infections.[28,29] Many patients develop benign infections of the skin and upper respiratory tract. Some patients develop mouth sores. Unlike children with other forms of neutropenia, patients with AIN can often mount a neutrophil response to bacteria and fungal infections. Patients who develop more severe infections should be screened for other comorbid immune deficiencies and other causes of neutropenia. Infectious risk can correlate with degree of neutropenia; however, most patients with AIN and absolute neutrophil counts less than $200/mm^3$ do not develop serious infections. Patients with AIN often have a monocytosis, and bone marrow evaluation usually shows normal to increased cellularity with myeloid hyperplasia. Mature neutrophils may be normal to decreased in bone marrow, and sometimes there is a maturational arrest.

Diagnosis of AIN can be difficult, because of the poor sensitivity and specificity of antineutrophil antibody testing.[26,29] Accordingly, it is recommended that 2 methods of testing be used to establish the diagnosis.[30] The most commonly used are the granulocyte indirect immunofluorescence test and the granulocyte agglutination test.

Most patients with AIN need no treatment. Preventive measures, including good oral hygiene and mouth rinses, are often used. Some centers use prophylactic antibacterial agents for these patients; however, there are no data to support this practice. For patients with serious or recurrent infections, granulocyte colony-stimulating factor (G-CSF, filgrastim) is the recommended first-line treatment.[28] Patients with AIN who are undergoing surgical procedures may also benefit from G-CSF. Some patients do not respond to G-CSF, and second-line therapies include granulocyte macrophage colony-stimulating factor (GM-CSF), a combination of G-CSF and GM-CSF, or other medicines used for immune-mediated cytopenias. Patients with single-lineage primary AIN rarely need these other therapies, whereas patients with multi-lineage cytopenias that include AIN or secondary AIN more commonly need immune modulation (see later discussion).

ES

The diagnosis and management of children with multi-lineage autoimmune cytopenias are more complex. ES is a diagnosis of exclusion, defined by idiopathic autoimmune destruction of multiple cell lineages. Patients with ES tend to have chronic disease and present at a young age (median 7–8 years) with symptoms based on the affected cell lineages.[31,32] Different definitions for ES exist in the literature, making study comparison challenging.[31–34] Some investigators and clinicians consider any patient with autoimmune disease affecting 2 or more cell lineages as having ES. Others restrict the definition to patients with autoimmune destruction of red cells and platelets with or without neutrophil destruction. Some studies restrict the diagnosis to patients with clinically relevant destruction of multiple lineages, whereas others include patients with ITP and a positive DAT without obvious hemolysis. Patients often present with splenomegaly with or without lymphadenopathy and may have an increased risk of secondary lymphomas.[31,32,34,35] The true risk of subsequent cancer development is difficult to determine, because studies are small, the disease is rare, definitions vary, and patients with autoimmune cytopenias caused by other, potentially more cancer-prone, diseases are often erroneously labeled ES. The term ES should be restricted to patients who have no identifiable underlying cause for multi-lineage autoimmune cell destruction. For example, autoimmune destruction of blood cells can occur as a consequence of systemic lupus erythematosus (SLE), but patients with SLE with multi-lineage autoimmune cytopenias do not have ES. The distinction is important, because the treatment and prognosis for idiopathic ES and secondary multi-lineage autoimmune cytopenias syndromes can be different.

Children with ES must have a thorough diagnostic evaluation for underlying causes of autoimmune cytopenias, especially for those that would lead to different therapy. Often the history and physical may suggest that a patient has an underlying immune deficiency, lymphoproliferative syndrome, malignancy, or rheumatologic disorder. At minimum, children with ES should be screened for ALPS, common variable immune deficiency (CVID), and SLE (**Box 1**). Patients with significant lymphadenopathy or splenomegaly may require imaging (positron emission tomography or computed to-mography) or biopsy to eliminate the possibility of an underlying malignancy. Testing for human immunodeficiency virus should be considered, especially in teenagers.[35] It is also important to reexamine for secondary causes of autoimmune disease period-ically, because multi-lineage autoimmune cytopenias can be an initial presentation of SLE, and other disease manifestations can appear with time.[36]

Our group reported in single-institutional and multi-institutional trials that 30% to 40% of children diagnosed with ES have forme fruste ALPS (described later).[33,37] We evaluated 45 children with ES and found that increased immunoglobulin levels, increased vitamin B_{12} levels, and isolated lymphadenopathy without splenomegaly were predictive of ALPS, although there was likely a selection bias, because not all children with ES were captured at each institution. A recent large study from France of childhood AIHA,[35] which included 99 patients with ES, did not find a high incidence of ALPS among children with ES. This study identified children with undiagnosed ALPS, and many patients were not tested for ALPS. Also, the definition of ES was restricted to patients diagnosed with AIHA. Because ALPS is a genetic disease, there is likely heterogeneity in the frequency in different populations. Several studies have screened patients with ES for CVID, making the diagnosis in a high percentage of patients.[38,39] Most of these studies were single-institution evaluations, with a small number of patients. In contrast, the frequency of CVID among patients with de novo single-lineage autoimmune cytopenias, including newly diagnosed ITP, is low.[40]

Childhood ES is often a chronic disease, with a waxing and waning course. Some patients require therapy only with disease flares and others need chronic therapy. Cor-ticosteroids are the first choice for acute flares and newly diagnosed patients. Based on the chronic nature of the illness and significant side effects of prolonged corticoste-roid use (see later discussion), we recommend alternative therapies early in the ther-apeutic course. Unlike single-lineage autoimmune cytopenias, splenectomy is often ineffective in ES. Several studies have shown remarkable efficacy using rituximab in ES. Because ES is a chronic disease, many patients relapse, typically 1 to 2 years after treatment.[41,42] Accordingly, we have a low threshold to transfer patients to single-agent oral immune suppression, using MMF or sirolimus, and have seen marked response in several patients (David Teachey, 2013, unpublished data). The risks with a single-agent are low (see later discussion). Anecdotal series and case reports

> **Box 1**
> **Secondary autoimmune cytopenias in children**
>
> *Diseases associated with autoimmune cytopenias in children*
>
> Lymphoproliferative disorders
>
>   ALPS[a]
>
>   Rosai-Dorfman disease
>
>   Castleman disease
>
>   Ras-associated leukoproliferative disorder
>
> Immune deficiencies
>
>   Common variable immune deficiency[a]
>
>   Selective IgA deficiency
>
>   Chromosome 22q11.2 deletion (DiGeorge or velocardiofacial syndrome)
>
>   Severe combined immunodeficiency
>
> Rheumatologic conditions
>
>   SLE[a]
>
>   Antiphospholipid antibody syndrome[a]
>
>   Juvenile idiopathic arthritis/juvenile rheumatoid arthritis
>
>   Sjögren syndrome
>
>   Sarcoid
>
> Malignancies
>
>   Non-Hodgkin lymphoma
>
>   Acute lymphoblastic leukemia
>
>   Myelodysplastic syndrome
>
>   Hodgkin lymphoma
>
> Chronic infections
>
>   Epstein-Barr virus
>
>   Human immunodeficiency virus[b]
>
>   *Helicobacter pylori*
>
>   Cytomegalovirus
>
>   Hepatitis C virus
>
> Other
>
>   Celiac disease
>
>   Inflammatory bowel disease
>
> *Recommended evaluation for children with chronic single-lineage autoimmune cytopenias or multi-lineage autoimmune cytopenias[a]*
>
> Flow cytometry for double-negative T cells (ALPS)
>
> Antinuclear antibodies (SLE)
>
> Antiphospholipid antibodies
>
> Quantitative immunoglobulins (CVID)
>
> Specific antibody titers (CVID)

T-cell subsets (CD3/CD4, CD3/CD8)

Human immunodeficiency virus[b]

[a] Consider screening for these conditions in children with chronic single-lineage autoimmune cytopenias or multi-lineage autoimmune cytopenias.

[b] Consider also screening for human immunodeficiency virus in adolescents with chronic single-lineage or multi-lineage autoimmune cytopenias. Other diseases should be considered if the history or physical are suggestive of the underlying condition. It is rare for the other conditions to present with autoimmune cytopenias and no other signs or symptoms suggestive of the underlying disease. Thus, the usefulness of routine screening is low.

have described success with a variety of immune suppressants, using both single-agent and combination therapy (see later discussion).

SECONDARY AUTOIMMUNE CYTOPENIA SYNDROMES

The diagnosis and management of secondary autoimmune cytopenias can be complex. A careful history and physical examination may identify a secondary cause in the acutely presenting patient; however, autoimmune cytopenias can be the only disease manifestation in some children with underlying immunodeficiency, rheumatologic, or lymphoproliferative disease. Splenomegaly and lymphadenopathy can often be found in children with idiopathic autoimmune cytopenias, making it difficult to use these findings to determine which patients should undergo more extensive evaluation. Nevertheless, we recommend that patients with chronic single-lineage disease and lymphadenopathy or splenomegaly undergo a bone marrow aspirate and biopsy. Also, imaging for mediastinal mass and lymph node biopsy may be indicated.

Many conditions (see **Box 1**) and medications can lead to comorbid autoimmune cytopenias. If possible, the primary goal is to treat the underlying cause of the autoimmunity. Patients with SLE with autoimmune cytopenias should be treated with medications active against other SLE disease manifestations. Patients with CVID often respond to increasing the dose of IVIgG replacement dosing from 400 mg/kg every 3 to 4 weeks to treatment dosing (800–1000 mg/kg every 3–4 weeks). Often, there are not disease-specific medications, and patients with secondary autoimmune cytopenia syndromes are treated similarly to patients with primary disease. It is beyond the scope of this article to discuss all of these conditions in detail; however, ALPS is described in detail as an example of how understanding disease biology can lead to better therapeutic options.

Patients who undergo solid organ transplant or HSCT rarely develop autoimmune cytopenias, a serious complication because these patients are often refractory to standard treatments and escalating immune suppression can increase the risk of opportunistic infection. Because transplant patients who develop immune cytopenias can be difficult to treat, aggressive multi-agent therapy, including rituximab, is often used.[43,44] In addition, the trigger in many patients is calcineurin inhibitor–mediated immune dysregulation. In this case, an effective treatment strategy can be to move to alternative immune suppression, such as sirolimus.[45,46]

ALPS

ALPS is a rare disorder of abnormal lymphocyte survival caused by dysregulation of the FAS apoptotic pathway (**Fig. 1**).[47] Normally, as part of the downregulation of the immune response, activated B and T lymphocytes upregulate Fas, and activated

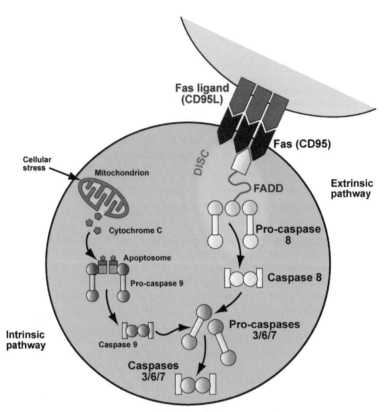

Fig. 1. Fas apoptotic pathway. Normally, as part of the downregulation of the immune response, activated B and T lymphocytes upregulate FAS and activated T lymphocytes upregulate FAS-ligand. These lymphocytes interact and trigger the caspase cascade, leading to proteolysis, DNA degradation, and apoptosis. This FAS-mediated pathway is part of the extrinsic apoptotic pathway. In contrast, mitochondrial-induced apoptosis after cellular stress is part of the intrinsic apoptotic pathway. Patients with ALPS have a defect in the FAS apoptotic pathway, leading to abnormal lymphocyte survival. (*Courtesy of* Sue Seif.)

T lymphocytes upregulate Fas ligand. Fas and Fas ligand interact to trigger the caspase cascade, leading to proteolysis, DNA degradation, and apoptosis. Patients with ALPS have a defect in this apoptotic pathway, leading to abnormal lymphocyte survival and subsequent lymphoproliferation, autoimmune disease, and cancer.[48] ALPS is classified by mutation type: germline mutations in *FAS* (ALPS-FAS) occur in 70% of patients; somatic mutations in *FAS* limited to the double-negative T cells (DNT) compartment (see later discussion; ALPS-sFAS) occur in 10%; rare patients have mutated *FASL* or *CASP10*, and approximately 20% have no identifiable genetic abnormality (ALPS-U).[49,50]

Most patients with ALPS present at a young age (median age 11.5 months).[51] Lymphoproliferation is ubiquitous and presents as lymphadenopathy, splenomegaly, or hepatomegaly, ranging from mild to massive. Lymphadenopathy rarely requires medical intervention; however, some patients have organ compromise from bulky disease, and others develop splenic sequestration. Autoimmunity is the second most common clinical manifestation, affecting more than 70% of patients; these disease manifestations most commonly require medical intervention. Most commonly seen are mild to severe autoimmune cytopenias affecting 1 or more cell lineages. Some patients require treatment of periodic disease flares after infections, and others need chronic therapy. Similar to SLE, patients with ALPS can also develop autoimmune disease affecting virtually any organ system.[52] Patients with ALPS may have an increased risk of secondary cancers, most commonly EBER+ non-Hodgkin lymphoma.[53] This risk is approximately 5% to 10% and is most common in patients with *FAS* mutations.

Until recently, in order for a patient to be diagnosed with ALPS, the patient had to meet 3 mandatory diagnostic criteria: (1) chronic nonmalignant lymphoproliferation (lymphadenopathy or splenomegaly >6 months); (2) increased peripheral blood DNTs; and (3) in vitro evidence of defective Fas-mediated apoptosis. These diagnostic criteria were revised in 2010 based on an international consensus conference.[49] The first 2 criteria continue to be mandatory under the new diagnostic algorithm. All patients with ALPS have increased peripheral blood DNTs, T cells that are CD3+/CD4−/CD8− and are positive for T-cell receptor α/β.[54] The third criterion, Fas-mediated apoptosis testing, is still used for diagnosis in some patients; however, it is not needed for most patients. This testing is labor intensive and performed in only a few specialized laboratories in the world. In addition, this testing is negative in the second most common form of ALPS: ALPS-sFAS.[50] Most patients can be diagnosed with genetic testing or by measuring biomarkers that are highly predictive of ALPS, including increased levels of vitamin B_{12}, interleukin 10 (IL-10), soluble Fas ligand (sFASL), and IL-18 or a combination of hypergammaglobulinemia and autoimmune cytopenias.[55,56]

The new diagnostic algorithm (**Box 2**) categorizes ALPS as definitive or probable.[49] Definitive ALPS is defined as meeting the 2 required criteria of lymphoproliferation and increased DNTs with either a genetic mutation in an ALPS causative gene or defective FAS-mediated apoptosis in vitro. Probable ALPS is defined as meeting the 2 required criteria and the presence of a biomarker, positive family history, or histopathologic finding of ALPS. Patients with probable and definitive ALPS should be counseled that they have ALPS and subsequently managed using the same approaches, with the probable distinction used only for consistency in the medical literature and for clinical trials.

Corticosteroids are the first-line agent of choice for acute flares.[57] ALPS is a chronic disease, and many patients need chronic treatment. IVIgG is usually ineffective in ALPS except for patients with single-lineage autoimmune thrombocytopenia.[58] The second-line therapies most commonly used in idiopathic ES, rituximab and splenectomy, are relatively contraindicated in ALPS.[59,60] Thus, it is important to distinguish ES from ALPS. Patients with ALPS who undergo splenectomy have a markedly increased lifetime risk of pneumococcal sepsis ($\sim$30%) even with vaccination and antimicrobial prophylaxis.[58,61] Rituximab can be useful in treating cytopenias in ALPS, but some patients never recover B-cell function, leading to lifelong IVIgG replacement.[62]

The 2 most commonly used second-line therapies for ALPS are MMF (Cellcept) and sirolimus (rapamycin, Rapamune). MMF has been shown to be effective in improving autoimmune cytopenias in approximately 80% of patients with ALPS based on clinical trial results from the National Institutes of Health.[63] Although many patients respond, these were frequently partial responses; some patients needed continued corticosteroid treatment, and some patients relapsed. MMF is not effective against lymphoproliferation and does not reduce DNTs. We have studied the activity of the mTOR inhibitor sirolimus in ALPS. We hypothesized that targeting the PI3K/Akt/mTOR

Box 2
ALPS diagnostic criteria

Old diagnostic criteria (before 2010)

Required

1. Chronic (>6 months) nonmalignant lymphoproliferation (lymphadenopathy or splenomegaly)

2. Increased DNTs in peripheral blood

3. Laboratory evidence of defective Fas-mediated apoptosis in vitro

New diagnostic criteria

Required

1. Chronic nonmalignant lymphoproliferation

2. Increased DNTs in peripheral blood

Accessory

  Primary

  1. Laboratory evidence of defective Fas-mediated apoptosis (on 2 separate assays)

  2. Mutation in ALPS causative gene (FAS, FASL, CASP10) (somatic or germline)

  Secondary

  1. Increased biomarkers (one or more of the following)

     a. Plasma or serum vitamin B_{12} level greater than 1500 ng/L

     b. Plasma sFASL level greater than 200 pg/mL

     c. Plasma IL-10 level greater than 20 pg/mL

     d. Plasma IL-18 level greater than 500 pg/mL

  2. Histopathologic findings on biopsy consistent with ALPS

  3. Autoimmune cytopenias and polyclonal hypergammaglobulinemia

  4. Family history of ALPS or nonmalignant lymphoproliferation

Definitive diagnosis: both required criteria plus 1 primary accessory criteria.
Probable diagnosis: both required criteria plus 1 secondary accessory criteria.
Patients with probable and definitive ALPS should be treated the same.

---

signaling pathway with sirolimus would be effective in ALPS. We tested this hypothesis first in a murine model and found rapid improvement in all disease manifestations and superior activity compared with other drugs, including MMF.[64] Abnormal DNTs were eliminated and other lymphocyte subsets were relatively spared. Furthermore, the PI3K/Akt/mTOR signaling pathway was abnormally activated in the DNT compartment, suggesting that sirolimus is a targeted therapy for the disease (David Teachey, 2013, unpublished data). Based on these results, we currently have an open clinical trial of sirolimus in pediatric ALPS (NCT00392951). The results of the first cohort of 5 patients have been published.[65] Most patients in the clinical trial (as well as 50 international patients for whom we have assisted with sirolimus management) had a rapid, complete, and durable response with resolution of autoimmune cytopenias and other autoimmune disease manifestations and elimination of lymphoproliferation and DNTs, results confirmed by other groups.[66,67] Most children were refractory to or intolerant of other therapies, including MMF.

Table 2
Immunosuppressive agents used for childhood autoimmune cytopenias and association with progressive multifocal leukoencephalopathy (PML)

Drugs Associated With PML	Drugs Not Associated With PML
Azathioprine	Everolimus
Cyclosporine	Methotrexate
Cyclophosphamide	Sirolimus
MMF	
Rituximab	
Tacrolimus	

Data from Schmedt N, Andersohn F, Garbe E. Signals of progressive multifocal leukoencephalopathy for immunosuppressants: a disproportionality analysis of spontaneous reports within the US Adverse Event Reporting System (AERS). Pharmacoepidemiol Drug Saf 2012;21:1216–20.

Box 3
Immune modulators for autoimmune cytopenias

Corticosteroids (prednisone and dexamethasone)

Mechanism of action: (multifactorial) downregulates inflammatory cytokine production at transcriptional and translational level; decreases leukocyte trafficking, including neutrophil migration; decreases dendritic cells; depletes T cells and B cells (T>>B); also, affects T-lineage commitment[70]

Lymphocytes targeted: B, T, natural killer cells, monocytes, macrophages, neutrophils, and eosinophils

Pros: most active drug for most patients with autoimmune cytopenias; fast acting; ability to titrate dose to response; lots of data on its use in combination with other drugs

Cons: short-term toxicities: mild (hypertension, hyperglycemia, irritability, weight gain); long-term toxicities: potentially severe (avascular necrosis, cataracts, growth delay)

Infectious risk: single-agent: low; combination therapy: higher risk than most other oral agents; pneumocystis pneumonia prophylaxis should be strongly considered when steroids combined with other immune suppressants; antifungal prophylaxis may also be needed

IVIgG

Mechanism of action: (multifactorial); poorly defined but proposed hypotheses include[71]

1. Competition with pathogenic IgGs for activating FcγRs (neonatal Fc receptor)

2. Saturation of FcRn by very high levels of IgG leads to breakdown of pathogenic IgGs

3. Exogenous IgG binds to targets cells, which triggers effector cells to downregulate immune response

Pros: active against ITP in most patients; well tolerated; quick acting (<48 hours)

Cons: short duration of activity; patients with chronic disease may need frequent retreatment; limited activity against AIHA or AIN; aseptic meningitis and severe allergic reactions

Infectious risk: none with current products; protective against certain infections

Anti-D immunoglobulin (anti-D)[72]

Mechanism of action: works only in patients who are Rh+ by saturating FcγRs in spleen

Pros: active against ITP in a most patients; well tolerated; quick acting (<48 hours)

Cons: may cause hemolytic anemia; recommended only for children with ITP who are Rh+, have a negative DAT, no anemia, and have not undergone splenectomy[6]; can also cause headache, fever, and chills; rarely, can cause life-threatening disseminated intravascular coagulation (DIC); not for children with AIHA or AIN

Infectious risk: none reported

TREATMENT OF SINGLE-LINEAGE AND MULTI-LINEAGE AUTOIMMUNE CYTOPENIAS

As mentioned earlier, the treatment of autoimmune cytopenias is heterogeneous and complex. Until recently, options were limited, and the initial management for patients with acute or chronic disease, single-lineage or multi-lineage, and primary or secondary disease was IVIgG or corticosteroids followed by splenectomy for intolerant or refractory patients. Recently, this paradigm has added rituximab early into therapy for many patients. Next-line treatments varied widely because of the lack of randomized trials and preclinical data, preventing disease-specific target identification. As described earlier with TPO-RAs in ITP and sirolimus in ALPS, disease biology can often lead to superior therapies. The genomic age may lead to a better understanding of the biology of autoimmune cytopenias.

Box 4
Monoclonal antibodies for autoimmune cytopenias

Rituximab[73]

Mechanism of action: anti-CD20 monoclonal antibody

Lymphocytes targeted: B cells

Pros: very active drug for many patients with autoimmune cytopenias; studied in randomized trials; does not require a patient to take daily medication

Cons: very long half-life, with B-cell depletion lasting up to a year in most patients; thus, nonresponders have continued B-cell depletion yet no benefit

Infectious risk: single-agent: low; risk of viral reactivation

Alemtuzumab (Campath)

Mechanism of action: anti-CD52 monoclonal antibody

Lymphocytes targeted: B, T, and natural killer cells

Pros: very active against many autoimmune diseases, including cytopenias

Cons: limited data for childhood idiopathic autoimmune cytopenias (most of the data in adults with autoimmune cytopenias secondary to chronic lymphocytic leukemia); very long half-life with B, T, and natural killer depletion lasting many months; very high infectious risk; no consistent recommendations on best dose or schedule; can be immunoablative at high doses, requiring stem cell rescue for immune recovery

Infectious risk: very high as a single-agent; risk of viral and fungal infections; prophylactic antifungal and antiviral medications should be considered; routine viral monitoring needed especially for cytomegalovirus reactivation; consider IVIgG replacement therapy

Antithymocyte globulin (ATG) and antilymphocyte globulin (ALG)

Mechanism of action: horse (ATG) or rabbit (ALG) antibodies against human T cells

Lymphocytes targeted: T cells

Pros: very active against many autoimmune diseases, including cytopenias

Cons: limited data on childhood idiopathic or secondary autoimmune cytopenias; most data anecdotal; however, numerous studies showing activity in autoimmune aplastic anemia and for prevention and treatment of graft-versus-host disease in children; high infectious risk; long half-life; severe infusional toxicities and risk for serum sickness

Infectious risk: high. Largely unknown as single-agent because most commonly combined with other drugs. Pneumocystis pneumonia, antifungal, and antiviral prophylaxis should be considered, especially if combined with other agents

Medication choice is often based on the experience of the practicing physician instead of evidence or biological rationale. In addition, there are considerable misconceptions surrounding the safety of several oral immune suppressants. Drugs such as MMF, sirolimus, tacrolimus, and mercaptopurine are often used as part of a multi-agent immunosuppressant backbone after organ or marrow transplant or as a part of a chemotherapy regimen for lymphoid malignancies. The risk of infection is markedly higher with multi-agent therapy compared with single-agent therapy. Some practitioners falsely assume that these drugs are more immunosuppressive and carry a higher infectious risk than corticosteroids. The posttransplant literature has clearly established that the agents most likely to predispose to opportunistic infection are corticosteroids.[68,69] Chronic corticosteroid use also has significant long-term morbidity, especially on bone health, because its use leads to osteoporosis and

---

Box 5
Antimetabolites for autoimmune cytopenias

Purine analogues (mercaptopurine [6MP], azathioprine, and thioguanine)

Mechanism of action: inhibits purine synthesis; azathioprine is metabolized into 6MP; this class of drugs also includes fludarabine, pentostatin, and cladribine; however, these are almost never used for autoimmune cytopenias in children

Lymphocytes targeted: B, T, and natural killer cells

Pros: well-tolerated agents with proven activity in children; numerous studies on childhood cancer have shown can be safely combined with other drugs

Cons: often takes 1 to 3 months for response[74,75]; polymorphisms in the enzyme thiopurine methyltransferase (TPMT) can lead to decreased activity of enzyme, inability to metabolize the drugs and markedly increased toxicity; can cause myelosuppression and hepatic toxicity

Infectious risk: single-agent low except in patients with absent TPMT activity

Methotrexate

Mechanism of action: inhibits folate synthesis, which is needed for thymidine synthesis; inhibits purine metabolism

Lymphocytes targeted: B, T, and natural killer cells (T>B)

Pros: well-tolerated agent with proven activity in children, especially in children with rheumatologic autoimmune diseases with secondary autoimmune cytopenias; can be given by oral, subcutaneous injection, or intravenous route; numerous studies in childhood cancer have shown can be safely combined with other drugs

Cons: dose-dependent myelosuppression, liver, neurologic, and renal toxicity; these side effects rare if dosed for autoimmune diseases (compared with dosing for cancer)

Infectious risk: single-agent low when dosed for autoimmune diseases

MMF

Mechanism of action: inhibits iosine monophosphate dehydrogenase in purine synthesis

Lymphocytes targeted: B, T, and natural killer cells

Pros: well tolerated with proven activity in children

Cons: often results in partial responses; side effects include diarrhea and neutropenia

Infectious risk: single-agent low; recently, the US Food and Drug Administration released a black-box warning because of the risk of progressive multifocal leukoencephalopathy; prescribers now need Risk Evaluation and Mitigation Strategies certification because of potential risks to the fetus in pregnant women

avascular necrosis. Among oral immune suppressants, the degree of immune suppression varies, as is shown by development of progressive multifocal leukoence-phalopathy with some drugs but not others (**Table 2**).

Rituximab has been shown to be effective against autoimmune cytopenias in several trials, as described earlier. Whether it is a better drug than the myriad of available oral immune suppressants is not known, and, based on the rarity and heterogeneity of childhood autoimmune cytopenia syndromes, it is unlikely that there will be randomized trials for many of these drugs. This situation raises the question: how should the child who fails standard front-line therapy be treated? One approach is to tailor the therapy based on response to medication. A patient who has no response to rituximab should be approached differently from a patient who has a partial response yet is unable to wean off corticosteroids or a patient who has a complete response and relapses 1 year later. Rituximab exclusively targets B cells. If a patient has no response to rituximab, it is likely that B cells are not the principal driver of the autoimmune disease, and T-cell–directed therapy, for example with a calcineurin inhibitor, could be considered. In contrast, the patient with a partial response to rituximab may benefit from a drug that suppresses both B and T cells, such as MMF.

Box 6
Signaling pathway inhibitors for autoimmune cytopenias

Calcineurin Inhibitors

Tacrolimus and cyclosporine (CSA)

Mechanism of action: prevents T-cell activation and cytokine release by inhibiting calcineurin; calcinuerin normally dephosphorylates the nuclear factor of activated T cells

Lymphocytes targeted: T cells only

Pros: well tolerated; anecdotal reports showing activity in childhood autoimmune cytopenias

Cons: can cause autoimmune cytopenias and microangiopathic hemolytic anemia (MAH); CSA has more side effects than tacrolimus and it is not more effective; nephrotoxic; can cause seizures from combination of hypomagnesemia and hypertension; requires therapeutic drug monitoring

Infectious risk: single-agent low; consider Pneumocystis pneumonia prophylaxis

mTOR Inhibitors

Sirolimus (rapamycin)

Mechanism of action: targets mTORC1 complex in PI3K/Akt/mTOR signaling pathway; other mTOR inhibitors, including everolimus, are being studied in autoimmune disease

Lymphocytes targeted: B and T cells; spares Tregs

Pros: well tolerated; very active in ALPS-associated autoimmune cytopenias; proven activity and arguably treatment of choice for post–solid organ transplant autoimmune cytopenias; least potential for secondary cancers with chronic use based on preclinical data; one of a few immune suppressants shown not to be associated with progressive multifocal leukoencephalopathy

Cons: requires therapeutic drug monitoring; significant drug-drug interactions; has few side effects; however, inhibits endothelial and epithelial healing and tends to magnify the side effects of other drugs; for example, does not cause MAH; however, when combined with drugs that cause MAH (eg, calcineurin inhibitors), greatly increases the risk over the other drug alone; can cause mucositis and hyperlipidemia

Infectious risk: single-agent very low; may have activity against Epstein-Barr virus, cytomegalovirus, and fungi

---

Box 7
Cytotoxic chemotherapeutics for autoimmune cytopenias

Cyclophosphamide

  Mechanism of action: alkylates DNA

  Lymphocytes targeted: B, T and natural killer cells; eliminates Tregs

  Pros: long and established track record of use in rheumatologic autoimmune disease, including autoimmune cytopenias

  Cons: toxicity (dose dependent); short-term: myelosuppression, GI toxicity, alopecia; long-term: associated with increased risk of monosomy 7 (AML) or myelodysplastic syndrome/acute myeloid leukemia; infertility in men; duration of response often limited to a few months

  Infectious risk: dose dependent; low risk with doses used commonly for autoimmune disease; very high risk with myeloablative dosing

Vincristine and vinblastine

  Mechanism of action: mitotic inhibitor

  Lymphocytes targeted: B, T, and natural killer cells

  Pros: long and established track record of use and documented efficacy

  Cons: infrequently used because of development of newer agents; side effects for vincristine include neuropathy and constipation; side effects for vinblastine include myelosuppression, GI toxicity, and alopecia; duration of response often limited to a few months

  Infectious risk: low with monotherapy; higher when combined with other drugs

---

Box 8
Other therapies for autoimmune cytopenias

Splenectomy[76]

  Mechanism of action: removes main site of platelet destruction and site of antiplatelet antibody production

  Lymphocytes targeted: not applicable

  Pros: curative in most patients with ITP; often effective in AIHA; well-characterized risks; does not affect fertility or harm fetus if pregnant

  Cons: removing a healthy organ and cannot predict who will respond; not very effective for AIN, or multi-lineage cytopenias; risk of infection with encapsulated organisms; increased risk of venous thromboembolism and artherosclerosis (?); increased risk of portal hypertension and pulmonary arterial hypertension

  Infectious risk: encapsulated organisms; relatively contraindicated in patients with ALPS

TPO mimetics (TPO-RAS, romiplostim and eltrombopag)[76]

  Mechanism of action: agonists for TPO receptor, the major regulator of megakaryocytopoiesis and platelet formation

  Lymphocytes targeted: not applicable

  Pros: only second-line agent studied in randomized placebo-controlled trials (adults) showing clear efficacy; high rates of response and most durable

  Cons: likely need long-term chronic treatment; abrupt discontinuation of drug can cause rebound thrombocytopenia; theoretic risk of bone marrow fibrosis and leukemic transformation; increased risk of venous thromboembolism; eltrombopag is hepatotoxic

  Infectious risk: none

HSCT[77–79]

Mechanism of action: allogeneic replaces all blood-producing cells with donor cells; mechanism of activity of autologous HSCT may be secondary to intensive immune suppression or because of immune reset

Lymphocytes targeted: all

Pros: can be curative

Cons: very toxic; ~10% to 50% mortality and significant morbidity; often ineffective ~50% response rates; should be reserved for patients with severe and refractory autoimmune cytopenias and proven success; most commonly used for secondary autoimmune cytopenias (immune deficiency, cancer, some lymphoproliferative disorders, some rheumatologic conditions); can worsen autoimmune disease

Infections: extremely high risk; bacteria, fungi, viruses, others

Plasmapheresis

Mechanism of action: mechanical plasma filtration to remove antibodies

Lymphocytes targeted: not applicable

Pros: very rapid onset; effective for IgG-mediated autoimmune cytopenias

Cons: improvements short-lived and often see relapse after stopping; often used in conjunction with immune suppression; requires central venous catheters in young children; limited activity against IgM-mediated disease; hypotension, hypocalcemia; removes beneficial antibodies too and medications

Infections: biggest risk is from the central line

Mercaptopurine and azathioprine are metabolized into the same active compound. Accordingly, it is likely ineffective to use mercaptopurine in a patient who fails azathioprine. Some agents require therapeutic drug monitoring, whereas others do not. Toxicity profiles are vastly different between agents and should be considered in the context of each patient's comorbidities. Some agents take time to be effective, occasionally up to 2 to 3 months. Thus, time and patience are a must and patients should be given a chance to respond to a new drug before switching therapies. **Boxes 3–8** list and describe the various immunosuppressive compounds that have been used to treat autoimmune cytopenias. A basic understanding of the drugs, their mechanism of action, the cells targeted, and the side effects of the drugs can help a clinician make rational choices when it comes to choosing the best agent to use for a given patient.

SUMMARY

The diagnosis, management, and treatment of childhood autoimmune cytopenias can be complex. The past 10 years have seen the discovery and use of new agents that have improved efficacy. The genomic era will certainly lead to novel insights into disease biology, allowing for the rational selection of targeted therapies, better determination of which patients need treatment, and improved prediction of which patients will have short-term disease.

REFERENCES

1. Neunert CE, Buchanan GR, Imbach P, et al. Severe hemorrhage in children with newly diagnosed immune thrombocytopenic purpura. Blood 2008;112:4003–8.

2. McMillan R. Antiplatelet antibodies in chronic immune thrombocytopenia and their role in platelet destruction and defective platelet production. Hematol Oncol Clin North Am 2009;23:1163–75.
3. Yazdanbakhsh K, Zhong H, Bao W. Immune dysregulation in immune thrombocytopenia. Semin Hematol 2013;50(Suppl 1):S63–7.
4. Bussel JB, Kuter DJ. New thrombopoietic agents: introduction. Semin Hematol 2010;47:211.
5. Rodeghiero F, Stasi R, Gernsheimer T, et al. Standardization of terminology, definitions and outcome criteria in immune thrombocytopenic purpura of adults and children: report from an international working group. Blood 2009;113:2386–93.
6. Neunert C, Lim W, Crowther M, et al. The American Society of Hematology 2011 evidence-based practice guideline for immune thrombocytopenia. Blood 2011;117:4190–207.
7. Aronis S, Platokouki H, Avgeri M, et al. Retrospective evaluation of long-term efficacy and safety of splenectomy in chronic idiopathic thrombocytopenic purpura in children. Acta Paediatr 2004;93:638–42.
8. Patel VL, Mahevas M, Lee SY, et al. Outcomes 5 years after response to rituximab therapy in children and adults with immune thrombocytopenia. Blood 2012;119:5989–95.
9. Hedlund-Treutiger I, Henter JI, Elinder G, et al. Randomized study of IVIg and high-dose dexamethasone therapy for children with chronic idiopathic thrombocytopenic purpura. J Pediatr Hematol Oncol 2003;25:139–44.
10. Kaushansky K, Lok S, Holly RD, et al. Promotion of megakaryocyte progenitor expansion and differentiation by the c-Mpl ligand thrombopoietin. Nature 1994;369:568–71.
11. Vadhan-Raj S, Murray LJ, Bueso-Ramos C, et al. Stimulation of megakaryocyte and platelet production by a single-dose of recombinant human thrombopoietin in patients with cancer. Ann Intern Med 1997;126:673–81.
12. Li J, Yang C, Xia Y, et al. Thrombocytopenia caused by the development of antibodies to thrombopoietin. Blood 2001;98:3241–8.
13. Arnold DM, Nazi I, Kelton JG. New treatments for idiopathic thrombocytopenic purpura: rethinking old hypotheses. Expert Opin Investig Drugs 2009;18:805–19.
14. Bussel JB, Buchanan GR, Nugent DJ, et al. A randomized, double-blind study of romiplostim to determine its safety and efficacy in children with immune thrombocytopenia. Blood 2011;118:28–36.
15. Letsky EA, Greaves M. Guidelines on the investigation and management of thrombocytopenia in pregnancy and neonatal alloimmune thrombocytopenia. Maternal and Neonatal Haemostasis Working Party of the Haemostasis and Thrombosis Task Force of the British Society for Haematology. Br J Haematol 1996;95:21–6.
16. Roberts IA. The changing face of haemolytic disease of the newborn. Early Hum Dev 2008;84:515–23.
17. Seve P, Philippe P, Dufour JF, et al. Autoimmune hemolytic anemia: classification and therapeutic approaches. Expert Rev Hematol 2008;1:189–204.
18. Bussel JB, Cunningham-Rundles C, Abraham C. Intravenous treatment of autoimmune hemolytic anemia with very high dose gammaglobulin. Vox Sang 1986;51:264–9.
19. Petz LD. Treatment of autoimmune hemolytic anemias. Curr Opin Hematol 2001;8:411–6.

20. Michel M. Classification and therapeutic approaches in autoimmune hemolytic anemia: an update. Expert Rev Hematol 2011;4:607–18.
21. Chertkow G, Dacie JV. Results of splenectomy in auto-immune haemolytic anaemia. Br J Haematol 1956;2:237–49.
22. Pignon JM, Poirson E, Rochant H. Danazol in autoimmune haemolytic anaemia. Br J Haematol 1993;83:343–5.
23. Berentsen S. How I manage cold agglutinin disease. Br J Haematol 2011;153: 309–17.
24. Petz LD. Cold antibody autoimmune hemolytic anemias. Blood Rev 2008;22: 1–15.
25. Maheshwari A, Christensen RD, Calhoun DA. Immune-mediated neutropenia in the neonate. Acta Paediatr 2002;91:98–103.
26. Bussel JB, Abboud MR. Autoimmune neutropenia of childhood. Crit Rev Oncol Hematol 1987;7:37–51.
27. Bruin MC, von dem Borne AE, Tamminga RY, et al. Neutrophil antibody specificity in different types of childhood autoimmune neutropenia. Blood 1999;94: 1797–802.
28. Capsoni F, Sarzi-Puttini P, Zanella A. Primary and secondary autoimmune neutropenia. Arthritis Res Ther 2005;7:208–14.
29. Bux J, Behrens G, Jaeger G, et al. Diagnosis and clinical course of autoimmune neutropenia in infancy: analysis of 240 cases. Blood 1998;91:181–6.
30. Bux J, Chapman J. Report on the second international granulocyte serology workshop. Transfusion 1997;37:977–83.
31. Mathew P, Chen G, Wang W. Evans syndrome: results of a national survey. J Pediatr Hematol Oncol 1997;19:433–7.
32. Wang WC. Evans syndrome in childhood: pathophysiology, clinical course, and treatment. Am J Pediatr Hematol Oncol 1988;10:330–8.
33. Seif AE, Manno CS, Sheen C, et al. Identifying autoimmune lymphoproliferative syndrome in children with Evans syndrome: a multi-institutional study. Blood 2010;115:2142–5.
34. Savasan S, Warrier I, Ravindranath Y. The spectrum of Evans' syndrome. Arch Dis Child 1997;77:245–8.
35. Aladjidi N, Leverger G, Leblanc T, et al. New insights into childhood autoimmune hemolytic anemia: a French national observational study of 265 children. Haematologica 2011;96:655–63.
36. Miescher PA, Tucci A, Beris P, et al. Autoimmune hemolytic anemia and/or thrombocytopenia associated with lupus parameters. Semin Hematol 1992;29:13–7.
37. Teachey DT, Manno CS, Axsom KM, et al. Unmasking Evans syndrome: T-cell phenotype and apoptotic response reveal autoimmune lymphoproliferative syndrome (ALPS). Blood 2005;105:2443–8.
38. Savasan S, Warrier I, Buck S, et al. Increased lymphocyte Fas expression and high incidence of common variable immunodeficiency disorder in childhood Evans' syndrome. Clin Immunol 2007;125:224–9.
39. Heeney MM, Zimmerman SA, Ware RE. Childhood autoimmune cytopenia secondary to unsuspected common variable immunodeficiency. J Pediatr 2003; 143:662–5.
40. George JN, Woolf SH, Raskob GE, et al. Idiopathic thrombocytopenic purpura: a practice guideline developed by explicit methods for the American Society of Hematology. Blood 1996;88:3–40.
41. Bader-Meunier B, Aladjidi N, Bellmann F, et al. Rituximab therapy for childhood Evans syndrome. Haematologica 2007;92:1691–4.

42. Rao A, Kelly M, Musselman M, et al. Safety, efficacy, and immune reconstitution after rituximab therapy in pediatric patients with chronic or refractory hematologic autoimmune cytopenias. Pediatr Blood Cancer 2008;50:822–5.
43. Miloh T, Arnon R, Roman E, et al. Autoimmune hemolytic anemia and idiopathic thrombocytopenic purpura in pediatric solid organ transplant recipients, report of five cases and review of the literature. Pediatr Transplant 2011;15:870–8.
44. Li M, Goldfinger D, Yuan S. Autoimmune hemolytic anemia in pediatric liver or combined liver and small bowel transplant patients: a case series and review of the literature. Transfusion 2012;52:48–54.
45. Acquazzino MA, Fischer RT, Langnas A, et al. Refractory autoimmune hemolytic anemia after intestinal transplant responding to conversion from a calcineurin to mTOR inhibitor. Pediatr Transplant 2013;17(5):466–71.
46. Teachey DT, Jubelirer T, Baluarte HJ, et al. Treatment with sirolimus ameliorates tacrolimus-induced autoimmune cytopenias after solid organ transplant. Pediatr Blood Cancer 2009;53:1114–6.
47. Rieux-Laucat F, Le Deist F, Fischer A. Autoimmune lymphoproliferative syndromes: genetic defects of apoptosis pathways. Cell Death Differ 2003;10: 124–33.
48. Bleesing JJ. Autoimmune lymphoproliferative syndrome: a genetic disorder of abnormal lymphocyte apoptosis. Immunol Allergy Clin 2002;22:339–49.
49. Oliveira JB, Bleesing JJ, Dianzani U, et al. Revised diagnostic criteria and classification for the autoimmune lymphoproliferative syndrome (ALPS): report from the 2009 NIH International Workshop. Blood 2010;116:e35–40.
50. Holzelova E, Vonarbourg C, Stolzenberg MC, et al. Autoimmune lymphoproliferative syndrome with somatic Fas mutations. N Engl J Med 2004;351:1409–18.
51. Jackson CE, Puck JM. Autoimmune lymphoproliferative syndrome, a disorder of apoptosis. Curr Opin Pediatr 1999;11:521–7.
52. Sneller MC, Wang J, Dale JK, et al. Clinical, immunologic, and genetic features of an autoimmune lymphoproliferative syndrome associated with abnormal lymphocyte apoptosis. Blood 1997;89:1341–8.
53. Straus SE, Jaffe ES, Puck JM, et al. The development of lymphomas in families with autoimmune lymphoproliferative syndrome with germline Fas mutations and defective lymphocyte apoptosis. Blood 2001;98:194–200.
54. Bleesing JJ, Brown MR, Dale JK, et al. TcR-alpha/beta(+) CD4(-)CD8(-) T cells in humans with the autoimmune lymphoproliferative syndrome express a novel CD45 isoform that is analogous to murine B220 and represents a marker of altered O-glycan biosynthesis. Clin Immunol 2001;100:314–24.
55. Magerus-Chatinet A, Stolzenberg MC, Loffredo MS, et al. FAS-L, IL-10, and double-negative CD4- CD8- TCR alpha/beta+ T cells are reliable markers of autoimmune lymphoproliferative syndrome (ALPS) associated with FAS loss of function. Blood 2009;113:3027–30.
56. Caminha I, Fleisher TA, Hornung RL, et al. Using biomarkers to predict the presence of FAS mutations in patients with features of the autoimmune lymphoproliferative syndrome. J Allergy Clin Immunol 2010;125:946–9.e6.
57. Bleesing JJ, Straus SE, Fleisher TA. Autoimmune lymphoproliferative syndrome. A human disorder of abnormal lymphocyte survival. Pediatr Clin North Am 2000; 47:1291–310.
58. Rao VK, Oliveira JB. How I treat autoimmune lymphoproliferative syndrome. Blood 2011;118(22):5741–51.
59. Teachey DT. Autoimmune lymphoproliferative syndrome: new approaches to diagnosis and management. Clin Adv Hematol Oncol 2011;9:233–5.

60. Teachey DT. New advances in the diagnosis and treatment of autoimmune lymphoproliferative syndrome. Curr Opin Pediatr 2012;24:1–8.

61. Neven B, Magerus-Chatinet A, Florkin B, et al. A survey of 90 patients with autoimmune lymphoproliferative syndrome related to TNFRSF6 mutation. Blood 2011;118(18):4798–807.

62. Rao VK, Price S, Perkins K, et al. Use of rituximab for refractory cytopenias associated with autoimmune lymphoproliferative syndrome (ALPS). Pediatr Blood Cancer 2009;52:847–52.

63. Rao VK, Dugan F, Dale JK, et al. Use of mycophenolate mofetil for chronic, refractory immune cytopenias in children with autoimmune lymphoproliferative syndrome. Br J Haematol 2005;129:534–8.

64. Teachey DT, Obzut D, Axsom KM, et al. Rapamycin improves lymphoproliferative disease in murine autoimmune lymphoproliferative syndrome (ALPS). Blood 2006;108(6):1965–71.

65. Teachey DT, Greiner R, Seif A, et al. Treatment with sirolimus results in complete responses in patients with autoimmune lymphoproliferative syndrome. Br J Haematol 2009;145:101–6.

66. Janic MD, Brasanac CD, Jankovic JS, et al. Rapid regression of lymphadenopathy upon rapamycin treatment in a child with autoimmune lymphoproliferative syndrome. Pediatr Blood Cancer 2009;53:1117–9.

67. Tommasini A, Valencic E, Piscianz E, et al. Immunomodulatory drugs in autoimmune lymphoproliferative syndrome (ALPS). Pediatr Blood Cancer 2012;58:310 [author reply: 311].

68. Mikulska M, Raiola AM, Bruno B, et al. Risk factors for invasive aspergillosis and related mortality in recipients of allogeneic SCT from alternative donors: an analysis of 306 patients. Bone Marrow Transplant 2009;44:361–70.

69. Bodro M, Sabe N, Gomila A, et al. Risk factors, clinical characteristics, and outcomes of invasive fungal infections in solid organ transplant recipients. Transplant Proc 2012;44:2682–5.

70. Van Molle W, Libert C. How glucocorticoids control their own strength and the balance between pro- and anti-inflammatory mediators. Eur J Immunol 2005; 35:3396–9.

71. Nimmerjahn F, Ravetch JV. The antiinflammatory activity of IgG: the intravenous IgG paradox. J Exp Med 2007;204:11–5.

72. Despotovic JM, Lambert MP, Herman JH, et al. RhIG for the treatment of immune thrombocytopenia: consensus and controversy (CME). Transfusion 2012;52:1126–36 [quiz: 1125].

73. Grace RF, Bennett CM, Ritchey AK, et al. Response to steroids predicts response to rituximab in pediatric chronic immune thrombocytopenia. Pediatr Blood Cancer 2012;58:221–5.

74. Boruchov DM, Gururangan S, Driscoll MC, et al. Multiagent induction and maintenance therapy for patients with refractory immune thrombocytopenic purpura (ITP). Blood 2007;110:3526–31.

75. Sobota A, Neufeld EJ, Lapsia S, et al. Response to mercaptopurine for refractory autoimmune cytopenias in children. Pediatr Blood Cancer 2009;52:80–4.

76. Ghanima W, Godeau B, Cines DB, et al. How I treat immune thrombocytopenia: the choice between splenectomy or a medical therapy as a second-line treatment. Blood 2012;120:960–9.

77. Rabusin M, Snowden JA, Veys P, et al. Long-term outcomes of hematopoietic stem cell transplantation for severe treatment-resistant autoimmune cytopenia in children. Biol Blood Marrow Transplant 2013;19:666–9.

78. Snowden JA, Pearce RM, Lee J, et al. Haematopoietic stem cell transplantation (HSCT) in severe autoimmune diseases: analysis of UK outcomes from the British Society of Blood and Marrow Transplantation (BSBMT) data registry 1997-2009. Br J Haematol 2012;157:742–6.
79. Pession A, Zama D, Masetti R, et al. Hematopoietic stem cell transplantation for curing children with severe autoimmune diseases: is this a valid option? Pediatr Transplant 2012;16:413–25.

HUS and TTP in Children

Howard Trachtman, MD

KEYWORDS

- Thrombotic microangiopathy (TMA) • Hemolytic uremic syndrome (HUS)
- Thrombotic thrombocytopenic purpura (TTP) • Shiga toxin (Stx)
- Alternative pathway of complement (APC)

KEY POINTS

- Thrombotic microangiopathy is a histopathological lesion that is present in all patients with hemolytic uremic syndrome (HUS) or thrombotic thrombocytopenic purpura.
- HUS is usually caused by antecedent infection with Shiga toxin producing strains of bacteria. Most patients recover with intensive medical care and less than 25% develop chronic kidney injury.
- Familial forms of atypical HUS are linked to genetic mutations in proteins that regulate the activity of the alternative pathway of complement. Eculizumab, a monoclonal antibody to C5a, is the standard of care for these patients.
- Thrombotic thrombocytopenic purpura is rare in children and responds well to treatment with plasmapheresis.

INTRODUCTION

Hemolytic uremic syndrome (HUS) and thrombotic thrombocytopenic purpura (TTP) are 2 rare clinical entities. They share a common underlying pathologic process termed thrombotic microangiopathy (TMA), characterized by endothelial cell injury, intravascular platelet-fibrin thrombi, and vascular damage. The 2 illnesses can occur as sporadic cases, in epidemic outbreaks, or in a genetic/familial pattern. Although HUS and TTP are orphan diseases, they remain among the most common causes of acute kidney injury (AKI) in nonhospitalized infants and children. Although most children exhibit recovery of renal function after an episode of TMA, some patients are left with permanent residual sequelae or progress to end-stage kidney disease (ESKD).

The pivotal involvement of endothelial cells in both HUS and TTP was clear from the start based on histopathological examination of biopsy and autopsy material. However, the underlying basis of these disorders remained obscure for several decades after the original description of HUS by Gasser in 1955 and TTP by Moschcowitz in 1925.[1] The landmark article by Karmali and coworkers[2] linking diarrhea-associated

Division of Nephrology, Department of Pediatrics, CTSI, NYU Langone Medical Center, 227 East 30th Street, Room #110, New York, NY 10016, USA
E-mail address: howard.trachtman@nyumc.org

Pediatr Clin N Am 60 (2013) 1513–1526
http://dx.doi.org/10.1016/j.pcl.2013.08.007
0031-3955/13/$ – see front matter © 2013 Elsevier Inc. All rights reserved.

HUS to antecedent gastrointestinal infection by strains of *Escherichia coli* that elaborate a toxin to cultured Vero cells was the first step that advanced the understanding of the cause of TMA. Subsequent studies indicated that the Vero toxin was, in fact, closely related to Shiga toxin (Stx), and were followed by studies that established a role of ADAMTS13 in the processing of von Willebrand factor (VWF) multimers. Moake and colleagues[3,4] demonstrated that TTP was caused by abnormally high levels of ultralarge VWF multimers due to congenital or acquired reductions in ADAMTS13 activity. In 1998, Warwicker and colleagues[5] confirmed a linkage of atypical HUS (aHUS) to the region on chromosome 1 that contained the genes for several complement regulatory proteins; this was followed by the sequential demonstration that mutations in factor H, factor I, membrane cofactor protein (MCP, CD46), factor B, C3, and thrombomodulin can cause familial cases of aHUS and contribute to all forms of TMA.[6,7] These advances in molecular genetics began to unravel the cause of hereditary forms of HUS and TTP and led to the development of targeted therapies for both of these causes of TMA.

Thus, there has been substantial progress in the understanding of the pathogenesis and treatment of TMA. This article focuses on both HUS and TTP, with an emphasis on HUS because it is more common than TTP in children. Several excellent reviews of diarrhea-associated HUS, aHUS, and TTP have been published in the last few years. As a consequence, this article details work done during the last decade, from 2000 to the present, and highlights key advances in diagnostic and therapeutic aspects of this fascinating group of disorders.

CLASSIFICATION

HUS and TTP are characterized by the triad of microangiopathic anemia with red blood cell fragmentation, thrombocytopenia, and AKI. TTP has the same 3 features plus the presence of fever and neurologic symptoms, creating a pentad. HUS and TTP share a histopathological phenotype called TMA. This pattern of injury is characterized by primary damage to the vascular endothelial cell. The endothelium initially becomes detached from the underlying basement membrane and the subendothelial space is filled with amorphous material and fibrin. Within the vascular lumen, there are platelet-fibrin thrombi that can occlude the vessel completely. Fibrin predominates in HUS and platelets are more prominent in patients with TTP.[8] There are 4 clinical categories of TMA, as follows:

1. Typical, diarrhea-associated HUS
2. Atypical, nonfamilial HUS
3. Atypical, familial HUS
4. TTP

In the past, episodes of HUS that developed after a prodromal gastrointestinal illness were called diarrhea-associated or D+HUS. However, in view of the close linkage between infections with Stx-producing strains of *E coli* (STEC) in most cases of HUS, the term STEC-HUS has become the preferred nomenclature for this category of TMA.[9] Clinical studies verify that episodes of STEC-HUS can be associated with significant neurologic manifestations and TTP can be triggered by gastrointestinal illnesses, suggesting overlap between these 2 illnesses. However, the distinction between the entities is now on much more solid footing because the contribution of Stx, defective regulation of the alternative complement pathway, and disordered release of VWF in STEC-HUS, aHUS, and TTP, respectively, has been well established by basic science and clinical investigations.

PATHOPHYSIOLOGY
STEC-HUS

There are 2 main variants of Stx produced by STEC. Stx2 is more likely to be associated with HUS.[10] The diarrhea and colitis that occur during the prodromal illness probably reflect direct damage to gastrointestinal cells and ischemia from the disseminated microangiopathy. When a person becomes infected with an STEC strain, bacteremia does not result. Instead, Stx is elaborated by the microorganism, crosses the gastrointestinal epithelium via a transcellular pathway, and enters the bloodstream.[11] Stx binds to polymorphonuclear leukocytes, which may enable the toxin to be delivered and unloaded in the peripheral vasculature. Neutrophil-associated Stx is detectable in 60% of patients with STEC-HUS and the amount of cell-bound toxin correlates with the extent of kidney injury.[12] After entering the circulation, Stx rapidly binds to the glycosphingolipid, globotriaosylceramide, which is found on glomerular endothelial cells, mesangial cells, podocytes, and tubular epithelial cells. It also binds to globotriaosylceramide on the endothelium in other organs, especially the brain.[10] Once Stx binds, it is internalized via a retrograde pathway to the Golgi apparatus, where it inhibits protein synthesis and causes damage to endothelial cells.[13] The intracellular trafficking of Stx is blocked by manganese and administration of this cation protects against Stx-induced disease in experimental animals.[14] The vascular damage leads to the release of thrombin and increased fibrin concentrations. In addition to the increased fibrin, increased levels of plasminogen activator inhibitor-1 block fibrinolysis and potentiate the thrombotic cycle.[10,15] Increased shear stress within occluded vessels leads to perturbations in the processing of VWF multimers with uncoiling of the molecule and fragmentation. Both of these alterations activate platelets and promote thrombus formation. Although HUS only develops in 15% of people infected, microangiopathy and microvascular thrombi occur whether or not a diagnosis of HUS is made.[10,16]

In addition to its direct effects on the endothelium, Stx induces an inflammatory response that is triggered by much lower levels of Stx than the amount needed to inhibit protein synthesis. This process includes a ribotoxic stress response, upregulation of adhesion molecules for leukocytes, and promotion of a prothrombotic state in blood vessels.[15] Stx also directly leads to the release of multiple cytokines such as interleukin-8 and fractalkine and chemokines, which contribute to cell damage.[15] Recent findings indicate that Stx increases endothelial cell expression of the chemokine receptor CXCR4 and its ligand stromal cell-derived factor 1. Specific blockade of this ligand–receptor system ameliorated STEC-HUS in mice.[17] Plasma levels of stromal cell-derived factor 1 are nearly 4-fold higher in children with STEC enteritis who progress to HUS than in children who do not.[17] Finally, there is activation of the alternative pathway of complement in children with STEC-HUS, evidenced by high circulating levels of activated factor B (Bb) and the soluble membrane attack complex (SC5b-9), both of which normalize within 4 to 7 days after the onset of the illness.[7,18]

aHUS

The injury to endothelial cells in aHUS is direct and is due to medications, infections, or systemic illnesses. In patients with nonfamilial aHUS, the provoking disturbance is generally severe in nature, leading to overt TMA. In contrast, in children with familial aHUS, even slight endothelial damage during a mild viral upper respiratory illness can trigger TMA because of defective regulation of the alternative complement pathway. The alternative complement cascade is constitutively active because binding of C3 to factor B generates a catalytically active complex that leads to continued formation of C3bBb, the pivotal alternative pathway C3 convertase. Several circulating (factors B, H, and I) and membrane-bound (MCP, thrombomodulin) molecules interact to prevent continuous activation of the pathway and endothelial injury.[19] Both inactivating (factors H and I) and activating mutations (factor B) have been linked to increased activity of the complement cascade and the development of aHUS.[7]

TTP

VWF is synthesized by endothelial cells and megakaryocytes and stored as ultralarge VWF multimers in Weibel-Palade bodies in the endothelium and as α granules in platelets. Ultralarge VWF is proteolytically degraded by ADAMTS13 (a disintegrin-like and metalloprotease domain with thrombospondin type-1 motif, number 13) after it is secreted by endothelial cells, preventing accumulation in the bloodstream. In addition, in vitro experiments in the absence of ADAMTS13 have demonstrated that a proportion of these ultralarge VWF multimers remain anchored to the activated endothelium. These multimers unravel, bind platelets, and wave in the direction of the flow. Inadequate ADAMTS13 activity on the cell surface and in the circulation promotes platelet aggregation and the formation of intravascular platelet-fibrin thrombi that are associated with episodes of TTP.[20] In patients with TTP, there can be congenital deficiency (Upshaw-Schulman syndrome) inherited as an autosomal trait with disease onset in the neonatal period. Alternatively, there can be an acquired or idiopathic reduction in the synthesis of ADAMTS13 as a consequence of autoantibodies that disrupt protease activity. Antibody synthesis can be secondary to autoimmune diseases, systemic inflammation, or medications such as clopidogrel.[8,21] ADAMTS13 proteolytic function declines to undetectable levels during episodes of overt TTP and normalization with resolution of the acute event.[22]

EPIDEMIOLOGY

Because the onset of all forms of TMA is usually abrupt and severe and occurs in previously healthy children, most cases rapidly come to medical attention with prompt diagnosis. There have been case reports of unusual presentations in which one target organ was disproportionately affected, obscuring the systemic nature of the illness and delaying recognition of the underlying TMA. However, STEC infection is included in infectious disease surveillance programs sponsored by the Centers for Disease Control. Moreover, in most states in the United States, STEC-HUS is a reportable disease that yields accurate epidemiologic information about this form of TMA.

The incidence of STEC-HUS ranges from 6:100,000 in children under the age of 5 years to 1–2:100,000 in the overall population, including adults over 18 years of age.[10,15,23] The incidence of STEC-HUS has been steady despite increased public awareness and efforts by governments and the food industry to reduce the risk of food-borne and waterborne transmission of STEC. Girls are affected more often than boys for no apparent reason. It occurs globally and in all racial/ethnic groups, except for African Americans, among whom the disease is distinctly less common than in whites. Again, there is no explanation for this observation. STEC-HUS is primarily seen in children except in epidemics when it may occur in patients with a wider age spectrum. For example, from May 2011 until July 2011, several European countries, particularly Northern Germany, experienced one of the largest STEC-HUS outbreaks ever reported. The E coli strain O104:H4 caused a unique multinational epidemic with 3816 patients who suffered from enterohemorrhagic E coli infection, 845 HUS cases, and 54 deaths.[24,25] The illness predominately affected adults who experienced severe renal and neurologic complications.

The incidence of both nonfamilial aHUS and familial aHUS is lower than STEC-HUS, and, taken together, they occur at a rate that is at most 10% of that for STEC-related forms of HUS.[23] These 2 subcategories of TMA have been documented in virtually every country without an increased susceptibility by gender or racial group. TTP is as rare as aHUS, with an annual incidence in the range of 1 to 2 cases per million population. Like STEC-HUS, it is more common in girls (3:2) and in whites more than in blacks (3:1). However, in contrast to STEC-HUS, the incidence of TTP peaks during the third and fourth decades of life and is uncommon in pediatric patients.[8,21]

CLINICAL CAUSES
STEC-HUS

E coli O157:H7 remains the most common strain that causes STEC-HUS with a minority of cases because of other serotypes such as O111 and O26.[10] The causative strains vary with time and region. Non-O157 strains of *E coli* are an increasingly common cause of STEC-HUS. In a report about the microbiology of STEC-HUS during the period 2000 to 2006, these strains accounted for half of all STEC infections and the same percentage of isolates produced Stx2 as O157 strains,[26] underscoring the importance of tests to detect Stx directly and that do not rely on stool culture to make the microbiological diagnosis.

Nonfamilial aHUS

The most common infectious trigger is *Streptococcus pneumoniae*, linked to neuraminidase production by the microorganism.[23,27,28] The incidence has been fairly steady, despite widespread use of pneumococcal vaccines with reduced overt disease rates in children. In fact, when serologic studies are performed in a timely manner, it can be demonstrated that pneumococcal-related HUS is caused by bacterial strains that are not included in the 7-valent or 23-valent vaccines, such as serotype 19A. Affected children with pneumococcal HUS tend to be young, with a mean age of 1 to 2 years. In general, the disease is more severe compared with STEC-related disease. Up to 80% of affected patients require dialysis, compared with 40% in STEC-HUS, and there is a higher frequency of serious extrarenal complications; however, despite the initial intensity of the episode, most children recover from the acute illness and have normal kidney function at long-term follow-up.[23] Other infections, medications, and miscellaneous medical conditions can cause aHUS. HIV, *Mycoplasma pneumoniae*, histoplasmosis, and Coxsackie virus are among the well-recognized infectious causes of sporadic aHUS. The most commonly prescribed drug class associated with TMA is calcineurin inhibitors (eg, cyclosporine and tacrolimus). Chemotherapeutic agents, such as mitomycin C, cytosine arabinoside, cisplatinum, and gemcitabine, have also been implicated in this complication. Antiplatelet drugs, such as ticlopidine and clopidogrel, can cause aHUS. Anti-angiogenesis treatment of malignancies can also provoke TMA. This complication has been reported after treatment with biologic agents that block the activity of vascular endothelial growth factor (VEGF; bevacizumab) or the tyrosine kinase VEGF receptor.[29] The range of malignancies that can cause TMA and aHUS includes solid organ tumors and the various forms of leukemia. Systemic lupus erythematosus and the anti-phospholipid syndrome can lead to aHUS, especially in women. When TMA occurs in the context of pregnancy, it is described by the acronym HELLP (hemolysis, elevated liver enzymes, and low platelet count). In its milder form, it is characterized by hypertension and proteinuria (ie, pre-eclampsia). The full-blown syndrome is associated with increased maternal and infant mortality and high circulating levels of the soluble VEGF receptor (sFlt1) or endoglin that inhibit the activity of VEGF.[30]

The most common causes of nonfamilial HUS in pediatric patients are summarized in **Table 1**.

Familial aHUS

A genetic mutation in one or more of the complement regulatory proteins can be documented in 44% to 61% of patients with hereditary aHUS—a single mutation is present in most patients with combined mutations in less than 10% of cases.[31,32] The genetic defects in patients with aHUS generally demonstrate incomplete penetrance, indicating that additional factors are needed for the disease to be manifest. Multiple mutations are 3-fold more common in patients with a defect in the MCP or factor I genes compared with patients with a mutation factor H, factor B, or C3. The presence of combined mutations or single mutations along with risk haplotypes is most significant for patients with MCP mutations because that subgroup has an increased risk of progression to ESKD and less favorable outcomes after kidney transplant.[31] The gene that has been most recently linked to aHUS is diacylglycerol kinase ε, an enzyme present in endothelial cells. Using exome sequencing, recessive mutations were detected in 9 unrelated kindreds with aHUS. The altered diacylglycerol kinase ε protein activated protein kinase C and caused a prothrombotic state.[33]

TTP

This form of TMA shares the same etiologic factors as HUS. For example, systemic lupus erythematosus is a trigger for TTP in both pediatric and adult patients, and recent reports suggest that up to 18% of individuals with this rheumatologic disorder will develop TMA.[34] Because of the higher prevalence of TTP in adults versus children, the underlying causes reflect disorders seen in older patients, such as pregnancy, anti-phospholipid syndrome, antiplatelet and anti-arrhythmic drugs, cryoglobulinemia, and solid organ malignancies. Patients with cancer-induced and/or chemotherapy-induced TTP generally have a poor prognosis despite treatment.

DIAGNOSIS

HUS is defined as the triad of hemolytic anemia with erythrocyte fragmentation, thrombocytopenia, and AKI occurring after a prodromal infection by a Stx-producing strain of bacteria. Some recent reports have made a diagnosis of "incomplete" HUS if only 2 of 3 criteria are present.[35] This less stringent definition may introduce variability into the incidence of the disease in different locales. The criterion

Table 1
Causes of nonfamilial aHUS in children

Category	Examples
Medications	Ticlopidine, tacrolimus, bevacizumab
Infections	S pneumoniae, HIV
Systemic disease	Systemic lupus erythematosus
Malignancy	Acute lymphoblastic leukemia Bone marrow transplantation
Pregnancy	HELLP (hemolytic anemia, elevated liver enzymes, low platelets) syndrome

for anemia is age-dependent and gender-dependent and the confirmation of the microangiopathic character is based on a microscopic review of the peripheral smear and detection of schistocytes. The combination of hemolysis and tissue ischemia results in high-serum lactic acid dehydrogenase levels in all patients with HUS or TTP. The direct antiglobulin test (Coombs test) is normal. The platelet count that is diagnostic is less than $150 \times 10^9/mm^3$. In contrast to patients with disseminated intravascular coagulation, the prothrombin time/international normalized ratio, partial prothrombin time, and fibrinogen levels are normal in patients with HUS and TTP. However, there can be activation of the fibrinolytic pathway with increased circulating levels of fibrin degradation products. Complement levels are usually normal except for select patients with aHUS, in whom hypocomplementemia may be a clue to an underlying disturbance in complement metabolism.

The definition of renal dysfunction varies in different reports and ranges from abnormalities in urinalysis to an elevation in the serum creatinine concentration above the 95th percentile for age and gender. Variations in the stringency of the definition of kidney disease may account for some of the variation in the severity of HUS.[25]

Patients with STEC-HUS have an antecedent episode of hemorrhagic enterocolitis, within 2 to 12 days before the onset of TMA. The diarrhea becomes bloody in 80% to 90% of cases as the colitis worsens. Among children with STEC enteritis, 5% to 15% will develop HUS, whereas the rest will have complete resolution of symptoms. Methods to prove STEC infection include stool culture, assays for free Stx in the stool, PCR assay to detect Stx genes in the stool, and serologic tests to confirm an increase in antibody titer to the STEC strain. Less than 50% of patients with STEC-HUS shed the bacteria in their stool at the time of diagnosis. Assays for free Stx or the toxin gene are more sensitive but are not routinely performed in all microbiology laboratories. In current practice, most clinical laboratories use only culture-based methods to detect STEC infection; however, the use of Stx assay kits increased nearly 2-fold, from 6% in 2003 to 11% in 2007.[36] Demonstration of an increase in antibody titer confirms the bacterial infection but the information is usually unavailable at the time of the acute episode and cannot be used in making the diagnosis in real time.

Nonfamilial forms of HUS occur sporadically and are diagnosed based on the complete history and physical examination with laboratory testing to confirm the suspected cause.

Patients with familial aHUS generally have disease that occurs throughout the year, that develops after an upper respiratory infection, and that follows a recurrent pattern with rapidly deteriorating kidney disease. Patients with aHUS secondary to a genetic mutation in a complement regulatory protein are just as likely to present during childhood and adulthood.[32] The current recommendation is to measure the levels of complement components and to perform genetic testing for all known complement regulatory protein in patients who present with aHUS.[6,28] The complete genetic profile helps delineate the short-term response and outcome after kidney transplantation if needed.

Patients with TTP have the same 3 features seen in children with HUS but also have fever and neurologic findings. The diagnosis is made by assaying ADAMTS13 activity. This test requires care to standardize the assay procedure to ensure the accuracy and validity of the results. Recent reports have suggested that documentation of ADAMTS13 deficiency may not be sufficient to diagnose TTP. Instead it may be critical to assay enzymatic activity and to quantitate levels that are less than 10%.[37] This residual ADAMTS13 may be a major determinant of the clinical manifestations of TTP and account for disease heterogeneity.

CLINICAL FEATURES

All of the forms of TMA are characterized by diffuse endothelial injury and can have adverse effects on every body organ. The kidney and brain are the primary targets in HUS and TTP,[38] but other organs can be impacted as well, and the percentage and severity will vary depending on the subcategory of TMA. Severe complications include seizures, cortical blindness, hemiparesis, adult respiratory distress syndrome, myocardial dysfunction, pancreatitis, and liver failure.[39] The frequency of major target organ involvement in the 4 categories of TMA is summarized in **Table 2**.

Mortality is generally higher in adults compared with children with STEC-HUS. The situation is reversed in those with familial aHUS, in which children have a nearly 9-fold higher mortality compared with adults.[32]

TREATMENT
STEC-HUS

Optimal care of children with STEC enteritis involves removal from their home environment to prevent spread of the disease to other household contacts. In addition, provision of adequate amounts of sodium-containing intravenous fluids may prevent activation of the coagulation cascade within the glomerular microcirculation and prevent the progression of the disease to full-blown HUS.[40,41]

There is no proven therapy for STEC-HUS and, therefore, treatment centers on supportive management of renal failure, anemia, hypertension, and fluid-electrolyte imbalances. Renal replacement therapy is advised if there is anuria for at least 24 hours or oliguria (<0.5 mL/kg/h) for at least 72 hours.[42] This guideline is probably relevant to all forms of TMA. Clinical trials have failed to demonstrate a significant benefit, namely, reduced need for dialysis support or occurrence of serious extrarenal complications, for any of the following therapeutic options: antibiotics, antiplatelet drugs, intravenous immunoglobulin G, corticosteroids, anticoagulants, fibrinolytic agents, plasma infusion, plasmapheresis, and oral administration of a Stx-binding agent.

The agent that has received the most attention recently as a potential treatment of STEC-HUS is eculizumab, a monoclonal antibody to C5a. During the peak of the large German outbreak in 2011, a Letter to the Editor in the *New England Journal of Medicine* was published describing 3 children, all 3 years of age, with severe STEC-HUS who were treated with eculizumab.[43] The patients already required dialysis and 2 of them had been unresponsive to plasmapheresis. The neurologic status as well as the platelet count and lactic acid dehydrogenase improved dramatically after the first dose of eculizumab. Dialysis was discontinued within 16 days and all 3 children were discharged without neurologic findings.[43] Based on this limited experience, German

Table 2				
Major target organ involvement in TMA				
	STEC-HUS (%)	Non-familial aHUS (%)	Familial HUS (%)	TTP (%)
Kidney involvement	100	100	100	80–90
Need for acute dialysis	40	50	50	10
Brain	40	20	40	85
Cardiovascular	30	10–20	30–40	20
Pancreas	25	10	20	10
Liver	10	10	10	10
Mortality	2–3	5–30	25	10

nephrologists approached the manufacturer of eculizumab (Alexion Pharmaceuticals, Inc, Cheshire, CT, USA) and received authorization to provide the antibody for "off-label" compassionate use during the outbreak of STEC-HUS to patients with the most severe clinical symptoms. At the Paul Ehrlich Institute, a multicenter, single-arm, open-label 28-week clinical study was conducted to test the safety and efficacy of eculizumab on clinical markers of TMA and the serious complications in STEC-HUS. The protocol involved intravenous administration of the monoclonal antibody, 900 mg weekly for 4 weeks, then 1200 mg biweekly, for a total of 7 doses, based on prior experience in treating aHUS. Treatment could be extended for an additional 8 weeks. A total of 328 patients with STEC-HUS received eculizumab during the outbreak. The study included 198 patients from 25 centers.[38,44] The report of Loos and colleagues[45] focuses on the clinical disease in 90 children who were treated at centers that participated in the German HUS Registry. Seventy-one percent of the patients (64/90) required at least temporary renal replacement therapy and 23/90 (26%) had neurologic symptoms. Most of the patients (77/90, 74%) received supportive care only; 17 received plasma exchange, and 13 were given eculizumab (together with plasma exchange therapy in 7 cases). Most patients recovered and only one child died. After a median follow-up of 4 months, all but 4 patients had returned to normal kidney function and only 5 had residual neurologic deficits that were slowly improving in all cases. Based on their findings, the authors conclude that the clinical profile of O104:H4 STEC is comparable to the disease caused by the O157 serotype and that there is no need for novel treatments such as plasmapheresis, besides intensive supportive care.[46] However, regardless of the findings of the effect of eculizumab during the outbreak, it will be important to evaluate this agent in a randomized clinical trial. Extended follow-up of all patients of all ages is needed to document the incidence of long-term renal and neurologic sequelae comparable to what has been done after the outbreak in Walkerton, Ontario.[47]

Atypical HUS

Following Food and Drug Administration approval of eculizumab in September 2011, the monoclonal antibody has become the standard of care for all patients with aHUS.[48] Plasma infusion or plasmapheresis may be implemented temporarily until the drug is received.[49] However, prompt initiation of eculizumab therapy is associated with more rapid control of the disease and better outcomes. Eculizumab is currently prescribed regardless of the underlying genetic defect. The drug is usually given weekly until there is normalization of the platelet count and microangiopathic anemia. The frequency can then be reduced to every 2 to 4 weeks based on the clinical response. Discontinuation of eculizumab has been associated with recurrence of disease (unpublished observations). Therefore, Alexion recommends maintaining antibody therapy indefinitely. However, in view of the high cost of the drug and the logistical issues involved in long-term intravenous administration of the agent, further clinical investigation is needed to determine the minimum dosage and frequency of eculizumab infusion that results in stable kidney function and prevention of relapses. There are no data about efficacy in relationship to specific genetic causes or rescue therapy in patients who do poorly on eculizumab therapy.

TTP

Unlike HUS, in patients with TTP, prompt implementation of plasmapheresis yields an overall response rate of 60% to 90%. Controlled trials have confirmed the superiority of plasma exchange therapy compared to plasma infusion. The usual protocol involves daily one plasma volume exchange; however, the regimen can be intensified with an increased exchange volume or frequency of treatment in patients with a suboptimal response. Because children have a greater likelihood of responding to supportive care, plasmapheresis is often reserved for patients with poor prognostic indicators. Corticosteroids can induce a remission in up to 30% of patients. Other immunosuppressive agents, such as vincristine, azathioprine, cyclophosphamide, intravenous IgG, can be implemented as primary therapy. The most recent biologic agent that has been tried in patients with TTP is rituximab, the monoclonal antibody to CD20 on the surface of B cells.[50] Splenectomy and prostacyclin infusions have been tried as last-resort approaches to prevent repeated relapses of TTP in patients who are refractory to the standard of care. An overall approach to treatment of the various forms of TMA is summarized in **Table 3**.

PROGNOSIS
STEC-HUS

The prognosis of STEC-HUS is generally good and most children recover fully from the acute episode without subsequent relapses.[51] The mortality in children with STEC-HUS is less than 5%.[39] Most patients have normal renal function 5 years after their illness. The short-term risk factors for decreased renal function and poor outcomes (including death) are the severity of the initial disease (eg, oligo-anuria, fever, leukocytosis, colitis) and the need for dialysis.[52,53] A more accurate assessment of kidney outcomes is possible 1 year after resolution of the episode. Those children with persistent proteinuria (ie, urine protein:creatinine ratio >1) or hypertension are at greater risk of progression to chronic kidney disease (CKD).[49] In a recent meta-analysis of the long-term outcome of children with STEC-HUS, up to 25% of children have evidence of CKD including hypertension, proteinuria, or reduced glomerular filtration rate.[54] Children with STEC-HUS who require kidney transplantation are not at risk for recurrent disease in the allograft.

aHUS

The outcome in children with nonfamilial aHUS is determined by the underlying disease. In addition, because the patients do not usually experience recurrences, the prognosis will reflect the degree of renal damage and the severity of any extrarenal complications that developed during the diagnostic episode of TMA. In most cases, there is recovery of renal function without permanent loss of renal function. Nonetheless, in general, the prognosis in these cases as a group is worse than in children with STEC-HUS.

The overall prognosis for children with familial aHUS is much worse than in children with STEC-HUS. Nearly 25% of patients die of CKD stage 5 or other serious

Table 3
Overall approach to treatment of children with TMA

	STEC-HUS	Non-familial aHUS	Familial aHUS	TTP
Supportive care	+	+	+	+
Treat triggering illness	−	+	−	−
Eculizumab	?	−	+	−
Plasmapheresis	+	?	Temporarily until start of eculizumab treatment	+

+, treatment is effective; −, treatment is ineffective; ?, effect of treatment is unproven and of uncertain value.

complications of the disease. In addition, up to 70% to 80% progress to ESKD and require permanent dialysis. A higher percentage of adults compared with children with aHUS progress to ESKD after their first episode of disease.[32] There is a substantial risk of recurrent disease after transplantation that is highest for factor H and I and lowest with MCP mutations.[32]

TTP

Although most patients with TTP respond to initial therapy, nearly 40% will have relapses that occur at a mean interval of 20 months from the initial episode. The long-term mortality with current therapy is much less than 10%. Patients with malignancy-related TTP have a worse prognosis (74% 1-year survival), especially those who have actively treated cancer (22% 1-year survival).

SUMMARY

TMA is a rare but important manifestation of disease in pediatric patients. Although the clinical syndromes—STEC-HUS, aHUS, and TTP—overlap, there are significant differences in the pathogenesis of these illnesses. The basis of treatment in most cases is reversal of the abnormality triggering the episode of TMA coupled with intensive supportive care. In some cases, improved understanding of disease has resulted in marked improvements in care (eg, eculizumab) in familial aHUS and plasmapheresis in TTP. However, the mortality and morbidity resulting from the TMA syndromes continue to be substantial. It is anticipated that future research in HUS and TTP will result in more sensitive diagnostic methods to detect disease earlier in the course of the illness and the design of therapeutic agents that target the causative step in each subtype of TMA.

REFERENCES

1. Moake JL. Moschcowitz, multimers, and metalloprotease. N Engl J Med 1998; 339:1629–31.
2. Karmali MA, Petric M, Lim C, et al. The association between idiopathic hemolytic uremic syndrome and infection by verotoxin-producing Escherichia coli. J Infect Dis 1985;151:775–82.
3. Moake JL, Rudy CK, Troll JH, et al. von Willebrand factor abnormalities and endothelial cell perturbation in a patient with acute thrombotic thrombocytopenic purpura. Am J Med Sci 1986;291:47–50.
4. Moake JL, Turner NA, Stathopoulos NA, et al. Involvement of large plasma von Willebrand factor (vWF) multimers and unusually large vWF forms derived from endothelial cells in shear stress-induced platelet aggregation. J Clin Invest 1986;78:1456–61.
5. Warwicker P, Goodship TH, Donne RL, et al. Genetic studies into inherited and sporadic hemolytic uremic syndrome. Kidney Int 1998;53:836–44.
6. Kavanagh D, Goodship T. Genetics and complement in atypical HUS. Pediatr Nephrol 2010;25:2431–42.
7. Noris M, Mescia F, Remuzzi G. STEC-HUS, atypical HUS and TTP are all diseases of complement activation. Nat Rev Nephrol 2012;8:622–33.
8. Chapman K, Seldon M, Richards R. Thrombotic microangiopathies, thrombotic thrombocytopenic purpura, and ADAMTS-13. Semin Thromb Hemost 2012;38: 47–54.
9. Copelovitch L, Kaplan BS. The thrombotic microangiopathies. Pediatr Nephrol 2008;23:1761–7.

10. Tarr PI, Gordon CA, Chandler WL. Shiga-toxin-producing Escherichia coli and hemolytic uremic syndrome. Lancet 2005;365:1073–86.

11. Philpott DJ, Ackerley CA, Kiliaan AJ, et al. Translocation of verotoxin-1 across T84 monolayers: mechanism of bacterial toxin penetration of epithelium. Am J Physiol 1997;273(6 Pt 1):G1349–58.

12. Brigotti M, Tazzari PL, Ravanelli E, et al. Clinical relevance of shiga toxin concentrations in the blood of patients with hemolytic uremic syndrome. Pediatr Infect Dis J 2011;30:486–90.

13. Sandvig K, Bergan J, Dyve AB, et al. Endocytosis and retrograde transport of Shiga toxin. Toxicon 2010;56:1181–5.

14. Mukhopadhyay S, Linstedt AD. Manganese blocks intracellular trafficking of Shiga toxin and protects against Shiga toxicosis. Science 2012;335:332–5.

15. Petruzziello-Pellegrini TN, Marsden PA. Shiga toxin-associated hemolytic uremic syndrome: advances in pathogenesis and therapeutics. Curr Opin Nephrol Hypertens 2012;21:433–40.

16. King LA, Nogareda F, Weill FX, et al. Outbreak of Shiga toxin-producing Escherichia coli O104:H4 associated with organic fenugreek sprouts, France, 2011. Clin Infect Dis 2012;54:1588–94.

17. Petruzziello-Pellegrini TN, Yuen DA, Page AV, et al. The CXCR4/CXCR7/SDF-1 pathway contributes to the pathogenesis of Shiga toxin-associated hemolytic uremic syndrome in humans and mice. J Clin Invest 2012;122:759–76.

18. Thurman JM, Marians R, Emlen W, et al. Alternative pathway of complement in children with diarrhea-associated hemolytic uremic syndrome. Clin J Am Soc Nephrol 2009;4:1920–4.

19. Java A, Atkinson J, Salmon J. Defective complement inhibitory function predisposes to renal disease. Annu Rev Med 2013;64:307–24.

20. De Ceunynck K, De Meyer SF, Vanhoorelbeke K. Unwinding the von Willebrand factor strings puzzle. Blood 2013;121:270–7.

21. Clark WF. Thrombotic microangiopathy: current knowledge and outcomes with plasma exchange. Semin Dial 2012;25:214–9.

22. Lotta LA, Wu HM, Cairo A, et al. Drop of residual plasmatic activity of ADAMTS13 to undetectable levels during acute disease in a patient with adult-onset congenital thrombotic thrombocytopenic purpura. Blood Cells Mol Dis 2013;50:59–60.

23. Constantinescu AR, Bitzan M, Weiss LS, et al. Non-enteropathic hemolytic uremic syndrome: causes and short-term course. Am J Kidney Dis 2004;43:976–82.

24. Final report and analysis of the epidemiology of the 2011 O104:H4 EHEC-HUS outbreak in Germany. Berlin: Robert Koch Institut; 2011.

25. Tarr PI, Karpman D. Escherichia coli O104:H4 and the hemolytic uremic syndrome: the analysis begins. Clin Infect Dis 2012;55:760–3.

26. Hedican EB, Medus C, Besser JM, et al. Characteristics of O157 versus non-O157 Shiga toxin-producing Escherichia coli infections in Minnesota, 2000-2006. Clin Infect Dis 2009;49:358–64.

27. Banerjee R, Hersh AL, Newland J, et al, Emerging Infections Network Hemolytic-Uremic Syndrome Study Group. Streptococcus pneumoniae-associated hemolytic uremic syndrome among children in North America. Pediatr Infect Dis J 2011;30:736–9.

28. Taylor CM, Machin S, Wigmore SJ, et al, Working party from the Renal Association, the British Committee for Standards in Haematology and the British

Transplantation Society. Clinical practice guidelines for the management of atypical haemolytic uraemic syndrome in the United Kingdom. Br J Haematol 2010;148:37–47.

29. Eremina V, Jefferson JA, Kowalewska J, et al. VEGF inhibition and renal thrombotic microangiopathy. N Engl J Med 2008;358:1129–36.

30. Venkatesha S, Toporsian M, Lam C, et al. Soluble endoglin contributes to the pathogenesis of preeclampsia. Nat Med 2006;12:642–9.

31. Bresin E, Rurali E, Caprioli J, et al, European Working Party on Complement Genetics in Renal Diseases. Combined complement gene mutations in atypical hemolytic uremic syndrome influence clinical phenotype. J Am Soc Nephrol 2013;24:475–86.

32. Fremeaux-Bacchi V, Fakhouri F, Garnier A, et al. Genetics and outcome of atypical hemolytic uremic syndrome: a nationwide French series comparing children and adults. Clin J Am Soc Nephrol 2013;8:554–62.

33. Lemaire M, Frémeaux-Bacchi V, Schaefer F, et al. Recessive mutations in DGKE cause atypical hemolytic-uremic syndrome. Nat Genet 2013;45(5):531–6. http://dx.doi.org/10.1038/ng.2590.

34. Wu LH, Yu F, Qu Z, et al. Inclusion of renal vascular lesions in the 2003 ISN/RPS system for classifying lupus nephritis improves renal outcome predictions. Kidney Int 2013;83:715–23.

35. Yoshioka K, Yagi K, Moriguchi N. Clinical features and treatment of children with hemolytic uremic syndrome caused by enterohemorrhagic Escherichia coli O157:H7 infection: experience of an outbreak in Sakai City, 1996. Pediatr Int 1999;41:223–7.

36. Hoefer D, Hurd S, Medus C, et al, Emerging Infections Program FoodNet Working Group. Laboratory practices for the identification of Shiga toxin-producing Escherichia coli in the United States, FoodNet sites, 2007. Foodborne Pathog Dis 2011;8:555–60.

37. Lotta LA, Wu HM, Musallam KM, et al. The emerging concept of residual ADAMTS13 activity in ADAMTS13-deficient thrombotic thrombocytopenic purpura. Blood Rev 2013;27:71–6.

38. Trachtman H, Austin C, Lewinski M, et al. Renal and neurological involvement in typical Shiga toxin-associated HUS. Nat Rev Nephrol 2012;8:658–69.

39. Trachtman H, Cnaan A, Christen E, et al. Effect of an oral Shiga toxin-binding agent on diarrhea-associated hemolytic uremic syndrome in children: a randomized controlled trial. JAMA 2003;290:1337–44.

40. Ake JA, Jelacic S, Ciol MA, et al. Relative nephroprotection during Escherichia coli O157:H7 infections: association with intravenous volume expansion. Pediatrics 2005;115:e673–80.

41. Hickey CA, Beattie TJ, Cowieson J, et al. Early volume expansion during diarrhea and relative nephroprotection during subsequent hemolytic uremic syndrome. Arch Pediatr Adolesc Med 2011;165:884–9.

42. Schulman SL, Kaplan BS. Management of patients with hemolytic uremic syndrome demonstrating severe azotemia but not anuria. Pediatr Nephrol 1996;10:671–4.

43. Lapeyraque AL, Malina M, Fremeaux-Bacchi V, et al. Eculizumab in severe Shiga-toxin–associated HUS. N Engl J Med 2011;364(26):2561–3.

44. European Centre for Disease Prevention and Control. Shiga toxin-producing E coli (STEC): update on outbreak in the EU. 2011. Available at: http://www.ecdc.europa.eu/en/healthtopics/escherichia_coli/whats_new/Pages/epidemiological_updates.aspx. Accessed August 9, 2011.

45. Loos S, Ahlenstiel T, Kranz B, et al. An outbreak of Shiga-toxin producing E. coli O104:H4 hemolytic uremic syndrome in Germany: presentation and short-term outcome in children. Clin Infect Dis 2012;55:753–9.

46. Colic E, Dieperink H, Titlestad K, et al. Management of an acute outbreak of diarrhoea-associated haemolytic uraemic syndrome with early plasma exchange in adults from southern Denmark: an observational study. Lancet 2011;378:1089–93.

47. Clark WF, Sontrop JM, Macnab JJ, et al. Long term risk for hypertension, renal impairment, and cardiovascular disease after gastroenteritis from drinking water contaminated with Escherichia coli O157:H7: a prospective cohort study. BMJ 2010;341:c6020.

48. Legendre CM, Licht C, Muus P, et al. Terminal complement inhibitor eculizumab in atypical hemolytic uremic syndrome. N Engl J Med 2013;368:2169–81.

49. Lou-Meda R, Oakes RS, Gilstrap JN, et al. Prognostic significance of microalbuminuria in postdiarrheal hemolytic uremic syndrome. Pediatr Nephrol 2007;22: 117–20.

50. Westwood JP, Webster H, McGuckin S, et al. Rituximab for thrombotic thrombocytopenic purpura: benefit of early administration during acute episodes and use of prophylaxis to prevent relapse. J Thromb Haemost 2013;11:481–90.

51. Spinale JM, Ruebner RL, Copelovitch L, et al. Long-term outcomes of Shiga toxin hemolytic uremic syndrome. Pediatr Nephrol 2013. [Epub ahead of print].

52. Oakes RS, Siegler RL, McReynolds MA, et al. Predictors of fatality in postdiarrheal hemolytic uremic syndrome. Pediatrics 2006;117:1656–62.

53. Oakes RS, Kirkham JK, Nelson RD, et al. Duration of oliguria and anuria as predictors of chronic renal-related sequelae in post-diarrheal hemolytic uremic syndrome. Pediatr Nephrol 2008;23:1303–8.

54. Garg AX, Suri RS, Barrowman N, et al. Long-term renal prognosis of diarrhea-associated hemolytic uremic syndrome: a systematic review, meta-analysis, and meta-regression. JAMA 2003;290:1360–70.

Transfusion and Hemovigilance in Pediatrics

Paula H.B. Bolton-Maggs, DM, FRCP, FRCPath

KEYWORDS

- Hemovigilance • Pediatric transfusion • SHOT • Root cause analysis
- Complications of transfusion

KEY POINTS

- Transfusion is very safe with a low risk of viral or other infection; the most common pathologic event is a febrile/allergic transfusion reaction.
- Adverse event reporting (hemovigilance) has resulted in changes in transfusion practice, which have reduced pathologic events such as transfusion-related acute lung injury.
- Errors in basic procedures have been identified as the most common cause of adverse transfusion incidents (correct identification of the patient is essential).
- Every transfusion should be assessed for appropriateness to avoid unnecessary exposure to blood components.

Questions about the safety of transfusion arose in the 1980s and 1990s with evidence of transmission of hepatitis viruses and the emergence of human immunodeficiency virus (HIV) in the blood supply. People with hemophilia were particularly susceptible because factor concentrates were manufactured from pools of plasma containing up to 20,000 donations, and hepatitis transmission was suspected soon after their introduction.[1] Transfusion-transmission of acquired immunodeficiency was recognized in 1983 when a 14-month-old infant developed unusual infections; this child had been transfused with blood from a donor who, although well at the time of donation, had subsequently died of acquired immunodeficiency.[2] Transfusion-transmission was soon confirmed in several other cases.[3,4] Screening of blood donations for HIV started in 1985.[5] Fortunately, the steps taken by Blood Centers, a combination of donor exclusion together with viral screening of donations, have been very effective. The residual risk of HIV and hepatitis C virus among all allogeneic donations in the United States is currently less than 1 per 1 million donations. Only 20 HIV transmissions have occurred in the United States since 1988,[6] the most recent in 2008. The

Disclosure: The author acts as a consultant to LFB and receives fees in relation to work on FXI concentrate, which has no bearing on this article.
Serious Hazards of Transfusion (SHOT), Manchester Blood Centre, Plymouth Grove, Manchester M13 9LL, UK
E-mail address: paula.bolton-maggs@nhsbt.nhs.uk

risk of viral infection is now very low, and most recent estimates in the United Kingdom are shown in **Table 1**.

At that time there was no systematic surveillance of blood transfusion recipients for these infections or other complications of transfusion. Continued surveillance of infections in the blood supply is very important as shown by the emergence of West Nile virus[7] and other agents. Different countries have different mechanisms and policies for surveillance.[8] Some transfusion specialists were also concerned that there was no surveillance for other adverse outcomes or errors such as wrong transfusions. A survey of 400 UK hematology departments reported 111 wrong blood incidents (6 deaths and 12 instances of major morbidity due to ABO incompatibility) from 245 respondents, and the authors recommended setting up a national reporting scheme.[9] Hence, hemovigilance was born.

HEMOVIGILANCE: DEFINITION

Surveillance procedures cover the whole transfusion chain, from collection of blood and its components, intended to collect and assess information on unexpected or undesirable effects resulting from the therapeutic use of labile blood products and to prevent their occurrence or recurrence (International Society of Blood Transfusion).

Hemovigilance is a recent addition to transfusion practice. National programs were developed in several European countries, most notably in France from 1991 and the United Kingdom in 1996. The UK system is described as a model of hemovigilance to demonstrate the benefits of hemovigilance. In addition, the UK system is unique in reporting data from pediatric transfusion. Although overall most transfusion recipients are older adults,[10] premature infants are a particularly highly transfused group with a long life expectancy.

In the United States, the Food and Drug Administration requires reporting of serious adverse reactions and deaths. Between 2008 and 2012, 200 deaths were reported. The Center for Disease Control has developed a national reporting scheme with Internet-based entry (a Hemovigilance Module in the National Healthcare Safety Network). This reporting system is voluntary and anonymous; by 2012 more than 140 institutions had enrolled, but this probably reflects surveillance of less than 5% of transfusions. Baseline data collected by the most recently reported National Blood Collection and Utilization Survey (NBCUS) for 2008 in the United States suggested that the reported adverse reaction rate was 2.6 events per 1000 units transfused compared with 3 to 7 events in other national schemes, suggesting underreporting.[11] Pediatric transfusions made up 2.6% of all red cell transfusions in this NBCUS.

In Europe, data collection is mandated by European Union law since 2002 and this has driven the development of several national systems. A recent review noted wide

Table 1
Estimated risk of infection from transfusion in the UK (Public Health England, 2013). The risk estimates in the UK, 2010–2011

Agent	Risk Per Million Donations (95% Confidence Interval)
Hepatitis B	0.76 (0.22–1.61)
Hepatitis C	0.036 (0.015–0.07)
HIV	0.15 (0.09–0.32)

Data from Public Health England. Available at: http://www.hpa.org.uk/Topics/InfectiousDiseases/InfectionsAZ/BIBD/EpidemiologicalData/bibd020EstfreqofinfecteddonenteringUKbloodsupply/.

variations in data quality assurance and that it is therefore difficult to make comparisons between countries.[12]

HEMOVIGILANCE: AIMS

- To identify trends in adverse reactions and events
- To inform transfusion policy
- To target areas for improved practice
- To stimulate research
- To raise awareness of transfusion hazards
- To provide early warning of new complications
- To improve transfusion safety for patients

The UK hemovigilance scheme, Serious Hazards of Transfusion (SHOT), was launched in 1996, funded by the UK blood services. All UK National Health Service hospitals were invited to register for participation. Definitions of what to report have been refined over the 16 years of reporting (**Table 2**)[13] and are comparable to those of the International Society of Blood Transfusion.[14] The reporting categories can be divided into pathologic reactions and those caused by error that should be completely preventable. Some pathologic incidents are probably preventable by better pre-transfusion assessment and better monitoring (eg, some instances of transfusion-associated circulatory overload, and some hemolytic transfusion reactions by better selection of red cells). SHOT does not collect donor events.

Table 2
Adverse incidents related to transfusion reported to SHOT

Group	Category
Pathologic incidents	Acute transfusion reactions (allergic, hypotensive, severe febrile)
	Hemolytic transfusion reactions (immediate or delayed)
	Transfusion-associated graft vs host disease
	Transfusion-related acute lung injury (TRALI)
	Posttransfusion purpura
	Transfusion-associated circulatory overload
	Transfusion-associated dyspnea
	Transfusion-transmitted infection
	Autologous transfusion or cell salvage incidents
	Uncategorized complications of transfusion
Incidents resulting from errors	Incorrect blood component transfused (wrong component or without specific requirements such as CMV negative or irradiated)
	Handling and storage errors (eg, out of cold storage for too long, or transfused over more than 4 h)
	Incidents where a patient received the right component but where one or more errors were made
	Inappropriate, unnecessary, or delayed transfusions (eg, transfused for iron deficiency, avoidable use of emergency O RhD negative units)
	Reporting errors in the administration of anti-D immunoglobulin to women during and after pregnancy
Incidents where no harm was done but from which lessons can be learned	Near miss events

In the first year (1996/7) 196 reports were received from 94 (22%) hospitals, but the reporting is now almost universal, with 99.5% registered to report, and 97.8% submitting greater than 3000 reports in 2012. Because the number of red cell units and components issued are known, it is possible to calculate risk estimates from the number of reports.

LOCAL INCIDENT REVIEW

An important part of hemovigilance, or any scheme of adverse incident reporting, is the local review of the incident as well as the national reporting of serious events. The purpose of hemovigilance is to improve practice by understanding what went wrong and why. All organizations should be encouraged to develop reporting with a view to corrective and preventive actions and not to look for blame. The level of investigation will vary depending on the severity of the incident and the risk that it will recur.

CASE STUDY: A GOOD ROOT CAUSE ANALYSIS

A 15-year-old boy regularly transfused for β-thalassemia major received a small amount of an incompatible red cell transfusion. His blood type was O and the transfused blood was group A. The transfusion was stopped and he suffered no adverse clinical consequences, although he was kept in hospital overnight for observation.

The root cause analysis demonstrated the following:

- The nurse was a lone worker and 3 children required transfusion; she therefore collected 3 units at one time because of staffing constraints despite that this was against hospital and national policy (which is to collect a single unit at a time).
- She borrowed a nurse from the next ward and checked each unit at the bedside with the correct patient, placing the units on tables between the beds.
- The first patient had a central line and required sterile access. The assisting nurse passed the unit to the first nurse; the unit was not checked again at the bedside as it was hung. The assisting nurse then returned to her own ward.
- The nurse realized the mistake as soon as she went to hang the blood unit for the next patient.

The case review established that this was a serious event that was likely to recur (scoring high on the risk matrix). Audit of practice demonstrated lone working on this ward occurred 74% of the time, and that transfusion observations were incomplete 47% of the time. The solution was to employ an additional nurse because it was clear that working alone had contributed to the potentially lethal error. The nurse involved needed revision of her competency assessment, but was supported for the manner in which she had dealt with the incident.

HEMOVIGILANCE CONTRIBUTES TO A REDUCTION IN PATHOLOGIC INCIDENTS

Annual reporting of incidents to SHOT has contributed to changes in practice at donor collection, resulting in fewer complications.

Reduction in Bacterial Infections

Bacterial infections from blood components are rare, but in the first 6 years of reporting 24 were described (6 fatal) with most contamination events caused by skin organisms contaminating platelet transfusions. SHOT and others[15] recommended that strategies be developed to reduce this complication. Diversion of the first 20 mL of the donation was introduced in 2002, together with better techniques for skin cleansing, and bacterial screening of platelet concentrates in recent years. These better techniques resulted in fewer bacterial infections; there have been none since 2010.

Reduction in Cases of Transfusion-Related Acute Lung Injury

These cases were observed to be associated with plasma-containing components, particularly platelets, and most often from female donors. The reaction is usually related to antineutrophil antibodies in donor plasma. SHOT recommended in 2002[16] that female donors be excluded for production of fresh frozen plasma (FFP) and platelets, and this strategy, applied to plasma and as far as possible to platelets, has led to a reduced incidence of transfusion-related acute lung injury (TRALI) from a maximum of 36 cases with 7 deaths in 2003, to 11 with no deaths in 2012. Interestingly, the NBCUS for 2008 noted no difference in reports of TRALI despite the introduction of several TRALI reduction strategies (principally "to minimize the preparation of high plasma-volume components from donors known to be leukocyte-immunized or at increased risk of leukocyte immunization" and also to ensure that all transfusions are appropriate).[17]

Observation of a reduction in events demonstrates the effectiveness of other strategies introduced by the blood services:

Transfusion-associated Graft Versus Host Disease

Universal leukodepletion was introduced in the United Kingdom in 1999. Following this, there have been no cases of transfusion-associated graft versus host disease since 2001 in patients who have received leukodepleted components, despite at least 800 recipients at risk receiving nonirradiated components, including children after hemopoietic stem cell transplants, those with immune deficiency, or those who had previously received intrauterine transfusion. The 2009 NBCUS reported that 80.4% of red cell units and 47.1% of platelets were leukodepleted in the United States in 2008[11] but leukocyte-reduced made up 68.6% of units transfused. Reports of post-transfusion purpura have also reduced since the introduction of leukodepletion.

HEMOVIGILANCE LEADS TO RECOGNITION OF PARTICULAR AT-RISK GROUPS
Patients Undergoing Hemopoietic Stem Cell Transplant

Individuals undergoing hemopoietic stem cell transplant may not receive appropriate components if the supplying transfusion laboratory is unaware that the transplant has taken place. Errors have been made with blood groups and failure to provide irradiated products. Good communication is the key to this.

Mistakes with Anti-D Administration to Pregnant Women

Failures may put women at risk of immune anti-D development with the possibility of hemolytic disease in future babies. Most errors are made by midwives.[18]

Patients with Hemoglobinopathies

People with thalassemia major or sickle cell disease (SCD) have particular risks relating to both the disease and the fact that many have a different racial origin from the donor population, making it more likely that they will meet different red cell antigens.

- Patients with SCD were noted to be overrepresented among reports of hemolytic transfusion reactions. Many of these cases (69%) are associated with major morbidity and one child died. Alloimmunization is a well-recognized risk in SCD[19] and particular care is needed in making the decision to transfuse, and the optimal choice of red cells. Patients should have their red cell phenotype analyzed preferably before any transfusion takes place, and the minimum recommendation is that red cells should be Rh and Kell matched. It is essential that the transfusion laboratory (Blood Bank) is aware of the diagnosis.

- Patients with thalassemia major are usually on regular transfusions. They continue to be at risk for acute transfusion reactions (ATRs; allergic type or febrile) and must be properly monitored with each transfusion.

CASE STUDY: SEVERE DELAYED HEMOLYSIS WITH HYPERHEMOLYSIS AND DEATH IN SCD

A child with SCD and a hemoglobin (Hb) level of 8.1 g/dL received 1 unit of red cells before a tonsillectomy. Thirteen days later, she was admitted unwell with a Hb level of 5.4 g/dL. After receiving 2 more units, her Hb decreased to 4.8 g/dL and she continued to decline. She was transferred to a pediatric intensive care unit (ICU), receiving a further unit of emergency O RhD negative red cells, but developed multiorgan failure and died. This child had developed hyperhemolysis as part of the hemolytic transfusion reaction.

CASE STUDY: FAILURE TO INFORM THE LABORATORY ABOUT THE DIAGNOSIS OF SCD

A patient was admitted 7 days after a transfusion with symptoms of a hemolytic transfusion reaction. The antibody screen showed 5 different alloantibodies. She had been transfused at a different hospital where the diagnosis of SCD was not transmitted to the laboratory, so that the 3 units were not of appropriate red blood cell phenotype.

CASE STUDY: ROUTINE TRANSFUSION AUDIT DETECTS INADEQUATE IDENTITY AND MONITORING ISSUES IN CHRONICALLY TRANSFUSED PATIENT WITH THALASSEMIA

A 14-year-old boy with β-thalassemia major was transfused without an identity band, without the local hospital transfusion checklist being completed, without observations being performed, and with an incomplete prescription.

HEMOVIGILANCE REPORTING HAS RESULTED IN SEVERAL NATIONAL INITIATIVES TO IMPROVE PRACTICE

Errors in the transfusion process remain the most important cause of adverse incidents (more than 60% of all reports to SHOT). The safe transfusion of blood is a complex process involving several steps and professionals from several different professional groups. Every step in the transfusion cycle must be correct to ensure patient safety (**Fig. 1**). Errors put patient lives at risk, the most serious being those that result in an individual receiving an ABO-incompatible transfusion (now included on the Department of Health's list of events that should never happen, the "Never Events"[20] list). In the first year of SHOT reporting, there were 12 deaths caused by transfusion and although the number of reports has increased year on year, the proportion with major morbidity or death has decreased from 34% in the first year, to 7% to 8% in 2011 to 2012. As a result of highlighting the error rate in transfusion through hemovigilance reporting, the following steps were taken:

- Government recommendations: Initiatives to improve transfusion training and practice—the Department of Health 3 "Better blood transfusion" circulars[21–23] recommended actions for hospitals, such as the development of hospital transfusion committees, participation in SHOT reporting, and recommendations on

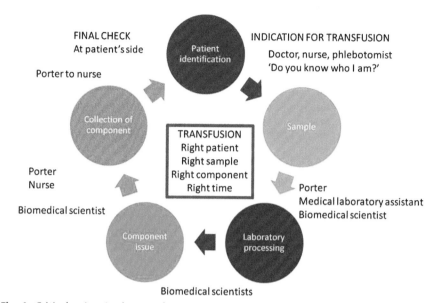

Fig. 1. Critical points in the transfusion process and different personnel involved.

education, training, and the development of a better evidence base. The third circular focused on safe and appropriate use of blood and encouraged the employment of transfusion safety officers (hospital transfusion practitioners) who would promote teaching, training and audit.

- A National Blood Transfusion Committee: The UK Chief Medical Officers mandated formation of a national blood transfusion committee in 2001, whose functions included facilitation of the recommendations in the better blood transfusion circulars for the establishment of a network of regional transfusion committees who were linked to their local hospitals.
- A National Audit Program produced its first report in 2003. This program has been valuable in establishing denominator data and benchmarking, because the hospitals are compared with one another (within their own region, and against the national overall results). Repeat audits can show improved practice.[24]
- Promotion of national transfusion guidelines: The results from hemovigilance reporting demonstrated areas for which additional or revised guidelines were required. National guidelines are produced for the United Kingdom through the British Committee for Standards in Hematology and can be viewed at www. bcshguidelines.com. Recent guidelines include those for the investigation of ATR,[25] and guidelines for pretransfusion compatibility testing.[26] Guidelines for transfusion of children and neonates were published in 2004[27] and are currently in revision, but it is notable how little good evidence there is to guide pediatric transfusion practice.

PEDIATRIC PATIENTS HAVE PARTICULAR RISKS

Children form a relatively small proportion of all transfused patients and there is a lack of standardization. Guidelines for pediatric transfusion in 2004[27] noted the lack of good evidence for many of the recommendations. There are still relatively few good studies. Neonates are the most transfused group in pediatrics, and patients with SCD are likely to be transfused in childhood, particularly now that transfusion-related benefit for management or prevention of cerebrovascular complications has been demonstrated.[28] A systematic review of randomized controlled trials examining the safety and efficacy of red cell transfusions in neonates found 27 trials[29] but only 2 of these examined neurodevelopmental outcome, with conflicting results.[30,31] The authors of these studies criticized the design of many prior trials and noted that they had not reported on outcomes likely to be of importance to clinicians. Some data on transfusion triggers in neonatal ICU have also been published that suggest, similar to findings in adult ICU, that a lower transfusion trigger of 7.0 g/dL is appropriate.[32,33]

WHAT DO WE KNOW ABOUT TRANSFUSION COMPLICATIONS IN PEDIATRICS?

- Information was gathered by a multi-institutional analysis in the United States using the Pediatric Health Information System, which collects discharge data.[34] Data were obtained from 35 hospitals. In more than 1 million discharges, 4.8% children (51,720) received transfusions. Neonates received 17.5% of the transfusions. There were 492 patients with 793 complications of transfusion. The overall rate of complications was 10.7 per 1000 products transfused, which is higher than in adults (2.5 per 1000 components transfused) but the complications were not well defined in this report. There were interesting differences between racial groups.
- Information from a UK National Blood Transfusion audit[35]: A national audit was conducted in the United Kingdom in 2010[35] to describe current red cell transfusion practice, to comment on the appropriateness of transfusions, to compare practice with national recommendations (in previous British Committee for Standards in Haematology guidelines[27,36]), and to identify areas where further studies are required. More than 2500 patients, with more than 4000 transfusion episodes, were monitored at 141 hospitals. Children transfused outside the neonatal unit (1302 patients) most often had cancer or leukemia (28%) or a hemoglobinopathy (20%), suggesting that there needs to be local transfusion guidelines for these groups. Prescribing by units of blood rather than by milliliters occurred in 39%, including small children. In the neonatal audit (1222 patients, 2718 transfusions) 73% were aged less than 1 month, and most transfusions were given for anemia with (60%) or without (21%) symptoms, and 75% were either mechanically ventilated or on continuous positive airway pressure at the time of transfusion (**Table 3**).

The results raised concern that infants were being prescribed excessive volumes; the mean was 18.7 mL/kg, and 24% received greater than 20 mL/kg. The recommended booster transfusion amount is 10 to 20 mL/kg.[27] These high volumes place infants at risk of transfusion-associated circulatory overload. The authors recommend improved education and training about safe prescribing and administration of red

Table 3 The number of transfusions was related to the gestational age at birth			
Number of Transfusions	<28 wk	23–32 wk	>32 wk
1–2	34%	60%	75%
3–4	22%	17%	6%
5–9	24%	8%	4%

Data from NCA. National Comparative Audit of the use of Red Cells in Neonates and Children 2010. Available at: http://hospital.blood.co.uk/library/pdf/NCA_red_cells_neonates_children.pdf.

cell transfusions for infants and for children. There was poor recording of the benefits of transfusion (18.5%), which should be documented rather than assumed. Anemia is the most common reason for transfusion, but this rationale is being challenged in the absence of symptoms.

- Information about transfusion complications from hemovigilance reporting: Many hemovigilance systems have not clearly reported incidents caused by errors, or near miss events. SHOT reports from pediatric patients make up 5% to 10% of reports each year (a total of 219 in 2011, and 203 in 2012). An initial SHOT analysis of pediatric incidents found that children were more likely to receive incorrect components (82.2%) than adults (63%).[37] The most frequently transfused group were neonates (29.9%). Nine children had hemolysis from ABO-incompatible transfusions. Children with SCD suffered delayed hemolytic transfusion reactions. Mistakes in identification of proper recipients continue to occur, particularly confusion in neonatal units, where the babies are unable to confirm their identity, may look similar, and may not be wearing identity bands. Each year SHOT receives reports whereby blood samples from twins have been confused and mislabeled. Maternal and cord blood samples may be mixed up. Infants transfused at birth in one hospital may then require a booster transfusion elsewhere, and information about the original group is confused, leading to an inappropriate choice of group.

CASE STUDY: ABO INCOMPATIBLE FFP TRANSFUSION

A 1-month-old preterm infant with a suspected bowel perforation was transferred urgently. A single transfusion sample was grouped as O RhD negative and the infant was given group O FFP. On testing a later blood sample, mixed field reactions were obtained; further inquiry established that the child had received multiple group O transfusions at the first hospital and that her original group was AB RhD positive. The local policy, when only a single grouping sample has been received, is to issue group O red cells and AB plasma only. This policy was not followed.

A further source of error in pediatrics relates to the volume transfused when the calculations are incorrect. In some instances, this is because pediatric patients are sometimes managed by doctors who usually see adults and are unfamiliar with the calculations. Such errors are more likely to occur where there is urgency associated with panic in emergency departments.

CASE STUDY: A MASSIVELY OVERTRANSFUSED INFANT

A 1-year-old child was admitted with suspected gastrointestinal bleeding and Hb was 9.8 g/dL. He was thought to have arterial bleeding. Emergency group O RhD negative units were supplied, and the transfusion was prescribed in units rather than milliliters (the child's weight was 10 kg). He received 4 units (1123 mL), 3 very rapidly over 20 minutes each. On transfer to the operating room, no source of bleeding was found. His Hb rose to 27.0 g/dL, and he required venesection and transfer to the pediatric ICU.

Uncategorized Complications of Transfusion

Uncategorized complications of transfusion is a reporting category for incidents that do not fit elsewhere. In 2011 there were 2 cases of transfusion-associated necrotizing enterocolitis (NEC) reported to SHOT. The association of this disease with transfusion is unclear and needs further research, but some evidence suggests that some infants are at risk.[38,39]

CASE STUDY: NEC ASSOCIATED WITH TRANSFUSION WITH A FATAL OUTCOME

A clinically stable nonventilated 6-week-old premature infant born at 26 weeks' gestation was transfused for anemia of prematurity Hb 9.3 g/dL. There were no adverse findings during transfusion and the posttransfusion Hb was 16.7 g/dL. Four hours later the baby developed signs consistent with NEC and subsequently deteriorated and died 36 hours after transfusion.

There is a national audit of cases of NEC in the United Kingdom, where transfusion data are also being collected that may help to clarify the association.

ATR (ALLERGIC, HYPOTENSIVE, AND SEVERE FEBRILE)

The number of reports of ATR has increased over recent years, comprising the largest group of pathologic incidents in both adults and children. The increase may partly be a result of the European Union legislation introduced into UK law in 2005, making hospitals more aware of their responsibility to report adverse events.

In the United Kingdom, because of the potential of infection with variant Creutzfeldt-Jakob disease from transfusion,[40] all children born since January 1, 1996 (by which time the variant Creutzfeldt-Jakob disease agent was no longer thought to be in the blood supply) are treated with pathogen-inactivated FFP, either methylene blue–treated (MB-FFP) (supplied by the UK blood services) or solvent detergent–treated (commercially available). MB-FFP has been withdrawn in France because of concerns that it was associated with more severe allergic reactions and variable fibrinogen concentration. SHOT reports of allergic reactions to FFP were reviewed to see if there was any excess of events related to MB-FFP in the UK experience and to date there is no evidence, and no change to current practice in the United Kingdom,[41] demonstrating an additional benefit of hemovigilance, the ability to perform surveillance for possibly emerging complications.

ATRs in pediatrics show some differences compared with adults. A higher proportion of pediatric ATRs occur after platelet transfusions than in adults where the reactions are more commonly occur with red cells.[42] Anaphylaxis can occur at any age (including in neonates) and is a reminder that closely monitoring the initiation and completion of all transfusions is an essential safety requirement. After careful review, SHOT has decided not to include minor transfusion reactions[13] that have no serious consequences. The total number of serious allergic reactions does not seem to be increased year on year.

"NEAR MISS" REPORTING

"Near miss" events are errors which, if undetected, could result in the determination of a wrong blood group or transfusion of an incorrect component. These errors make up a third of all reports made to SHOT; 1080 in 2011, and 981in 2012. "Near miss" reporting is valuable as lessons can be learned and practice altered before a patient comes to harm. Each year about half the near misses are sample errors and more than 90% of these are "wrong blood in tube" (ie, the sample is from the intended patient and labeled with the wrong patient's details, or is taken from the wrong patient and labeled with the intended patient's detailed). These errors happen because either the patient is not identified correctly or the sample is labeled away from the patient. These mistakes are most commonly made by doctors and rarely by phlebotomists. Such events also occur in pediatric practice and, of 25 "wrong blood in tube" incidents in 2012, 12 were related to infants less than 7 days old, and 13 of the 25 occurred because the patients were not identified correctly. Each year the same errors are identified, and confusion of neonates is a particular risk in pediatrics.

Hemovigilance reporting over 16 years in the United Kingdom consistently shows that the greatest risk to patients is that a mistake will be made somewhere in the transfusion process. This error in the transfusion process has not been reduced despite efforts to improve education, the introduction of competency assessments, and publication of several guidelines. The key points are correct identification of the patient at the time of sampling, and the final check at the patient's side where errors occurring earlier in the process may be detected. SHOT reports often show multiple errors.

CASE STUDY: NEAR MISS DETECTED AFTER SEVERAL ERRORS

Blood was prescribed for 2 patients being transfused in the same bay on a hematology ward. The prescriptions were at the nurses' station. The nurse instructed a health care assistant to collect blood for patient X but handed her the prescription for patient Y. When the unit arrived, the nurse checked the blood with the patient's identity band using the electronic bedside verification system, and the scanner audibly alarmed to warn of a mismatch. The nurse contacted the laboratory, who advised that a new identity band should be printed, and the nurse used the identity details on the blood bag, instead of confirmation with the patient, to generate the identity band. This band was then applied to the patient without any verbal identification checks, and the unit was rescanned and now was consistent with the band. Fortunately the patient asked why the unit was not irradiated and on investigation the nurse realized she had the blood bag for the other patient in the bay.

Errors are not unique to transfusion but occur across medicine and surgery at all levels, and indeed in other complex systems. The benefits of introduction of checklists in the aircraft industry are well known. Gawande notes that "the volume and complexity of what we know has exceeded our individual ability to deliver its benefits correctly, safely or reliably. Knowledge has both saved us and burdened us... we need a different strategy."[43] The introduction of a checklist before surgery has clearly improved patient safety[44] and SHOT recommends the use of a checklist in the transfusion process. A model checklist is available on the SHOT Web site at http://www.shotuk.org/wp-content/uploads/2010/03/SHOT-Transfusion-Process-Checklist-May-2012.pdf.

SUMMARY

Hemovigilance is an essential part of the transfusion process from which many lessons can be learned about pathologic reactions and why they occur, but also about errors that contribute to morbidity and mortality. Pediatric transfusion is relatively underresearched and systematic vigilance, together with audit, will result in improved practice and increased patient safety.

REFERENCES

1. Biggs R. Jaundice and antibodies directed against factors 8 and 9 in patients treated for haemophilia or Christmas disease in the United Kingdom. Br J Haematol 1974;26:313–29.
2. Ammann AJ, Cowan MJ, Wara DW, et al. Acquired immunodeficiency in an infant: possible transmission by means of blood products. Lancet 1983;1:956–8.
3. Curran JW, Lawrence DN, Jaffe H, et al. Acquired immunodeficiency syndrome (AIDS) associated with transfusions. N Engl J Med 1984;310:69–75.

4. Saulsbury FT, Wykoff RF, Boyle RJ. Transfusion-acquired human immunodeficiency virus infection in twelve neonates: epidemiologic, clinical and immunologic features. Pediatr Infect Dis J 1987;6:544–9.
5. Holland PV, Richards CA, Teghtmeyer JR, et al. Anti-HTLV-III testing of blood donors: reproducibility and confirmability of commercial test kits. Transfusion 1985;25:395–7.
6. Zou S, Dorsey KA, Notari EP, et al. Prevalence, incidence, and residual risk of human immunodeficiency virus and hepatitis C virus infections among United States blood donors since the introduction of nucleic acid testing. Transfusion 2010;50:1495–504.
7. Biggerstaff BJ, Petersen LR. Estimated risk of transmission of the West Nile virus through blood transfusion in the US, 2002. Transfusion 2003;43:1007–17.
8. O'Brien SF, Zou S, Laperche S, et al. Surveillance of transfusion-transmissible infections comparison of systems in five developed countries. Transfus Med Rev 2012;26:38–57.
9. McClelland DB, Phillips P. Errors in blood transfusion in Britain: survey of hospital haematology departments. BMJ 1994;308:1205–6.
10. Wells AW, Mounter PJ, Chapman CE, et al. Where does blood go? Prospective observational study of red cell transfusion in north England. BMJ 2002;325:803.
11. American Association of Blood Banks. The 2009 National Blood Collection and Utilization Survey Report. Available at: http://wwwaabborg/programs/biovigilance/nbcus/Documents/09-nbcus-reportpdf 2009. Accessed June 3, 2013.
12. Wiersum-Osselton JC, van Tilborgh-de Jong AJ, Zijlker-Jansen PY, et al. Variation between hospitals in rates of reported transfusion reactions: is a high reporting rate an indicator of safer transfusion? Vox Sang 2013;104:127–34.
13. Serious Hazards of Transfusion. SHOT Definitions. Available at: www.shotuk.org/wp-content/uploads/2010/03/SHOT-definitions-Nov012-finalpdf. Accessed June 6, 2013.
14. International Society of Blood Transfusion/International Haemovigilance Network, Haemovigilance Working Party. Proposed standard definitions for surveillance of non-infectious adverse transfusion reactions. Available at: http://www.isbtweb.org/fileadmin/user_upload/WP_on_Haemovigilance/ISBT_definitions_final_2011__4_.pdf 2011. Accessed September 30, 2013.
15. Wagner SJ. Transfusion-transmitted bacterial infection: risks, sources and interventions. Vox Sang 2004;86:157–63.
16. Love E, Soldan K, Jones H. SHOT annual report 2000/2001. Manchester; 2002. Available at: www.shotuk.org.
17. Strong DM, Lipton KS. AABB. Association Bulletin #06-07. Available at: http://www.bpro.or.jp/publication/pdf_jptrans/us/us200611en.pdf. Accessed September 30, 2013.
18. Bolton-Maggs P, Davies T, Poles D, et al. Errors in anti-D immunoglobulin administration: retrospective analysis of 15 years of reports to the UK confidential haemovigilance scheme. BJOG 2013;120:873–8.
19. Yazdanbakhsh K, Ware RE, Noizat-Pirenne F. Red blood cell alloimmunization in sickle cell disease: pathophysiology, risk factors, and transfusion management. Blood 2012;120:528–37.
20. DH. Never Events List 2012/13-Transfusion of ABO-incompatible blood components 2012;17:13. Available at: https://www.gov.uk/government/uploads/system/uploads/attachment_data/file/142013/Never_events_201213.pdf. Accessed September 30, 2013.

21. Department of Health. Health Service Circular: Better Blood Transfusion. 1998. Available at: http://webarchive.nationalarchives.gov.uk/20130107105354/http://www.dh.gov.uk/en/Publicationsandstatistics/Lettersandcirculars/Health servicecirculars/DH_4004262. Accessed September 30, 2013.
22. Department of Health. Health Service Circular: Better Blood Transfusion - the appropriate use of blood. 2002. Available at: http://webarchive.nationalarchives.gov.uk/20130107105354/http://www.dh.gov.uk/en/Publicationsandstatistics/Lettersandcirculars/Healthservicecirculars/DH_4004264. Accessed September 30, 2013.
23. Department of Health. Health Service Circular: Better Blood Transfusion - safe and appropriate use of blood. 2007. Available at: http://webarchive.nationalarchives.gov.uk/20130107105354/http://www.dh.gov.uk/prod_consum_dh/groups/dh_digitalassets/documents/digitalasset/dh_080803.pdf. Accessed September 30, 2013.
24. NCA. National Comparative Audit of Blood Transfusion - Re-audit of bedside transfusion practice 2011:1–75. Available at: http://hospital.blood.co.uk/library/pdf/NCA_2011_bedside_tx_re-audit_report.pdf. Accessed September 30, 2013.
25. Tinegate H, Birchall J, Gray A, et al. Guideline on the investigation and management of acute transfusion reactions Prepared by the BCSH Blood Transfusion Task Force. Br J Haematol 2012;159:143–53.
26. British Committee for Standards in Haematology, Milkins C, Berryman J, et al. Guidelines for pre-transfusion compatibility procedures in blood transfusion laboratories. Transfus Med 2013;23:3–35.
27. Gibson BE, Todd A, Roberts I, et al. Transfusion guidelines for neonates and older children. Br J Haematol 2004;124:433–53.
28. Verduzco LA, Nathan DG. Sickle cell disease and stroke. Blood 2009;114:5117–25.
29. Venkatesh V, Khan R, Curley A, et al. The safety and efficacy of red cell transfusions in neonates: a systematic review of randomized controlled trials. Br J Haematol 2012;158:370–85.
30. McCoy TE, Conrad AL, Richman LC, et al. Neurocognitive profiles of preterm infants randomly assigned to lower or higher hematocrit thresholds for transfusion. Child Neuropsychol 2011;17:347–67.
31. Whyte RK, Kirpalani H, Asztalos EV, et al. Neurodevelopmental outcome of extremely low birth weight infants randomly assigned to restrictive or liberal hemoglobin thresholds for blood transfusion. Pediatrics 2009;123:207–13.
32. Corwin HL, Carson JL. Blood transfusion–when is more really less? N Engl J Med 2007;356:1667–9.
33. Lacroix J, Hebert PC, Hutchison JS, et al. Transfusion strategies for patients in pediatric intensive care units. N Engl J Med 2007;356:1609–19.
34. Slonim AD, Joseph JG, Turenne WM, et al. Blood transfusions in children: a multi-institutional analysis of practices and complications. Transfusion 2008;48:73–80.
35. NCA. National Comparative Audit of the use of Red Cells in Neonates and Children 2010. Available at: http://hospital.blood.co.uk/library/pdf/NCA_red_cells_neonates_children.pdf. Accessed September 30, 2013.
36. British Committee for Standards in Haematology. Guideline on the Administration of Blood Components. 2010. Available at: http://www.bcshguidelines.com/documents/Admin_blood_components_bcsh_05012010.pdf. Accessed September 30, 2013.

37. Stainsby D, Jones H, Wells AW, et al. Adverse outcomes of blood transfusion in children: analysis of UK reports to the serious hazards of transfusion scheme 1996-2005. Br J Haematol 2008;141:73–9.

38. Christensen RD. Association between red blood cell transfusions and necrotizing enterocolitis. J Pediatr 2011;158:349–50.

39. Blau J, Calo JM, Dozor D, et al. Transfusion-related acute gut injury: necrotizing enterocolitis in very low birth weight neonates after packed red blood cell transfusion. J Pediatr 2011;158:403–9.

40. Ironside JW. Variant Creutzfeldt-Jakob disease: an update. Folia Neuropathol 2012;50:50–6.

41. JPAC. Methylene blue-treated Plasma: Joint UKBTS/HPA Professional Advisory Committee/Serious Hazards of Transfusion (SHOT) Position Statement. Available at: http://www.transfusionguidelines.org.uk/index.aspx?Publication=DL& Section=12&pageid=7737. Accessed September 30, 2013.

42. Bolton-Maggs PHB, Cohen H. The Annual SHOT Report (2011). 2012. Available at: www.shotuk.org.

43. Gawande A. The checklist manifesto. London: Profile Books Ltd; 2009.

44. Haynes AB, Weiser TG, Berry WR, et al. A surgical safety checklist to reduce morbidity and mortality in a global population. N Engl J Med 2009;360:491–9.

Blood Banking/ Immunohematology
Special Relevance to Pediatric Patients

Edward C.C. Wong, MD[a,b],*

KEYWORDS

- Transfusion medicine/blood banking • Immunohematology • Pediatrics

KEY POINTS

- Transfusion is part of the treatment plan of many children and adolescents.
- Pediatric licensed care providers should have a basic understanding of different components, including storage conditions, indications and contraindications, and procedures for administration.
- The rationale and indications for product modifications are necessary to provide appropriate blood and blood components.
- Immunohematological testing is critically important in providing appropriate blood and blood components for children.
- The decision to transfuse should involve careful consideration of the risks versus benefits.

DONOR SELECTION AND COLLECTION

Fig. 1 shows the overall schema and processes involved before and after the transfusion of blood and blood components.[1] In the United States, the Food and Drug Administration (FDA) regulates donor selection, collection, testing, component preparation, storage, and distribution of blood and blood components (Code of Federal Regulation under sections 211 and 606). Facilities that collect or manufacture blood components must register with the FDA and be licensed if the manufactured blood component is transferred across US state lines. In addition, AABB (formerly known as the American Association of Blood

Funding Sources: Sebia, Sysmex, Haemonetics (honorarium, educational, or investigative grants).
Conflict of Interest: Grant for "Use of Thromboelastography in Neonates" (Haemonetics).
[a] Division of Laboratory Medicine, Center for Cancer and Blood Disorders, Children's National Medical Center, Sheikh Zayed Campus for Advanced Children's Medicine, 111 Michigan Avenue, Northwest, Washington, DC 20010, USA; [b] Departments of Pediatrics and Pathology, George Washington University School of Medicine and Health Sciences, Washington, DC 20010, USA
* Division of Laboratory Medicine, Children's National Medical Center, 111 Michigan Avenue, Northwest, Washington, DC 20010.
E-mail address: ewong@childrensnational.org

Pediatr Clin N Am 60 (2013) 1541–1568
http://dx.doi.org/10.1016/j.pcl.2013.08.005
0031-3955/13/$ – see front matter © 2013 Elsevier Inc. All rights reserved.

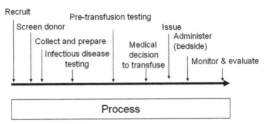

Fig. 1. The process of blood transfusion: from selection to transfusion. The complex process of recruiting, screening, collection, and testing of blood products as well as the decision to transfuse, issuing/administering the product, and performing posttransfusion monitoring are depicted. (*Modified from* Dzik WH. Emily Cooley Lecture 2002: transfusion safety in the hospital. Transfusion 2003;43:1190–9.)

Banks) regularly publishes *Standards for Blood Banks and Transfusion Services*, which are used by accrediting agencies.[2] Countries outside the United States have similar regulatory agencies that oversee manufacturing of their blood products.

Current infectious disease testing in the United States includes serologic testing for human immunodeficiency virus (HIV), hepatitis B and C, human T lymphotropic virus I/II, and syphilis, with nucleic amplification testing for HIV, hepatitis C, West Nile virus, and, in the future, for hepatitis B. Although not currently required by the FDA, testing for Chagas disease is required by the AABB. The FDA and the AABB implemented platelet product bacterial contamination testing because of the risk of bacterial contamination of platelets. This approach to bacterial detection has likely reduced the risk of bacterially contaminated platelets[3]; however, culture bottle detection systems with a minimal culture duration of 24 hours or using other less sensitive methods[4] still potentially allows the release of a product that has clinically significant bacterial growth. Hence, on January 31, 2011, the AABB standard 5.1.5.1.1 became effective, specifying that bacterial detection methods for platelet components use assays either approved by the FDA or validated to provide sensitivity equivalent to FDA-approved methods in order to further minimize the risk of sepsis.

COMPONENT PREPARATION
Whole Blood–Derived Products

Whole blood components, whole blood is collected into bags made of polyvinyl chloride containing di-(2-ethylhexyl) phthalate (DEHP) to make the bags pliable. DEHP is lipophilic and leaches into biologic fluids, including blood. DEHP is metabolized to mono-(2-ethylhexyl) phthalate. Animal in vitro toxicology studies and human epidemiologic studies have linked DEHP and its metabolites to proestrogenic effects. Despite small, long-term follow-up studies showing normal sexual development after early high exposure to DEHP,[5] DEHP-free medical devices, including blood bags, have been recommended for transfusion use in vulnerable patients, including infants and pregnant women, in many countries, including the United States. Most of the red blood cell (RBC) and plasma products (including fresh frozen plasma [FFP], thawed plasma, and so forth) are derived from the donation of whole blood.[6] In Canada and Europe, whole blood–derived platelets are derived using an alternative buffy coat method. **Fig. 2** shows the processes by which whole blood is separated into the various blood components. Depending on the type of processing, one whole blood unit can generate a unit each of packed RBCs, platelet concentrate, and plasma. In addition, subsequent thawing and precipitation of FFP at 1°C to 6°C generates a unit of cryoprecipitate (see **Fig. 2**).

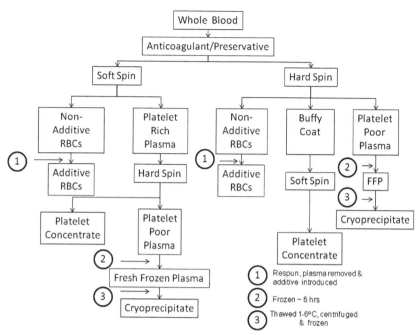

Fig. 2. Process of component preparation using US and European/Canadian preparation methodology. Detailed process flow of how whole blood products are processed in the United States and Europe/Canada. The major difference is in the production of whole blood–derived platelets. In the United States (*left arm*), a soft spin is used to generate platelet-rich plasma. This plasma, in turn, undergoes a hard spin to generate a platelet concentrate. In Europe and Canada (*right arm*), an initial hard spin is used to generate a buffy-coat layer, nonadditive RBCs, and platelet-poor plasma; the platelet-poor plasma is subsequently processed to FFP and cryoprecipitate. The buffy coat undergoes a soft spin to generate a platelet concentrate. In both arms, in the process of making additive units, nonadditive RBC units are respun with the removal of plasma and addition of additive solution.

The US National Blood Collection and Utilization Survey Report[6] reported that in 2008, 15 014 000 whole blood/RBC units and 1 300 000 whole blood–derived platelets, 4 484 000 units of plasma, and 1 109 000 units of cryoprecipitate were transfused in the United States. Of these transfusions, 383 000 whole blood/RBC units (2.6%) and 101 000 plasma units (2.3%) of total transfusions were given to children. No data were provided for the transfusion of whole blood–derived platelets (except for apheresis equivalent platelets, see later discussion) or cryoprecipitate to children.

Apheresis-Derived Products

Platelet, plasma, and RBCs can be obtained from whole blood processing and may also be obtained using apheresis techniques. Apheresis techniques provide the ability to obtain 4 to 6 equivalent donor whole blood platelet concentrates, a double unit of RBCs, or jumbo plasma (up to 500 or 600 mL depending on donor weight). Granulocytes can also be obtained.

The major impact of apheresis technology has been the improved ability to obtain platelets by apheresis. In 2008, 83.7% of platelets were derived from apheresis, with an increasing trend toward production of this product[6] with 7% of apheresis equivalent units (1 apheresis unit equals approximately 5 whole blood–equivalent units) transfused to pediatric patients.

RBC/Whole Blood Products

Whole blood is collected into bags containing anticoagulant/preservative solutions, which include acid citrate dextrose solution, citrate-phosphate-dextrose solution (CPD or CP2D), and citrate-phosphate-dextrose-adenine solution (CPDA-1). Additive solutions may be added to packed RBC units to increase the shelf life and include AS-1, AS-3, AS-5, and AS-7. In Europe, Canada, and other countries, an alternative additive solution is sodium chloride, adenine, glucose, mannitol (SAG-M) (**Table 1**). Toxic levels of the components of these anticoagulant/preservative and additive solutions are only reached in patients undergoing massive transfusion or extracorporeal membrane oxygenation (**Table 2**).[7]

Some centers prepare and store whole blood–equivalent units at colder temperatures (similar to RBC units) to decrease donor exposure and to provide a product with possible improved hemostatic capability in postcardiac surgery or trauma patients.[8,9] The data supporting the use of this blood component, however, are controversial because it is well known that refrigerated platelets stored for 72 hours have decreased in vivo survival.[10] However, the study by Manno and colleagues[8] showed that whole blood refrigerated up to 48 hours had an equivalent hemostatic effect platelet concentrates stored at 20°C to 24°C. However, logistically, whole blood stored for less than 48 hours is difficult to obtain given the turnaround time for results of transfusion-transmitted disease testing.

In some situations, whole blood units (reconstituted from packed RBCs and compatible plasma) may be necessary. Reconstituted whole blood may be needed for apheresis

Table 1
Contents of anticoagulant/preservative solutions (based on manufacturer's data)

Constituent	CPDA-1[a]	CPD	AS-1[b]	AS-3[b]	AS-5[b]	AS-7[b]	SAG-M[b]
Volume (mL)	100	63	100	100	100	100	100
Sodium Chloride (mg)	0	0	900	410	877	0	877
Dextrose (mg)	2000	1610	2200	1100	900	1585	820
Adenine	17.3	0	27	30	30	27	17
Mannitol	0	0	750	0	525	1000	0
Trisodium citrate (mg)	1660	1660	0	588	0	0	0
Citric acid	206	206	0	42	0	0	0
Sodium phosphate							
(Monobasic) (mg)	140	140	0	276	0	0	0
(Dibasic) (mg)	0	0	0	0	0	170	0
Shelf life of WBC units	35						
Shelf life of RBC units[c]	35	28	35–42	35–42	35–42	35–42	35–42

Abbreviation: AS, additive solution.
[a] Approximately 450 mL of donor blood is drawn into 63 mL CPDA-1. A unit of RBCs (hematocrit ~70%) is prepared after centrifugation and removal of most plasma.
[b] When AS-1, AS-5, AS-7, or SAG-M is used, approximately 450 mL of donor blood is drawn into CPD. When AS-3 is used, approximately 450 mL of donor blood is drawn into CP2D, which differs from CPD in containing double the amount of dextrose. After centrifugation and removal of plasma, the RBCs are resuspended in 100 mL of the additive solution with final hematocrit of 55% to 60%. Note: CPD solution used to make SAG-M units contains 525 mg sodium chloride/63 mL.
[c] Approved shelf life varies depending on the country's regulatory agency.

Table 2
Quantity of additives infused during transfusion of 15 mL/kg of representative CPDA-1, AS-1, AS-3, or SAG-M units in comparison with 2 units (AS-1) for pump prime during ECMO[a]

Additive	CPDA-1 (mg/kg)	AS-1 (mg/kg)	AS-3 (mg/kg)	SAG-M (mg/kg)	ECMO (2 units)	Toxic Dose[b] (g/kg/h)
NaCL	0	28.0	5.0	35.6	641	137
Dextrose	13.0	86.0	15.0	20.4	1982	240
Adenine	0.2	0.4	0.4	0.2	18	15
Citrate	12.0	6.5	8.4	6.5	148	180
Phosphate	9.0	1.3	3.7	1.3	31	>60
Mannitol	0	22.0	0	0	500	360

Abbreviation: ECMO, extracorporeal membrane oxygenation.
[a] Assuming 60% hematocrit for CPDA-1, AS-1, AS-3, and SAG-M units.
[b] Toxic dose actually difficult to predict because adenine, dextrose, and phosphate enter RBCs.
Data from Luban NL, Strauss RG, Hume HA. Commentary on the safety of red blood cells preserved in extended storage media for neonatal transfusions. Transfusion 1991;31:229–35.

procedures in very small patients or for whole blood exchange for hemolytic disease of the newborn to avoid iatrogenically induced coagulopathy. Reconstituted whole blood units are devoid of platelets and, thus, may lead to clinically significant iatrogenic thrombocytopenia requiring platelet transfusion to minimize bleeding risk.

Plasma Products

Plasma products include (1) FFP prepared after separation of whole blood and frozen at −18°C or less within 6 hours of preparation; (2) plasma frozen within 24 hours after phlebotomy (PF24) prepared from a whole blood or apheresis collection and stored at 1°C to 6°C within 8 hours of collection and frozen at −18°C or less; and (3) plasma frozen within 24 hours after phlebotomy, held at room temperature up to 24 hours after phlebotomy (PF24RT24), and prepared from either whole blood or apheresis collection.

All of these plasma products are considered to be equivalent in terms of clinical potency, with similar levels of coagulation factor proteins. However, because of the delayed freezing of PF24 and PF24RT24, the replacement of labile coagulation factors, such as factor V and VIII, is contraindicated with these products. In addition, PF24RT24 has significantly less protein S activity compared with PF24 and FFP and should not be used in patients with severely deficient protein S.[11,12]

All plasma products, thawed in an open system, must be discarded after 24 hours in order to minimize bacterial contamination. If the product has been thawed in a closed system, storage for up to 5 days at 1°C to 6°C is allowed, but the product must be relabeled as *thawed plasma*.

Platelet Products

Platelets can be either whole blood or apheresis derived. In the United States, whole blood–derived platelets are derived from a second hard spin of platelet-rich plasma (see **Fig. 2**). In Europe, Canada, and other countries, platelets are also derived from whole blood using the buffy coat method (see **Fig. 2**). The advantages of various platelet products are detailed in **Table 3**.[13] Clinical studies comparing the 3 different platelet preparations have been limited to comparisons of posttransfusion platelet increments, adjusting for patient blood volume and platelet product content (eg,corrected count increment). Studies have not consistently noted differences between the 3 products; thus, the products are thought to be equivalent in efficacy if given in equivalent doses.[13]

Table 3
Advantages of different platelet products

	Apheresis Platelets	Whole Blood–Derived Platelet (Platelet-Rich Plasma)	Whole Blood–Derived Platelets (Buffy Coat Method)
Donor exposure	Lower	Higher	Higher
Repeat donors (percentage)	Higher	Lower	Lower
Compatibility with cost-effective, sensitive bacterial detection methods	Yes	No (unless prestorage pooling)	No (unless prestorage pooling)
Compatibility with pathogen reduction technologies	Yes	No (unless prestorage pooling)	No (unless prestorage pooling)
Hospital preparation (pooling, point-of-care bacterial testing)	Less	More	More
Transfusion service Paperwork	Less	More	More
Wastage	Less	More	More
Febrile, nonhemolytic transfusion reactions	Fewer	More	More
Platelet activation	Lower	Highest	Lowest
Apheresis associated risk	Yes	No	No
Single-donor plasma exposure	Higher than whole blood derived	Reduced	Reduced
Cost of production	Higher	Significantly less than apheresis	Significantly less than apheresis, least expensive method
Availability during holiday and inclement weather	Less	More	More

Modified from Vassallo RR, Murphy S. A critical comparison of platelet preparation methods. Curr Opin Hematol 2006;13:323–30.

The FDA recently approved the use of a platelet additive solution (PAS) for apheresis platelets. PAS solutions contain acetate or glucose as a substrate for platelet metabolism, phosphate to buffer lactate production, citrate to prevent coagulation and lactate production, and potassium and magnesium to improve platelet function during storage. The theoretical advantages include improved in vivo and in vitro platelet quality, including improved platelet recovery and survival, increased total ATP content, improved hypotonic shock response/shape change, decreased transfusion reactions, improved bacterial detection, compatibility with pathogen inactivation methods, and potentially increased storage length.[14–16] It is likely that platelets in additive solutions will be increasingly used in the future.

Cryoprecipitate

Cryoprecipitate is prepared by thawing whole blood-derived FFP between 1°C and 6°C and recovering the precipitate via centrifugation. The cold-insoluble precipitate is placed in the freezer within 1 hour after removal from the refrigerated centrifuge and then thawed for use. Cryoprecipitate contains high levels of fibrinogen (>150 mg), factor VIII (>80 IU), factor XIII, von Willebrand factor (vWF), and fibronectin. The current indications include hypofibrinogenemia, both congenital and acquired, and factor XIII deficiency, if factor concentrates are not available. The remainder of this product, cryo-poor plasma, is another license product that is infrequently used as replacement fluid in thrombotic thrombocytopenic purpura.

Granulocytes

Granulocytes are an unlicensed product collected using apheresis technology. Donors are stimulated with dexamethasone or granulocyte colony-stimulating factor (G-CSF) and undergo apheresis to collect at least 1×10^{10} white blood cells (WBCs) per unit. Several studies have suggested that granulocytes may be indicated when there is anticipated WBC recovery in febrile patients who are neutropenic, have a bacterial or fungal infection, and have been unresponsive to antibiotics for several days.[17] Granulocytes may also be indicated in patients with a neutrophil function defect (eg, chronic granulomatous disease, leukocyte adhesion deficiency, and so forth) who are unresponsive to antibiotics.[18] Granulocytes collected from dexamethasone and G-CSF–stimulated donors have not undergone rigorous clinical trials for efficacy and are considered experimental. Thus, appropriate consent and/or approval by the local institutional review board must be obtained from both donors and recipients.

Pediatric patients who need granulocytes are often at risk for developing transfusion-transmitted or nosocomial cytomegalovirus (CMV) infection. Because LR is contraindicated, CMV serologically negative products may be required. In addition, patients receiving granulocytes are exposed to a large load of foreign human leukocyte antigens (HLA), which may increase the risk of HLA alloimmunization, development of subsequent platelet refractoriness, and/or a reduced likelihood for stem cell engraftment.

Granulocytes have high metabolic activity and need to be stored at 20°C to 24°C to be functionally active; the shelf life is limited to 24 hours, so completion of infectious disease testing must be waived, increasing the risk of transfusion-transmitted infections. Granulocytes contain a significant amount of RBCs (>30 mL, with the hematocrit generally between 5% and 15%) and, therefore, must be crossmatch compatible against a patient's specimen. The Resolving Infection in Neutropenia with Granulocytes Study is a phase IIII randomized study of adjunctive granulocyte transfusion in septic patients undergoing standard antimicrobial therapy and may answer whether transfusion of dexamethasone/G-CSF–stimulated granulocytes have added benefit in septic children and adults.[19]

In the United Kingdom, a phase I study is underway to determine whether transfused whole blood–derived granulocytes stored in additive solutions and plasma have a similar safety profile to whole blood–derived granulocytes. The potential advantages of using whole blood–derived granulocytes include the decreased cost of production, greater availability, and potentially longer storage, if stored in an additive solution. Clinical trials have yet to demonstrate the efficacy of this product.[20] This product is not available in the United States.

Storage and the Storage Lesion

Each blood component has its own unique storage requirements and storage lesion (**Tables 4** and **5**).[21–23] Based on ^{51}Cr labeling studies, the FDA requires that RBC products have at least 75% recovery and less than 1% hemolysis (24 hours after transfusion). The theoretical risk of worse outcomes with the transfusion of older blood has

Table 4
Storage conditions and usual indications of selected blood products

Component/Product (Volume)	Composition	Storage Length	Storage Conditions	Usual Indications
RBCs (in CPD, CP2D, CPDA-1, ~250 mL)	RBCs (~75% Hct); 50–70 mL plasma, 10^9–10^{10} WBCs and platelets (nonfunctioning)	28 d	1°C–6°C	Increase RBC mass in symptomatic anemia
RBCs (additive, ~300 mL)	RBCs (~60% Hct); 40 mL plasma, 10^9–10^{10} WBCs and platelets (nonfunctioning); 100 mL additive solution	35–42 d	1°C–6°C	Increase RBC mass in symptomatic anemia
RBCs leukocytes reduced (~300 mL with additive; ~225 mL without additive)	RBCs with Hcts as previous for additive and nonadditive solutions; <5 × 10^6 WBCs (United States) <1 × 10^6 WBCs (Europe), few dysfunctional platelets, 40 mL plasma; should contain ≥85% of original red cell content	28 d	1°C–6°C	Increase RBC mass in symptomatic anemia, decrease likelihood of febrile reaction, alloimmunization to leukocyte antigens, reduce CMV transmission
Washed RBCs (~180 mL)	RBCs with ~Hct 75%; <5 × 10^6 WBCs, no plasma	24 h	1°C–6°C	Increase RBC mass in symptomatic anemia, reduced potassium, additives, and pathologic antibody exposure
Whole blood (~500 mL)	RBCs (~Hct 40%); 200 mL plasma, (deficient in labile clotting factors V and VIII, platelets (dysfunctional at 72 h) 10^9–10^{10} WBCs	28 d	1°C–6°C	Increase RBC mass in symptomatic anemia, possible improved hemostatic ability, if given
48 h or less after collection
Whole blood–derived platelets (~50 mL)	Platelets >5.5 × 10^{10}/unit; ~50 mL plasma; RBCs; WBCs	5 d	Agitated, 20°C–24°C	Bleeding caused by thrombocytopathy or thrombocytopenia
Apheresis platelets (~300 mL)	Platelets >3 × 10^{11}/unit; ~300 mL plasma; RBCs; WBCs	5 d	Agitated, 20°C–24°C	As previous

Component	Content	Expiration	Storage	Indications
Platelets leukocytes reduced (~300 mL)	Platelets as previous; <5 × 10^6 WBCs	5 d	Agitated, 20°C–24°C	As previous; decrease likelihood of febrile reaction, alloimmunization to leukocyte antigens, reduce CMV transmission
FFP (~250 mL)	Plasma, all coagulation factors and complement (no platelets)	1 y	≤–18°C	Treatment of coagulation factor deficiency when a suitable derivative or recombinant product is not available or suitable; treatment of TTP
PF24 (~250 mL)	Plasma, all stable coagulation factors and complement (no platelets), decreased level of labile coagulation factors	1 y	≤–18°C	Clinically significant stable coagulation factor deficiencies; treatment of TTP[a]
PF24RT24 (~250 mL)	Plasma, all stable coagulation factors and complement (no platelets), decreased level of labile coagulation factors	1 y	≤–18°C	Clinically significant stable coagulation factor deficiencies[a]
Thawed plasma (derived from FFP, PF24, or PF24RT24, ~250 mL)	Plasma, all stable coagulation factors and complement (no platelets), variable level of other coagulation factors	See next box	See[b]	Clinically significant stable coagulation factor deficiencies[a] (including protein S deficiency, if prepared from PF24RT24)
Cryoprecipitate (~15 mL)	Fibrinogen ≥150 mg/unit; factor VIII ≥80 IU/unit; factor XIII, fibronectin, vWF	1 y	≤–18°C	Deficiency or dysfunction of fibrinogen or factor XIII; von Willebrand disease or hemophilia A if a safe alternative is not available
Apheresis granulocytes (~200–300 mL)	Granulocytes (>1 × 10^{10} PMN/unit; lymphocytes; platelets [>2.0 × 10^{11}/unit], some RBCs, 3–8 × greater content from G-CSF and dexamethasone stimulated donors)	24 h	Agitated, 20°C–24°C	Provide functional granulocytes for febrile, septic patients, with anticipated WBC recovery and unresponsive to antibiotics

Abbreviations: Hct, hematocrit; PMN, polymorphonuclear leukocytes; TTP, thrombotic thrombocytopenic purpura.

[a] Note: Not to be used for deficiencies of labile clotting factors, such as factor V and VIII; use as replacement for TTP.

[b] Thawed at 30°C to 37°C and maintained at 1°C to 6°C for 4 days after the initial 24-hour period.

Table 5
The RBC storage lesion

Biochemical and Biochemical Changes	In Vitro Findings	In Vivo Correlations with Stored RBCs/Potential Clinical Significance
2,3-DPG depletion	Left shift of oxygen-hemoglobin curve	Restoration of RBC 2,3-DPG within 24–72 h of transfusions; delay in oxygen delivery
ATP depletion	Rapid loss lead to reversible spheroechinocyte formation	Poor correlation of ATP levels with 24 h posttransfusion RBC survival
Increased intracellular calcium	Promotes RBC dehydration with echinocytosis and microvesiculation	Increased viscosity, reduced flow in capillary systems
Metabolic modulation	Increased glucose consumption via pentose phosphate pathway and increased O_2 saturation of RBC hemoglobin; progressive acidification and lactate buildup	Unknown
Decreased Na-K pump activity	Leakage of K from RBCs not returned to RBCs	Increased K levels in older RBCs, clinically significant hyperkalemia; worsened by irradiation
Depletion of SNO-Hb	Loss of SNO-Hb after 3 d of storage	No off loading of NO under hypoxic conditions to promote vasodilation and increased blood flow
Low-level hemolysis	Free hemoglobin scavenges NO; breakdown to free heme and iron	Decreased NO causes vasoconstriction; free heme can cause hypertensive crises in the pulmonary circulation and acute tubular injury in the kidney
Membrane phospholipid loss	Loss of RBC microvesicles correlates with spheroechinocyte formation and increased osmotic fragility	Decreased vesiculation associated with prolongation of viable storage time and increased survival of AS-1 preserved RBCs
Abnormal membrane phospholipid distribution	PS accumulates on outer membrane in acid pH or in presence of aminophospholipid translocase inhibitor; this loss is seen less with additive solutions and hypotonic solutions; however, no change during routine blood bank storage	Senescent RBCs and sickle RBCs have accumulation of PS on outer membrane Animal models show PS accumulation on RBCs associated with increased clearance Exposed PS potentially prothrombotic and proinflammatory

(continued on next page)

Table 5
(continued)

Biochemical and Biochemical Changes	In Vitro Findings	In Vivo Correlations with Stored RBCs/Potential Clinical Significance
Lipid peroxidation and protein oxidation	Depletion of glutathione Spectrin oxidation	Decreased lipid peroxidation associated with prolongation of viable storage time and increased survival of AS-1 preserved RBCs
	Abnormal spectrin-actin-protein 4.1 complex binding associated with phospholipid loss Rate of RBC lipid peroxidation slowed in donors taking antioxidants or addition of antioxidants to stored blood Addition of antioxidants to stored blood decreases lipid peroxidation, decreased osmotic fragility, and increased RBC deformability	Oxidative damage to lipids can result in lysophospholipid-induced TRALI and posttransfusion thrombotic events

Abbreviations: DPG, diphosphoglycerate; Hb, hemoglobin; Na-K, sodium-potassium; NO, nitric oxide; PS, phosphatidylserine; SNO-Hb, s-nitroso hemoglobin; TRALI, transfusion-related acute lung injury.

been suggested by a large retrospective study of adult patients undergoing cardiac surgery.[24] Prospective randomized clinical trials have not yet been completed.

Both whole blood–derived platelets and apheresis platelets must be stored on an agitator in a gas-permeable container (bag) for no more than 5 days (United States) at 20°C to 24°C because of the increased risk of bacterial growth causing clinical sepsis and decreased circulation of transfused platelets.[25] Some countries (eg, Netherlands, Sweden, and Switzerland), however, allow storage of up to 7 days. Studies of cold storage demonstrated platelet activation and decreased survival, so platelet concentrates are stored at 20°C to 24°C. In the future, new storage solutions may improve and permit the storage of platelets at colder temperatures for longer storage duration.[26]

Platelets are issued in their original gas-permeable transfer bags or in syringes. Syringes allow easy aliquoting of products for a precise administration rate using an infusion pump. Platelets stored in syringes undergo a switch to anaerobic respiration with declining pH, glucose levels, and platelet function resulting in a 4-hour outdate.[27–29] Aliquots of apheresis platelets stored in gas-permeable bags are offered as appropriate doses for transfusion in children; however, storage of less than 40 mL of apheresis platelets in gas-permeable bags is not recommended because this is associated with impaired platelet aggregation.[30] **Table 6** identifies the elements of the platelet storage lesion.[31] In the United States, there is no regulatory requirement for posttransfusion survival, which will likely change because new platelet products must be evaluated for quality.[32]

Table 6
The platelet storage lesion: correlation with in vitro and in vivo studies

Biochemical Changes	In Vitro Studies	Correlation with Recovery	Correlation with Survival
Platelet activation/ degranulation	Increased surface expression of CD62 P	Possibly[a]	Possibly[a]
	Release of β-thromboglobulin and platelet factor 4, reflecting release of alpha granules	No	No
Increased binding to anionic phospholipids	Increased annexin V binding	[b]	[b]
Shape change	Loss of swirling	Possibly[a]	No
	Decreased morphology score (decreased discoid shape)	No	No
	Decreased hypotonic shock response	Yes	Yes
	Decreased extent of shape change with ADP	Yes	Yes
Altered metabolism/ loss of buffering capacity	Decreased pH	Yes	Yes
	Decreased ATP content	No	No
	Decreased glucose consumption	No	No
	Increased Pco_2	No	No
	Decreased Po_2	No	Possibly[a]
	Increased lactate production	Yes (neg correlation)	Yes (neg correlation)

Abbreviation: neg, negative.
[a] Studies not consistent.
[b] Not assessed in Devine and Serrano[31].
Data from Devine DV, Serrano K. The platelet storage lesion. Clin Lab Med 2010;30:475–87.

BLOOD COMPONENT MODIFICATIONS
Leukoreduction

In Europe, Canada, and other countries (except in the United States), universal leukoreduction (LR) has been adopted as standard for all cellular blood components (except granulocytes). RBCs, which typically contain 1 or more to 10×10^9 white cells, can be leukoreduced by filtering whole blood at the beginning of processing (prestorage LR) or by attaching a filter with a sterile connecting device to a unit of packed RBC. Although the latter technique can be performed at the bedside, the procedure is usually performed in the blood bank because of the higher failure rates of bedside LR. Current LR filters reduce the number of WBCs 1000-fold so that the residual WBC count does not exceed 5×10^6 per packed RBC unit (United States) or 1×10^6 (Europe) while retaining 85% of the original red cell content.

The major indications for LR include reducing transfusion-associated CMV, bacteria, and prion transmission. In a prospective observational study of very low birth weight (VLBW) infants, although universal LR did not result in significant reduction of neonatal intensive care unit mortality or bacteremia, the adjusted odd ratios for bronchopulmonary dysplasia, retinopathy of prematurity, and necrotizing enterocolitis favored the use of leukoreduced RBCs.[33] It should be noted that LR should never be used as a strategy for the prevention of transfusion-associated graft-versus-host disease (TA-GVHD).

Irradiation

Irradiation is performed to prevent proliferation of donor lymphocytes, which may recognize recipient tissues as foreign and initiate TA-GVHD **Box 1**.[34] Irradiation

---

Box 1
Clinical indications for irradiated products

Fetus/Infant

   Intrauterine transfusion

   Premature infants

   Congenital immunodeficiency (identified or suspected)

   Those undergoing exchange transfusion for erythroblastosis

Child/Adult

   Congenital immunodeficiency (identified or suspected)

   Hematological malignancy or solid tumor (neuroblastoma, sarcoma, Hodgkin disease receiving ablative chemotherapy/radiotherapy)

   Recipient of peripheral blood stem cells, marrow, or cord blood

   Recipient of familial blood donation

   Recipient of HLA-matched products

   Lupus or any other condition requiring fludarabine, cyclophosphamide

Potential indications

   Term infant

   Recipient and donor pair from a genetically homogeneous population

   Other patient with hematological malignancy or solid tumor receiving immunosuppressive agents

Data from Wong EC. Irradiated products. In: Hillyer C, Strauss R, Luban NL, editors. Handbook of pediatric transfusion medicine. 1st edition. Amsterdam: Elsevier; 2004. p. 101–12.

---

practice varies tremendously between institutions. Some institutions selectively irradiate blood products based on the diagnosis, age (or weight) of patients, and/or the relationship of the donor to the recipient, whereas other institutions irradiate all blood products. Much of the practice variability depends on logistical issues, such as costs, wastage, irradiator and technologist availability, and patient population. FFP and cryoprecipitate do not require irradiation because these products are derived from thawed frozen plasma, which damages WBCs during the freezing process. In contrast, plasma products that have not been frozen should be irradiated before transfusion. Irradiation reduces RBC storage shelf life to 28 days after irradiation or actual outdate, whichever comes first, as a result of irradiation-induced increased potassium leakage.[35] To avoid wastage of these units, centers irradiate just before issue. Some centers will wash RBCs to reduce the amount of potassium present.

Instrumentation used for blood radiation includes (1) free-standing gamma source irradiators (^{137}Cs or ^{60}Co) and (2) linear accelerators that use x-ray irradiation. In the United States, most facilities use free-standing lead-shielded ^{137}Cs gamma irradiators, which allow irradiation of products within minutes.

Washed Cellular Components

Washing decreases the protein (RBC and platelet) and potassium content (RBC) of a blood product. The indications include (1) severe or recurrent allergic reactions to plasma proteins within cellular blood products, (2) anaphylaxis reaction caused by immunoglobulin A (IgA) antibodies in IgA-deficient recipients, and (3) patients with neonatal alloimmune thrombocytopenia receiving platelets from their mother. The last indication is recommended in order to remove the circulatory platelet-specific antibody responsible for the thrombocytopenia. In cases when patients have recurrent, severe allergic reactions, the use of RBC additive units and premedication may be considered because these units do not contain plasma. Another indication for washing is the removal of potassium from large-volume (>20–25 mL/kg) RBC transfusions. Other controversial indications for washing of RBCs include patients with T-activation (caused by the exposure of the cryptic T-antigen by neuraminidase from a bacterial infection) to remove IgM T antibody, which is present in all adult plasma, or to remove the small amount of ABO antibodies in the plasma of packed RBCs transfused to patients with paroxysmal nocturnal hemoglobinuria (ie, a non–O group patient transfused with O RBCs). However, based on experience at the author's institution and others and a lack of convincing evidence in the medical literature, washing of RBCs for these indications is not indicated.

Because the washing process is an open process, the outdate of washed cellular products is 24 hours for RBCs and 4 hours for platelets. Coordination is required between the ordering physician and the blood bank when a washed product is needed. Washed platelets have a significant loss of product during processing and may become activated with decreased platelet aggregation and potentially poorer in vivo survival and function.[36,37]

Volume Reduction

Volume reduction is a blood bank procedure whereby cellular products are concentrated with the simultaneous reduction of plasma in the product. Indications include (1) patients who need to restrict intake volume (eg, RBC and platelet transfusions in patients with renal failure) and (2) removal of plasma in patients who would benefit from removal of potentially pathologic antibodies (eg, ABO-incompatible platelets). In the case of ABO-incompatible platelets, some institutions have used isoagglutinin titer cutoffs instead of using washed or volume-reduced platelet products.[38] Volume reduction is associated with significant loss of product and increased activation after processing[37,39–41] and should be used for specific indications.

SPECIAL PEDIATRIC POPULATION NEEDS
Special Considerations for Neonates

The small blood volume of neonates mandates smaller aliquots of blood products. Issue containers typically include syringes or transfer bags with volumes of 25 to 50 mL or less, which requires special considerations for product labeling and handling, especially for platelets. Because a VLBW patient may need multiple, small transfusions during the entire hospital course, one or more RBC units may be dedicated for that patient.[42,43] Small-volume transfusions (≤15 mL/kg) of additive or nonadditive RBC units may be used up to the date of expiration without the risk of hyperkalemia.[44] However, if large volumes need to be transfused (>25 mL/kg), less than 5- to 7-day-old units are recommended with transfusion rates of no more than 0.5 mL/kg/h.[45] Strategies to estimate individual neonatal transfusion needs, allowing RBC transfusions from the same bag for multiple neonates, can decrease wastage while still minimizing donor exposure.[43] With the use of dedicated RBC units to minimize donor exposure, some centers also identify units with low lead levels for transfusion.[46]

Special Considerations for Patients on Extracorporeal Life Support and Other Critically Ill Patients

Older versus fresher RBCs

One large retrospective study in adult patients[24] and other retrospective studies in adult and pediatric surgery patients[47,48] suggest an increase in morbidity and mortality with the use of older RBCs. A major criticism of these retrospective studies is that they include confounders or biases associated with worse outcomes, which are not eliminated by multivariate analysis. Indeed, some small randomized controlled trials in adults[49,50] did not demonstrate harm from transfusion of prolonged storage of RBC units; in addition, these studies did not include pediatric patients undergoing cardiovascular surgery.

Because of the possible higher morbidity and mortality with the use of older RBCs, several randomized controlled clinical trials are underway. Recently, the Age of Red Blood Cells in Premature Infants study, a double-blind, randomized clinical trial of transfusion of RBCs less than 7 days old versus standard-age RBCs in VLBW Canadian infants, demonstrated no difference in clinical outcomes between the two groups.[51] The age of blood in children in the pediatric ICU (ABC-PICU), a randomized double-blind clinical trial of fresher versus older blood, is about to begin to answer whether fresher blood is associated with better clinical outcomes in critically ill pediatric patients.

Special Considerations for Hematopoietic Stem Cell Transplant Recipients

ABO minor and major mismatch hematopoietic stem cell transplant patients are subject to potential changes in ABO/Rh type, which can result in fatal hemolysis.[52] When to change a recipient's blood type depends on the patient's forward and reverse type, the DAT, and possibly other less well-defined parameters, including the degree of engraftment and risk of relapse. Blood type changes should be investigated by the blood bank and agreed on by the transfusion medicine and stem cell transplant services. Basic guiding principles include the following: (1) the product given must avoid hemolysis of the donor graft and recipient and (2) delayed RBC engraftment by the recipient (**Table 7**).[53]

Because platelets are frequently in short supply and have short outdates, Rh-positive (D+) platelets may be given to Rh-negative (D−) hematopoietic stem cell transplant or oncology patients. Adult and pediatric studies have shown that the use of Rh-positive (D+) apheresis platelets in these patients is associated with a zero or near zero risk of anti-D alloimmunization.[54,55] Since 2000, the author's experience at the Children's National Medical Center with transfusion of multiple D+ apheresis platelets to D-pediatric hematopoietic stem cell recipients and oncology patients has not shown the development of anti-D in these patients.

Special Considerations for Patients with Sickle Cell Disease

Patients with sickle cell disease (SCD) often require transfusions and have a high rate of RBC alloantibody development. The National Institutes of Health recommends that an RBC phenotype (ABO, Rh, Kell, Duffy, Kidd, Lewis, Lutheran, P, and MNS at a minimum) be obtained on all patients with SCD who are older than 6 months. In addition, patients should be transfused with leukocyte-reduced, phenotypically matched RBCs (RBCs matched for C, E, and K [unless there are other antibodies present]) to limit the development of antibodies.[56] However, these recommendations are not universally followed.

Special considerations for transfusion include providing sickle-negative, antigen-matched units per institutional protocol. Because of the chronicity of transfusion,

Table 7
Transfusion support for patients undergoing ABO mismatched allogeneic hematopoietic stem cell transplantation

Recipient	Donor	Mismatch Type	Pretransplant (Phase I)[a] All Components	Peritransplant (Phase 2)[b] RBCs	Peritransplant (Phase 2)[b] First-Choice Platelets	Peritransplant (Phase 2)[b] Next-Choice Platelets	Peritransplant (Phase 2)[b] FFP	Posttransplant (Phase 3)[c] All Components
A	O	Minor	Recipient	O	A	AB, B, O	A, AB	Donor
B	O	Minor	Recipient	O	B	AB, A, O	B, AB	Donor
AB	O	Minor	Recipient	O	AB	A, B, O	AB	Donor
AB	A	Minor	Recipient	A	AB	A, B, O	AB	Donor
AB	B	Minor	Recipient	B	AB	B, A, O	AB	Donor
O	A	Major	Recipient	O	A	AB, B, O	A, AB	Donor
O	B	Major	Recipient	O	B	AB, A, O	B, AB	Donor
O	AB	Major	Recipient	O	AB	A, B, O	AB	Donor
A	AB	Major	Recipient	A	AB	A, B, O	AB	Donor
B	AB	Major	Recipient	B	AB	B, A, O	AB	Donor
A	B	Minor & Major	Recipient	O	AB	A, B, O	AB	Donor
B	A	Minor & Major	Recipient	O	AB	B, A, O	AB	Donor

Data from Robitaille N, Hume HA. Blood components and fractionated plasma products: preparation, indications and administration. In: Arceci RJ, Hann IM, Smith OP. editors. Pediatric hematology. 3rd edition. Malden (MA): Blackwell Publishing; 2006. p. 693–723.

[a] Phase 1: Patient is prepared for transplantation until myeloablation (day -1).

[b] Phase 2: From the start of myeloablative therapy (day 0) until:

For RBCs: Direct antiglobulin test is negative and antidonor isohemagglutinins are no longer detectable.

For FFP: Recipient's erythrocytes are no longer detectable (ie, forward typing is consistent with donor's ABO group).

[c] Phase 3: After the forward and reverse type are consistent with the donor's ABO group.

several centers also have developed dedicated donor programs that target African American groups.[57–61] In the instance that a truly rare alloantibody is identified, appropriate antigen-negative units may be available through the American Rare Donor Registry or other similar types of registries.[62]

SPECIAL PRODUCTS
Recombinant Products/Plasma Derivatives

Blood banks may provide specialized coagulation products in addition to cellular blood components. The rationale for keeping these products (**Table 8**) in the blood bank includes (1) inventory control, (2) specialized handling to avoid waste, and (3)

Table 8
Factor derivative and recombinant products often kept in pediatric transfusion medicine service facilities

Concentrate	Source	Preparation	Indications
Factor VIII	Plasma derivative	Hemofil M, Monarc M, Monoclate P	Hemophilia A
		Humate P, Alphanate, Koate	Hemophilia A, Humate-P, and Alphanate are licensed in the United States for von Willebrand disease
	Recombinant	Recombinate Helixate FS Kogenate FS	Hemophilia A, generally considered product of choice
Factor IX	Plasma derivative	AlphaNine SD, Mononine	Hemophilia B
		3 factor PCC (Konyne, Profilnine SD)	Coagulation factor deficiencies, warfarin reversal; however, 4 factor PCC are more efficacious
		4 factor PCC (Proplex T, Octaplex, Kcentra)	Coagulation factor deficiencies; warfarin reversal
		FEIBA (activated PCC)	Thrombotic risk, used for patients with hemophilia with inhibitors
	Recombinant	BeneFix (third)	Hemophilia B, generally considered product of choice
Antithrombin III	Plasma derivative	Thrombate	Antithrombin deficiency (congenital and acquired)
	Recombinant	Atryn	Produced from transgenic goats; perioperative and peripartum venous thromboembolisms with congenital antithrombin III deficiency
Activated factor VII	Recombinant	NovoSeven	Patients with hemophilia A or B with high titer antibodies; patients who are factor VII deficient; Glanzmann thrombasthenia (Europe)

Abbreviation: PCC, prothrombin complex concentrate.

oversight of appropriateness of transfusion. Many of these products are produced without neonatal or pediatric patient dosing in mind. Only some products allow continuous infusion. Most products use defined formulas.

Recombinant factor VII is approved for patients with severe hemophilia A or B with high titer inhibitor, congenital factor VII deficiency, and Glanzmann thrombasthenia (Europe) but has been used in a variety of off-label bleeding conditions with variability in dosing and success.[63] Despite enthusiasm in controlling bleeding and perceived safety, randomized clinical trials have not permitted the expansion of approved indications. The use of the product often requires consultation and approval to gate keep inappropriate use.

IgA-Deficient Products

The use of IgA-deficient products may be required when there is evidence for posttransfusion anaphylaxis caused by the development of anti-IgA antibodies reacting with IgA present in the plasma of blood components. Any blood product may induce such a reaction. Because the diagnosis requires documentation of anti-IgA antibodies from a reference laboratory, communication between the licensed care provider and the blood bank is essential for timely provision of blood products. There have been reports of anaphylaxis with anti-IgA antibodies in the presence of low levels of IgA.[64] An alternative to IgA-deficient blood products includes washed cellular products. However, if plasma or cryoprecipitate is needed, IgA-deficient products must be sourced.

HLA-Matched/Crossmatch Compatible Platelets

Platelet alloimmunization to class I HLA antigen or platelet-specific antigens is a relatively common occurrence in transfused pediatric patients recovering from chemotherapy or undergoing allogeneic stem cell transplantation who require frequent platelet transfusions.[65] In a large Canadian adult study, alloimmunization was only reduced from 17% to 9% in patients with acute leukemia or undergoing hematopoietic stem cell transplantation despite the use of leukoreduced platelet products.[66] In a pediatric study, LR of platelets (using third-generation filters) did not reduce the HLA alloimmunization rate (24%). However, the investigators indicated several potential confounders, including the small size of the study and use of bedside filtration.[65]

Platelet alloimmunization is diagnosed by the lack of platelet increment as determined by a correct count increment (CCI) less than 7500 on 2 consecutive occasions despite using platelets that are ABO identical and 3 days or less in age.[67] The CCI is defined by the following equation:

$$CCI = (\text{plt count increment per mm}^3 \times \text{body surface area per m}^2 \times 10^{11})/\text{total plt transfused, where } plt \text{ is platelet}$$

For example, in a 1-hour posttransfusion platelet count increment of 40 000/mm^3 (40 × 10^9/L) in a patient with a body surface area of 0.9 m^2 who received 3 equivalent whole blood–derived platelet units (3 × 5.5 × 10^{10}), the platelets would have a CCI of 21 818.

Consecutive ABO identical platelet transfusions with CCIs less than 7500 are suggestive of platelet refractoriness and require the use of crossmatched or HLA-matched platelets. There are several tests that can identify platelet alloimmunization, including solid phase RBC adherence assay for the detection of IgG antibodies on platelets (Capture-P, Immucor, Norcross GA), platelet immunofluorescence test, monoclonal antibody immobilization of platelet antigen, and specific HLA antibody identification by a variety of methods.[68–70] Either crossmatch-compatible or HLA-compatible platelets may improve the CCI.

The HLA matchmaker software program can predict HLA compatibility by identifying immunogenic epitopes represented by amino acid triplets in antibody access regions of various HLA molecules; this has allowed a greater number of HLA compatible platelets to be identified compared with conventional cross-reactive group matching.[71] Another group has developed the antibody specificity prediction method to select platelets based on patients' HLA antibody specificity using an antiglobulin-enhanced microlymphocytotoxicity test modified by the addition of serum and a computer program.[72]

Antigen-Negative Platelet Products for Neonatal Alloimmune Thrombocytopenia

Neonatal alloimmune thrombocytopenia develops when the infant's paternally derived platelet antigens are seen as foreign by the mother's immune system and results in the production of IgG antibodies that cross the placental, causing fetal or neonatal thrombocytopenia. If platelets are urgently needed, nonantigen-matched platelets are the best product to use.[73,74] These platelet products should be leukoreduced to provide a CMV reduced risk product. Some institutions may also provide a CMV seronegative product.

When non-antigen matched platelets are ineffective, antigen negative platelets may be required, which require coordination with the local blood center with a request for HPA-negative units.[75] Specific donor recruitment, collection, testing, and shipping can take more than 72 hours. In cases when the specific antigen is not known (especially if the ethnicity is non-Caucasian), maternal whole blood–derived platelets or apheresis donation may be needed. Platelet products from the mother must be washed, irradiated, and leukoreduced. The ordering physician may waive infectious disease testing if there is a potential for life-threatening bleed and infectious disease testing cannot be completed in time.

Pathogen-Inactivated Blood Products

Pathogen-inactivated products have the potential for reducing current and emerging infectious disease risk because only a limited number of pathogens are currently tested for and donor history may not detect high-risk behaviors or exposures. Four processes (methylene blue plus visible light, amotosalen plus UV light, riboflavin plus UV light, and solvent detergent) have received the CE Mark in Europe for plasma, and 2 of these (amotosalen and riboflavin processes) have also received the CE Mark for platelets. Currently, only one solvent detergent–treated plasma product (Octaplas, Octapharma AB, Sweden) is licensed in the United States. Altered potency and toxicity have been reported.[76]

In 2013, the FDA allowed a premarket approval application for amotosalen plus UV light pathogen inactivated plasma and platelet product (INTERCEPT Blood System, Cerus, Concord, CA). This pathogen inactivation system for platelet and plasma products has had extensive clinical and safety studies both outside and within the United States. In this process, irreversible DNA/RNA cross-linking occurs when the synthetic psoralen is illuminated with UV light, inhibiting the replication of both microorganisms and WBCs. Studies have shown as much as a 10^5- to 10^7-log decrease of bacteria and viruses in these plasma-rich products.

Another pathogen inactivation system, Mirasol Pathogen Reduction Technology (PRT) system (Terumo BCT, Lakewood, CO), has been extensively studied in Europe and, like the INTERCEPT Blood System, it is currently approved for use in Europe for platelets and plasma. This system uses riboflavin and UV light to introduce irreparable lesions of nucleic acids, inhibiting pathogens and WBC replication. Both the INTERCEPT Blood and Mirasol PRT systems may also add further protection against TA-GVHD.[77]

Table 9
Commonly used techniques used in the blood bank

Test	Principle of the Test	Purpose
Group and Type TAT: 5–20 min	Mixing of known anti-A, anti-B, anti-AB reagent with patients' red cells (forward type) and mixing of patients' plasma or serum with red cells of known ABO and Rh (D) type (reverse type)	To determine ABO and Rh (D) type
Antibody Screen (IAT) TAT: 45–60 min	Mixing of patients' plasma or serum with single-donor reagent red cells with known antigenic phenotype (usually 2 or 3 reagent cells used); can be used with or without enhancement media (eg, low ionic strength solution, polyethylene glycol); can be performed at various incubation phases (eg, immediate spin, 37°C, antihuman globulin) and various incubation times	To detect IgG alloantibodies and/or autoantibodies in the patients' plasma and/or serum
Antibody Panel TAT: 45–60 min	Same as antibody screen but with a larger group of reagent red cells (11 or more reagent cells)	To detect IgG alloantibodies and/or autoantibodies in the patients' plasma and/or serum
Crossmatch TAT: 5–60 min	Mixing of patients' plasma or serum with selected donor red cells; can be used with or without enhancement media; can be performed at various incubation phase	To detect incompatibility between patient and donor red cells (eg, ABO and/or other antigens)
Direct Antiglobulin Test TAT: 20–30 min	Mixing of patients' red cells from EDTA sample with various antihuman globulin antisera (eg, anti-C3b; anti-C3d; anti-C3b, d; anti-IgG)	To detect in vivo sensitization of patients' red cells with IgG and/or complement
Elution TAT: 60–90 min	To release bound antibodies from patients' red cells to identify the antibody; various methods exist depending on the type of antibody to be recovered; some methods leave the patients' red cells intact so that they can be phenotyped	To identify the specificity of antibodies that are bound to patients' red cells and/or to phenotype patients' red cells after removal of bound antibodies

(continued on next page)

Table 9 (continued)		
Test	Principle of the Test	Purpose
Cold Antibody Screen TAT: 60–90 min	Mixing of patients' plasma or serum with single-donor reagent red cells with known antigenic phenotype (usually screening cells, A and B cells, and cord blood cells); can be performed at various incubation phases (ie, immediate spin, room temperature, 15°C, 4°C) and various incubation times	To detect IgM alloantibodies and/or autoantibodies in patients' plasma and/or serum
Cold Antibody Panel TAT: 60–90 min	Same as cold antibody screen but with a larger group of reagent red cells (11 or more reagent cells)	To detect IgM alloantibodies and/or autoantibodies in the patients' plasma and/or serum
Serologic RBC Antigen Typing TAT: 5–60 min (may take longer if full phenotyping required)	Mixing of patients' or donor's red cells with known antisera (eg, anti-A, anti-C, anti-D, and so forth)	To detect the presence or absence of specific antigens on patient or donor red cells

Abbreviations: EDTA, ethylenediaminetetraacetic acid; IAT, indirect antiglobulin test; TAT, turn around time.

In Octaplas, the only FDA-approved, human-pooled, solvent detergent–treated plasma product for use in the United States, coagulation factor activities in the final product are quality controlled to obtain levels within the range of normal human plasma. Protein S and alpha2-antiplasmin, which are labile to solvent/detergent treatment, are quality controlled to ensure levels of 0.4 IU/mL or more in the final product; however, the product is contraindicated in patients with severe protein S deficiency.[78]

Frozen Deglycerolized RBCs

RBCs can be frozen by adding the cryoprotective agent glycerol to the RBCs before freezing. RBCs are then thawed and deglycerolized by washing with successively lower concentrates of sodium chloride. This product contains 80% or more of the red cells present in the original unit of blood and has the same expected posttransfusion survival as RBCs. The deglycerolization process can take several hours, and the resulting unit must be transfused within 24 hours after thaw if prepared in an open system (within 2 weeks if a closed system is used). Use is restricted to situations in which standard transfusion components are inappropriate or unavailable, for example, for alloimmunized patients with SCD who need rare RBC antigen-negative units.

SPECIAL BLOOD BANK SITUATIONS
Massive Transfusion

Massive transfusion is defined as the replacement of a patient's total blood volume within a 24-hour period. There are several different approaches to managing massive transfusions.[79] One approach has a transfusion medicine specialist actively involved in the decision to transfuse and monitor the transfusion efficacy. Another approach uses laboratory testing to guide transfusion, whereas a third model uses a component-driven model. Retrospective studies have suggested a survival benefit in the component-driven model, especially in military studies, which incorporates fix ratios of RBCs, platelets, and FFP. However, single-institutional studies in pediatric patients have not demonstrated a survival advantage of a component-driven approach.[80,81] For an excellent review on this topic, see the review by Diab and colleagues.[82]

There has been recent interest in using rapid whole-blood analysis of coagulation (eg, thromboelastography) to aid in the appropriate choice of blood components during massive transfusion or trauma situations. Routine coagulation testing (ie, prothrombin, activated partial thromboplastin time, fibrinogen) addresses only certain aspects of coagulation; is performed at 37°C, which may not reflect the true hemostatic picture in hypothermic trauma patients; and is not timely. The thromboelastograph is now being studied to evaluate if it can provide directed hemostatic resuscitation strategy for patients with hemorrhagic shock.[83–86] Given the small volume of sample needed and the advantage of adjusting the temperature at which testing can take place, this strategy may be potentially useful in pediatric patients.[87]

Emergency Release Blood

Occasionally, patients require RBC transfusions before compatibility testing can be completed (eg, pediatric trauma, massive gastrointestinal bleeding, massive postoperative bleeding, bleeding on extracorporeal membrane oxygenation [ECMO], and rupture of an extracorporeal circuit). In these circumstances, an emergency blood pack of universal donor (O Rh negative [D−]) uncrossmatched red cells can be released. A blood sample from the patient should be collected for subsequent testing so that testing can confirm that the units transfused were compatible. Transfusion services routinely use an emergency release form signed by the attending physician that indicates that the RBCs are needed before the completion of testing.

IMMUNOHEMATOLOGY TECHNIQUES

Tables 9 and **10** identify commonly used and specialized immunologic techniques with a description of methodology, turnaround times, and purpose. These techniques identify the causes of incompatibility between recipient RBCs and patient plasma, underlying causes of hemolysis (eg, warm autoimmune hemolytic anemia, paroxysmal cold hemoglobinuria, and so forth), and the evaluation of potential transfusion reactions.

Neonatal Immunohematological Issues

Neonates do not develop significant isohemagglutinins until approximately 4 months of age. Therefore, neonatal samples do not require a crossmatch against donor RBCs unless there has been transfusion of plasma as seen in ECMO or massive transfusion. Initial testing should include one or more samples for ABO/D typing. ABO/D type (red cell, forward group) should be performed to document no misidentification of the sample; however, plasma typing (reverse group) is not required. In addition an antibody screen and testing for maternal IgG ABO isohemagglutinins for type-specific transfusion should be performed. Sequential testing for ABO/D type, antibody screen, or crossmatch is not required. However, if circulating maternal antibody is present on the initial screen, antigen-negative or crossmatch compatible RBC units are required.

Table 10
Uncommonly used (specialized) techniques in the blood bank

Test	Principle of the Test	Purpose
Donath-Landsteiner Test TAT: 2–3 h	Mixing of patient serum with known P positive reagent cell at cold temperature (ice water bath) and then incubating at warm temperature (37°C) resulting in visible hemolysis	To detect Donath-Landsteiner antibody (anti P) by demonstrating its unique hemolytic property
Minor Crossmatch TAT: 5–60 min	Mixing of donor plasma with patients' red cells	To detect incompatibility between patients' and donor's plasma
Lectin Panel TAT: 15–20 min	Mixing of patients' red cells with known lectins (ie, Arachis hypogaea, Glycine max)	To detect the exposure of crypt T antigens on the patients' red cells (polyagglutination)
Molecular RBC Phenotyping TAT: 8 h to 1 wk (depending on methodology and availability)	Extracting DNA from patients' or donor's white blood cells, amplifying specific targets, and detecting the amplified targets	To detect the presence or absence of specific polymorphisms to predict the patients' or donor's red cell antigenic phenotype
Adsorption for cold or warm antibodies TAT: ~8 h	Mixing of patients' plasma or serum with autologous treated red cells or reagent cells with known phenotype, followed by incubation to adsorb out the autoantibodies; may need to perform 2 or 3 times	To remove unwanted autoantibodies to facilitate the detection of alloantibodies

Abbreviation: TAT, turn around time.

SUMMARY

Blood component therapy plays a critical role in the treatment of pediatric patients. The ordering licensed care practitioner, who should have a firm understanding of the risks and benefits of transfusion, must specify product modifications. Newer blood and blood products transfused to children are likely to have an improved safety profile. Molecular immunohematologic testing will likely be more common in the future.

REFERENCES

1. Dzik WH. Emily Cooley Lecture 2002: transfusion safety in the hospital. Transfusion 2003;43:1190–9.
2. Carson TH. Standards for blood banks and transfusion service. 28th edition. Bethesda (MD): AABB Press; 2012.
3. Jenkins C, Ramírez-Arcos S, Goldman M, et al. Bacterial contamination in platelets: incremental improvements drive down but do not eliminate risk. Transfusion 2011;51:2555–65.

4. Brecher ME, Jacobs MR, Katz LM, et al, AABB Bacterial Contamination Task Force. Survey of methods used to detect bacterial contamination of platelet products in the United States in 2011. Transfusion 2013;53:911–8.
5. Rais-Bahrami K, Nunez S, Revenis ME, et al. Follow-up study of adolescents exposed to di (2-ethylhexyl) phthalate (DEHP) as neonates on extracorporeal membrane oxygenation (ECMO) support. Environ Health Perspect 2004;112:1339–40.
6. Report of the US Department of Health and Human Services. The 2009 national blood collection and utilization survey report. Washington, DC: US Department of Health and Human Services, Office of the Assistant Secretary for Health; 2011.
7. Luban NLC, Strauss RG, Hume HA. Commentary on the safety of red blood cells preserved in extended storage media for neonatal transfusions. Transfusion 1991;31:229–35.
8. Manno CS, Hedberg KW, Kim HC, et al. Comparison of the hemostatic effects of fresh whole blood, stored whole blood, and components after open heart surgery in children. Blood 1991;77:930–6.
9. Pidcoke HF, McFaul SJ, Ramasubramanian AK, et al. Primary hemostatic capacity of whole blood: a comprehensive analysis of pathogen reduction and refrigeration effects over time. Transfusion 2013;53(Suppl 1):137S–49S.
10. Kahn RA, Staggs SD, Miller WV, et al. Recovery, lifespan, and function of CPD-Adenine (CPDA-1) platelet concentrates stored for up to 72 hours at 4 C. Transfusion 1980;20:498–503.
11. 102nd meeting of the Blood Products Advisory Committee. Gaithersburg, MD. May 16th, 2012.
12. AABB Circular of Information Task Force. Circular of information. Bethesda (MD): AABB Press; 2013.
13. Vassallo RR, Murphy S. A critical comparison of platelet preparation methods. Curr Opin Hematol 2006;13:323–30.
14. Johnson L, Winter KM, Hartkopf-Theis T. Evaluation of the automated collection and extended storage of apheresis platelets in additive solution. Transfusion 2012;52:503–9.
15. Kacker S, Ness PM, Savage WJ, et al. The cost-effectiveness of platelet additive solution to prevent allergic transfusion reactions. Transfusion 2013. [Epub ahead of print]. http://dx.doi.org/10.1111/trf.12095.
16. Yomtovian R, Jacobs MR. A prospective bonus of platelet storage additive solutions: a reduction in biofilm formation and improved bacterial detection during platelet storage. Transfusion 2010;50:2295–300.
17. Quillen K, Wong E, Scheinberg P, et al. Granulocyte transfusions in severe aplastic anemia: an eleven-year experience. Haematologica 2009;94:1661–8.
18. Heim KF, Fleisher TA, Stroncek DF, et al. The relationship between alloimmunization and posttransfusion granulocyte survival: experience in a chronic granulomatous disease cohort. Transfusion 2011;51:1154–62.
19. Dale DC, Price TH. Granulocyte transfusion therapy: a new era? Curr Opin Hematol 2009;16:1–2.
20. Massey E, Harding K, Kahan BC, et al. The granulocytes in neutropenia 1 (GIN 1) study: a safety study of granulocytes collected from whole blood and stored in additive solution and plasma. Transfus Med 2012;22:277–84.
21. Tinmouth A, Chin-Yee I. The clinical consequences of the red cell storage lesion. Transfus Med Rev 2001;15:91–107.
22. Pavenski K, Saidenberg E, Lavoie M, et al. Red blood cell storage lesions and related transfusion issues: a Canadian Blood Services research and development symposium. Transfus Med Rev 2012;26:68–84.

23. Neal MD, Raval JS, Triulzi DJ, et al. Innate immune activation after transfusion of stored red blood cells. Transfus Med Rev 2013;27:113–8.
24. Koch CG, Li L, Sessler DI, et al. Duration of red-cell storage and complications after cardiac surgery. N Engl J Med 2008;358:1229–39.
25. Dumont LJ, Dumont DF, Unger ZM, et al, BEST Collaborative. A randomized controlled trial comparing autologous radiolabeled in vivo platelet (PLT) recoveries and survivals of 7-day-stored PLT-rich plasma and buffy coat PLTs from the same subjects. Transfusion 2011;51:1241–8.
26. Rumjantseva V, Hoffmeister KM. Novel and unexpected clearance mechanisms for cold platelets. Transfus Apher Sci 2010;42:63–70.
27. Diab Y, Wong E, Criss VR, et al. Storage of aliquots of apheresis platelets for neonatal use in syringes with and without agitation. Transfusion 2011;51:2642–6.
28. Pisciotto PT, Snyder EL, Napychank PA, et al. In vitro characteristics of volume-reduced platelet concentrate stored in syringes. Transfusion 1991;31:404–8.
29. Weiss S, Scammell K, Levin E, et al. In vitro platelet quality in storage containers used for pediatric transfusions. Transfusion 2012;52:1703–14.
30. Winkler AM, Sheppard CA, Culler EE, et al. Effects of storage duration and volume on the quality of leukoreduced apheresis-derived platelets: implications for pediatric transfusion medicine. Transfusion 2010;50:2193–8.
31. Devine DV, Serrano K. The platelet storage lesion. Clin Lab Med 2010;30:475–87.
32. Murphy S. Radiolabeling of PLTs to assess viability: a proposal for a standard. Transfusion 2004;44:131–3.
33. Fergusson D, Hébert PC, Lee SK, et al. Clinical outcomes following institution of universal leukoreduction of blood transfusions for premature infants. JAMA 2003;289:1950–6.
34. Wong EC. Irradiated products. In: Hillyer C, Strauss R, Luban NL, editors. Handbook of pediatric transfusion medicine. 1st edition. Amsterdam: Elsevier; 2004. p. 101–12.
35. Moroff G, Holme S, AuBuchon JP, et al. Viability and in vitro properties of AS-1 red cells after gamma irradiation. Transfusion 1999;39:128–34.
36. Schoenfeld H, Muhm M, Doepfmer U, et al. Platelet activity in washed platelet concentrates. Anesth Analg 2004;99:17–20.
37. Veeraputhiran M, Ware J, Dent J, et al. A comparison of washed and volume-reduced platelets with respect to platelet activation, aggregation, and plasma protein removal. Transfusion 2011;51:1030–6.
38. International forum: transfusion of apheresis platelets and ABO groups. Vox Sang 2005;88:207–22.
39. Schoenfeld H, Spies C, Jakob C. Volume-reduced platelet concentrates. Curr Hematol Rep 2006;5:82–8.
40. Schoenfeld H, Muhm M, Doepfmer UR, et al. The functional integrity of platelets in volume-reduced platelet concentrates. Anesth Analg 2005;100:78–81.
41. Moroff G, Friedman A, Robkin-Kline L, et al. Reduction of the volume of stored platelet concentrates for use in neonatal patients. Transfusion 1984;24:144–6.
42. Cook S, Gunter J, Wissel M. Effective use of a strategy using assigned red cell units to limit donor exposure for neonatal patients. Transfusion 1993;33:379–83.
43. Wang-Rodriguez J, Mannino FL, Liu E, et al. A novel strategy to limit blood donor exposure and blood waste in multiply transfused premature infants. Transfusion 1996;36:64–70.

44. Fasano RM, Paul WM, Pisciotto PT. Complications of neonatal transfusions. In: Popovsky MA, editor. Transfusion reactions. 4th edition. Bethesda (MD): AABB Press; 2012.

45. Strauss RG. RBC storage and avoiding hyperkalemia from transfusions to neonates and infants. Transfusion 2010;50:1862–5.

46. Criss VR, Luban NL, Paul W, et al. Utility of lead screening of whole blood donors to avoid lead exposure in children. Transfusion 2012;52(Suppl):233A.

47. Sanders J, Patel S, Cooper J, et al. Red blood cell storage is associated with length of stay and renal complications after cardiac surgery. Transfusion 2011;51:2286–94.

48. Manlhiot C, McCrindle BW, Menjak IB, et al. Longer blood storage is associated with suboptimal outcomes in high-risk pediatric cardiac surgery. Ann Thorac Surg 2012;93:1563–9.

49. Schulman CI, Nathe K, Brown M, et al. Impact of age of transfused blood in the trauma patient. J Trauma 2002;52:1224–5.

50. Walsh TS, McArdle F, McLellan SA, et al. Does the storage time of transfused red blood cells influence regional or global indexes of tissue oxygenation in anemic critically ill patients? Crit Care Med 2004;32:364–71.

51. Fergusson DA, Hébert P, Hogan DL, et al. Effect of fresh red blood cell transfusions on clinical outcomes in premature, very low-birth-weight infants: the ARIPI randomized trial. JAMA 2012;308:1443–51.

52. Bolan CD, Childs RW, Procter JL, et al. Massive immune haemolysis after allogeneic peripheral blood stem cell transplantation with minor ABO incompatibility. Br J Haematol 2001;112:787–95.

53. Robitaille N, Hume HA. Blood components and fractionated plasma products: preparation, indications and administration. In: Arceci RJ, Hann IM, Smith OP, editors. Pediatric hematology. 3rd edition. Malden (MA): Blackwell Publishing; 2006. p. 693–723.

54. Molnar R, Johnson R, Sweat LT, et al. Absence of D alloimmunization in D-pediatric oncology patients receiving D-incompatible single-donor platelets. Transfusion 2002;42:177–82.

55. Bartley AN, Carpenter JB, Berg MP. D+ platelet transfusions in D-patients: cause for concern? Immunohematology 2009;25:5–8.

56. National Institutes of Health. National Heart, Lung and Blood Institute. The management of sickle cell disease. 4th edition. Bethesda (MD): National Institutes of Health; 2002. Publication No. 02-2117.

57. Fasano RM, Paul WM, Siegal E, et al. Transfusion protocol for patients with sickle cell hemoglobinopathies at Children's National Medical Center. Immunohematology 2012;28:13–6.

58. Roberts DO, Covert B, Lindsey T, et al. Directed blood donor program decreases donor exposure for children with sickle cell disease requiring chronic transfusion. Immunohematology 2012;28:7–12.

59. Isaak EJ, LeChien B, Lindsey T, et al. The Charles Drew Program in Missouri: a description of a partnership among a blood center and several hospitals to address the care of patients with sickle cell disease. Immunohematology 2006;22:112–6.

60. Chou ST, Friedman DF. Transfusion practices for patients with sickle cell disease at the Children's Hospital of Philadelphia. Immunohematology 2012;28:27–30.

61. Hillyer KL, Hare VW, Josephson CD, et al. Partners for Life: the transfusion program for patients with sickle cell disease offered at the American Red Cross Blood Services, Southern Region, Atlanta, Georgia. Immunohematology 2006; 22:108–11.

62. Flickinger C. In search of red blood cells for alloimmunized patients with sickle cell disease. Immunohematology 2006;22:136–42.
63. Shander A, Goodnough LT, Ratko T, et al. Consensus recommendations for the off-label use of recombinant human factor VIIa (NovoSeven) therapy. Pharma Ther 2005;30:644–58.
64. Sandler SG, Zantek ND. Review: IgA anaphylactic transfusion reactions. Part II. Clinical diagnosis and bedside management. Immunohematology 2004;20:234–8.
65. Hogge DE, McConnell M, Jacobson C, et al. Platelet refractoriness and alloimmunization in pediatric oncology and bone marrow transplant patients. Transfusion 1995;35:645–52.
66. Seftel MD, Growe GH, Petraszko T, et al. Universal prestorage leukoreduction in Canada decreases platelet alloimmunization and refractoriness. Blood 2004; 103:333–9.
67. Schiffer CA, Anderson KC, Bennett CL, et al, American Society of Clinical Oncology. Platelet transfusion for patients with cancer: clinical practice guidelines of the American Society of Clinical Oncology. J Clin Oncol 2001;19:1519–38.
68. Friedman DF, Lukas MB, Jawad A, et al. Alloimmunization to platelets in heavily transfused patients with sickle cell disease. Blood 1996;88:3216–22.
69. Fontão-Wendel R, Silva LC, Saviolo CB, et al. Incidence of transfusion-induced platelet-reactive antibodies evaluated by specific assays for the detection of human leucocyte antigen and human platelet antigen antibodies. Vox Sang 2007; 93:241–9.
70. Bontadini A. HLA techniques: typing and antibody detection in the laboratory of immunogenetics. Methods 2012;56:471–6.
71. Nambiar A, Duquesnoy RJ, Adams S, et al. HLA matchmaker-driven analysis of responses to HLA-typed platelet transfusions in alloimmunized thrombocytopenic patients. Blood 2006;107:1680–7.
72. Petz LD, Garratty G, Calhoun L, et al. Selecting donors of platelets for refractory patients on the basis of HLA antibody specificity. Transfusion 2000;40:1446–56.
73. Bussel JB, Sola-Visner M. Current approaches to the evaluation and management of the fetus and neonate with immune thrombocytopenia. Semin Perinatol 2009;33:35–42.
74. Kiefel V, Bassler D, Kroll H, et al. Antigen-positive platelet transfusion in neonatal alloimmune thrombocytopenia (NAIT). Blood 2006;107:3761–3.
75. Allen D, Verjee S, Rees S, et al. Platelet transfusion in neonatal alloimmune thrombocytopenia. Blood 2007;109:388–9.
76. Lozano M, Cid J. Analysis of reasons for not implementing pathogen inactivation for platelet concentrates. Transfus Clin Biol 2013;20:158–64.
77. Mintz PD, Wehrli G. Irradiation eradication and pathogen reduction: ceasing cesium irradiation of blood products. Bone Marrow Transplant 2009;44:205–11.
78. Doyle S, O'Brien P, Murphy K, et al. Coagulation content of solvent/detergent plasma compared with fresh frozen plasma. Blood Coagul Fibrinolysis 2003; 14:283–7.
79. Shaz BH, Dente CJ, Harris RS, et al. Transfusion management of trauma patients. Anesth Analg 2009;108:1760–8.
80. Hendrickson JE, Shaz BH, Pereira G, et al. Coagulopathy is prevalent and associated with adverse outcomes in transfused pediatric trauma patients. J Pediatr 2012;160:204–9.
81. Hendrickson JE, Shaz BH, Pereira G, et al. Implementation of a pediatric trauma massive transfusion protocol: one institution's experience. Transfusion 2012;52: 1228–36.

82. Diab YA, Wong EC, Luban NL. Massive transfusion in children and neonates. Br J Haematol 2013;161:15–26.

83. Cotton BA, Faz G, Hatch QM, et al. Rapid thrombelastography delivers real-time results that predict transfusion within 1 hour of admission. J Trauma 2011;71: 407–17.

84. Holcomb JB, Minei KM, Scerbo ML. Admission rapid thrombelastography can replace conventional coagulation tests in the emergency department. Ann Surg 2012;256:476–86.

85. Schöchl H, Cotton B, Inaba K. FIBTEM provides early prediction of massive transfusion in trauma. Crit Care 2011;15:R265.

86. Schöchl H, Nienaber U, Maegele M, et al. Transfusion in trauma: thromboelastometry-guided coagulation factor concentrate-based therapy versus standard fresh frozen plasma-based therapy. Crit Care 2011;15:R83.

87. Forman KR, Wong E, Gallagher M, et al. Effect of temperature on thromboelastography (TEG) and implications for clinical use in neonates undergoing therapeutic hypothermia. E-PAS 2012: 3851.628 [abstract].

Pediatric Therapeutic Apheresis
Rationale and Indications for Plasmapheresis, Cytapheresis, Extracorporeal Photopheresis, and LDL Apheresis

Yeowon A. Kim, MD, MHS, Steven R. Sloan, MD, PhD*

KEYWORDS

- Pediatric • Apheresis • Plasmapheresis • Plasma exchange
- Extracorporeal photopheresis • Red cell exchange • Leukapheresis

KEY POINTS

- During apheresis, peripheral blood components are separated from each other. The selected component is isolated while the remainder is returned to the donor or patient.
- Apheresis is performed for a wide variety of medical indications. It is also used for peripheral hematopoietic progenitor cell collection.
- The decision to perform apheresis on pediatric patients is largely extrapolated from the adult experience.

INTRODUCTION/BACKGROUND

Apheresis refers to a group of medical technologies in which peripheral blood is processed by an instrument that separates blood into components. The selected component is isolated while the remainder is returned to the donor or patient. Modern apheresis instruments are fully automated and separation can be performed on the basis of density, size, and/or differential adsorption. Most apheresis instruments rely on density differences to separate blood into components by centrifugation. A notable exception is low-density lipoprotein (LDL) apheresis, in which LDL is selectively removed from plasma through filtration and/or adsorption.

Most forms of therapeutic apheresis are designed to remove the pathogenic components from the circulation. The therapeutic efficacy depends many factors including the importance of the substance removed in the pathophysiology of the disease,

Joint Program in Transfusion Medicine, Department of Laboratory Medicine, Boston Children's Hospital, Blood Bank–Bader 410, 300 Longwood Avenue, Boston, MA 02115, USA
* Corresponding author.
E-mail address: Steven.Sloan@childrens.harvard.edu

Pediatr Clin N Am 60 (2013) 1569–1580
http://dx.doi.org/10.1016/j.pcl.2013.08.006
0031-3955/13/$ – see front matter © 2013 Elsevier Inc. All rights reserved.

efficiency of removal of the pathogenic substance, and the presence of other complementary/adjunctive therapies. Therapeutic plasma exchange (TPE) or plasmapheresis is usually performed to remove toxic antibodies from the circulation. Cytapheresis is used to deplete leukocytes in the setting of hyperleukocytosis and leukostasis (specifically, leukapheresis) or platelets (plateletpheresis) in the setting of thrombocytosis and increased thrombotic or hemorrhagic risk. Leukapheresis is also used to collect peripheral hematopoietic progenitor cells (HPCs). Pathogenic red blood cells (RBCs) containing sickle hemoglobin can be removed and "exchanged" for donor RBCs with normal hemoglobin. Unlike other forms of therapeutic apheresis, the component removed during extracorporeal photopheresis (ECP), peripheral blood mononuclear cells, may not directly contribute to the disease process. During ECP the mononuclear cells are subjected to ultraviolet A light in the presence of psoralen and then reinfused to the patient.

The decision to perform apheresis on pediatric patients is often based on results of adult studies. The American Society for Apheresis (ASFA) guidelines, which assigns disease entities to 1 of 4 categories according to the strength of recommendations and quality of published evidence, does not distinguish between pediatric or adult-onset disease. The limited use of therapeutic apheresis in pediatric patients may be attributed to the lack of generally accepted indications and treatment course, as well as technical difficulty. Modifications of adult procedures to factor in smaller total blood volume and limit potential fluid shifts in pediatric patients, procedural anticoagulation regimens that minimize hypocalcemia, and improved options for vascular access have made therapeutic apheresis procedures safe to perform in most children.

Vascular Access

Peripheral access may be possible for older children with adequate vein size. If adequate peripheral access cannot be obtained (ie, 18-gauge or larger steel needle placed in the antecubital vein for the draw and a 22-gauge or larger needle placed in peripheral vein of opposite arm for return), central venous access is necessary. Catheters should be able to withstand negative pressure from blood withdrawal at high flow rates. Hence, most peripherally inserted central catheters (ie, most PICC lines) are not compatible to use for drawing but may be used for returning. Some institutions have had success with specific PICC lines designed to tolerate the flows and pressures of apheresis (eg, Power PICC). Femoral venous catheters are placed in urgent situations and are usually restricted for patients requiring only a few procedures or for temporary use until alternate central venous access is obtained. Femoral catheters are assumed to be associated with a higher risk of infection or thrombosis than other routes of access, although these beliefs have recently been challenged.

Procedural Risks

The major risks of apheresis are related to the need for peripheral access and include pain, infection, bleeding, and thrombosis. Complications associated with central venous access include pneumothorax, hemothorax, cardiac arrhythmias, and central vein stenosis. Sedation may be required for placement of the access device. In addition, femoral catheters impair the patient's mobility. Because of small pediatric total blood volumes, procedure-related fluid shifts, intraprocedural anemia, and iron deficiency anemia with chronic apheresis therapy are of a greater concern in children than adult patients.

Citrate and/or heparin prevent clotting of blood in the apheresis circuit. Citrate chelates calcium ions, thus preventing the calcium-dependent coagulation cascade. Citrate has a short half-life and is metabolized by the liver and excreted by the kidneys. Patients with renal or hepatic impairment undergoing lengthy procedures or receiving replacement fluids containing additional citrate (ie, plasma or RBCs) are at risk for developing symptomatic hypocalcemia. Signs and symptoms of hypocalcemia in adults begin with perioral or digital paresthesias and may progress to include nausea, vomiting, anxiety, diarrhea, lightheadedness, tremors, and muscle cramps. QT prolongation can occur, and in severe cases, the patient may develop tetany, seizures, and cardiac arrhythmias. Pediatric patients may not be able to communicate symptoms of hypocalcemia, which may present differently from adults, with abdominal pain, vomiting, pallor, and/or hypotension.[1] Indeed, hypotension, which can be due to both hypocalcemia and hypovolemia, is one of the leading adverse events in pediatric apheresis. To avoid the complications of hypocalcemia, heparin can be used for anticoagulation in pediatric apheresis, although prophylactic administration of divalent cations such as calcium and magnesium can prevent most citrate-related toxicities.[2] If blood products are used to prime the apheresis circuit and/or as replacement fluid, there will be additional risks related to blood component transfusion.

The remainder of the article provides an overview of the commonly encountered indications for apheresis and refers to ASFA categories. ASFA category I includes diseases in which therapeutic apheresis is primary or adjunct first-line therapy; category II denotes diseases for which apheresis is supportive or adjunctive therapy; category III includes diseases for which the existing evidence is insufficient to establish the efficacy of therapy; and category IV indicates disorders for which controlled trials have shown no benefit or anecdotal reports are discouraging.[3]

INDICATIONS
Hematologic

Hemoglobinopathies

RBC exchange is a procedure in which patient red cells are exchanged for donor red cells. RBC exchange in sickle cell disease or other heterozygous compound hemoglobinopathies (ie, HbSC disease) is performed to replace pathogenic RBCs for donor RBCs with wild-type hemoglobin, hence improving oxygen-carrying capacity, decreasing blood viscosity, and suppressing endogenous erythropoiesis. Advantages of RBC exchange over simple transfusion include rapid decrease in percentage of hemoglobin S (HbS), ability to more precisely control posttreatment hematocrit, and reduced risk of fluid overload. In sickle cell disease, RBC exchange associated with benefits of transfusion and also minimized tissue iron loading.[4] Disadvantages of RBC exchange include exposure to more blood units and increased venous access requirements. The increased number of transfused RBC units with RBC exchanges may increase alloimmunization but one report suggests this is not the case.[5]

Acute chest syndrome, which is defined by new radiographic infiltrate accompanied by respiratory signs and symptoms, is the second leading cause of sickle cell–associated mortality in children. In acute chest syndrome both simple and exchange transfusion (ASFA category II) can rapidly improve oxygenation. Exchange transfusion should be reserved for patients whose hematocrit is so high that simple transfusion would dangerously increase viscosity, with more severe hypoxia requiring mechanical ventilation, and/or failure to improve with simple transfusion.[6]

RBC exchange is first-line therapy for acute stroke (ASFA category I) and has been shown to be effective in decreasing both primary[7] and secondary strokes in children while reducing iron overload[4] (ASFA category II). RBC exchange (ASFA category III) may also be preferred over simple transfusion in the setting of acute multiorgan failure and higher hematocrit levels to avoid hyperviscosity while rapidly reducing HbS levels. RBC exchange may be indicated preoperatively in patients with high blood hemoglobin concentrations who are undergoing high-risk procedures.[8] Transfusion therapy, whether simple or exchange, has not been shown to benefit patients with frequent pain episodes, acute pain crisis, prevention of pulmonary hypertension, or priapism.

Immune-mediated cytopenias

Autoimmune hemolytic anemia (AIHA) and immune thrombocytopenic purpura are caused by production of autoantibodies that result in RBC and platelet destruction, respectively. The efficacy of TPE in treating immune thrombocytopenic purpura and warm AIHA has not been proven by (ASFA categories IV and III, respectively). Although cold AIHA is primarily a disease of the elderly, it can be seen in children. Cold AIHA is due to immunoglobulin M antibodies, most of which reside intravascularly and can be effectively removed by plasmapheresis. Thus severe life-threatening cold AIHA is an ASFA category II indication. Thombotic thrombocytopenic purpura, an important indication for plasmapheresis, and hemolytic uremic syndrome are discussed in the article by Trachtman elsewhere in this issue.

Oncologic

Hyperleukocytosis with or without leukostasis

Hyperleukocytosis can cause significant morbidity and mortality through inducing tumor lysis syndrome, leukostasis, and/or disseminated intravascular coagulopathy. In leukostasis, occlusion of the microcirculation by leukocyte aggregates may lead to endothelial damage, thrombosis, and/or hemorrhage. Leukostasis of cerebral and pulmonary vasculature are most likely to cause immediate symptoms. In acute myelogenous leukemia, the white blood cell (WBC) count threshold for symptomatic leukostasis is typically greater than $100,000/\mu L$, while it is often greater than $400,000/\mu L$ in acute lymphoblastic leukemia.[9] Because the type of acute leukemia is often unknown at presentation, leukapheresis should be considered in all patients with new onset acute leukemia whose WBC is greater than $100,000/\mu L$, especially if they are symptomatic. In addition to absolute WBC and blast count, blast-endothelial cell interactions likely play a role in the pathophysiology.

The management of hyperleukocytosis includes cytoreduction and supportive care. Mechanical cytoreduction by leukapheresis has been performed in the setting of symptomatic leukostasis as well as prophylaxis/bridge to definitive therapy. There is general consensus that symptomatic leukostasis is a valid indication for leukapheresis (ASFA category I). However, it is less clear whether prophylactic leukapheresis reduces complications of hyperleukocytosis. Although some analyses suggest that leukapheresis may reduce early mortality, this benefit does not extend to improvement in long-term prognosis.[10] Hence, prophylaxis of hyperviscosity has been designated as a category III indication by ASFA guidelines. Leukapheresis is particularly at risk in patients with acute promyelocytic leukemia as it may worsen associated disseminated intravascular coagulation.

Peripheral hematopoietic progenitor cell collection

Hematopoietic progenitor cells are used for hematologic reconstitution following myeloablative chemotherapy to eradicate underlying disease. Such diseases include both hematological and nonhematological malignancies and inherited metabolic and immune disorders. There are 3 sources of HPC: bone marrow, peripheral blood, and umbilical cord blood. Most autologous HPC transplants are peripheral blood-derived. Pediatric allogeneic HPC transplants are mostly bone marrow- and umbilical cord blood-derived.

Peripheral blood-derived HPCs are collected by leukapheresis following mobilization to increase the number of circulating HPCs. HPCs from autologous donors can be mobilized with cytotoxic chemotherapeutic agents and/or growth factors such as granulocyte - colony stimulating factor (G-CSF) and/or an agent that disrupts the attraction of the HPCs to the bone marrow such as plerixafor. G-CSF is most commonly used to mobilize allogeneic HPC donors. Peripheral access is often sufficient to collect peripheral HPCs from older donors. In contrast, young, small pediatric patients often require central venous access because of inadequate peripheral vascular access.

Graft-versus-host disease

Acute graft-versus-host disease (GVHD) occurs in 20% to 50% of patients after allogeneic hematopoietic stem cell transplantation and chronic graft-versus-host disease (cGVHD) affects 30% to 50% of engrafted survivors. cGVHD usually occurs greater than 100 days posttransplant, with fibrosis and sclerosis predominating. The cause of GVHD includes donor T-cell alloreactivity to recipient human leukocyte antigens (HLA). GVHD frequently requires long-term systemic immunosuppression and ECP is useful as adjunctive therapy for refractory disease (cutaneous GVHD ASFA category II, noncutaneous GVHD ASFA category III). The exact mechanisms behind ECP are unclear, but murine studies indicate that ECP leads to induction of CD4+, CD25+, Foxp+ regulatory T-cells that mediate immunologic tolerance[11] and human studies have demonstrated ECP allows for decreased steroid doses for patients with chronic cGVHD.

Neurologic

Acute inflammatory demyelinating polyneuropathy/Guillain-Barré syndrome

Acute inflammatory demyelinating polyneuropathy (AIDP)/Guillain-Barré syndrome is an acute progressive paralysis disorder resulting in both motor and sensory deficits. It is caused by antibodies against peripheral nerve myelin. Spontaneous recovery occurs in most cases, although severe cases may necessitate mechanical ventilation and intensive care. The efficacy of TPE has been demonstrated in randomized controlled trials[12] and is an ASFA category I designation. Although randomized controlled trials have not been performed in children, case series or retrospective reviews have shown a beneficial effect of TPE in pediatric patients with AIDP.[13] Intravenous immunoglobulin (IVIG) is equivalent to plasma exchange for patients with AIDP.

Chronic Inflammatory Demyelinating Polyneuropathy

Chronic inflammatory demyelinating polyneuropathy (CIDP) is a chronic demyelinating disorder of the peripheral nervous system resulting in motor and sensory deficits that is thought to be of an autoimmune nature and possibly antibody-mediated. TPE is effective in adults with CIDP (ASFA category I),[14] is comparable to IVIG,[15] and has been used in pediatric patients with CIDP.

Myasthenia Gravis

Myasthenia gravis is an autoimmune disorder typically caused by antibodies to the acetylcholine receptor that disrupts neuromuscular transmission resulting in muscle weakness. TPE is usually reserved for severe or refractory Myasthenia gravis, and is an ASFA category I indication in this setting.

Multiple Sclerosis and Neuromyelitis Optica

Multiple sclerosis (MS) is a demyelinating disorder of the central nervous system (CNS) white matter. The relapsing-remitting form is the most common clinical pattern, although others include primary progressive, secondary progressive, and relapsing progressive forms. Neuromyelitis optica (NMO), which is related to but distinct from MS, specifically involves demyelination of the optic nerve and/or spinal cord, although the brain may be involved in a minority of cases. The pathogenesis of both disorders is unclear but is thought to be immune-mediated. The T-cell-rich CNS lesions of MS point to a cellular-mediated process, although oligoclonal immunoglobulin in the CSF of MS patients suggests an additional humoral component. Immunoglobulin G antibodies to aquaporin-4 (a molecule found on CNS astrocytes) have been found in most NMO patients, although its pathogenesis remains unproven.

TPE has been explored in both steroid-refractory MS and NMO. TPE was shown to be effective in a randomized, sham-controlled trial of 22 patients with steroid-refractory acute CNS demyelination.[16] However, the study has been criticized because of the heterogeneous study population representing a variety of diagnoses (MS, NMO, transverse myelitis, acute disseminated encephalomyelitis) without subgroup analysis. There is general consensus that TPE has minimal benefit in treating chronic or progressive forms of MS, but may have a role in acute relapsing MS or NMO resistant to immunosuppressive therapies. Acute MS refractory to steroids and NMO are ASFA class II indications.

Acute Disseminated Encephalomyelitis

Acute disseminated encephalomyelitis is an acute inflammatory demyelinating disease of the CNS primarily affecting children and young adults postinfection or vaccination. It is thought to be due to an autoimmune response against CNS antigens. TPE may have a role in managing steroid-refractory cases (ASFA category II indication).[17]

Chronic Focal Encephalitis (Rasmussens Encephalitis)

Rasmussen encephalitis is a rare acquired disorder resulting in seizures refractory to anticonvulsant drugs and progressive dementia and hemiparesis. The cause is unclear, but autoantibodies to the glutamate receptor GluR3 and glutamic acid decarboxylase 65 have been reported. TPE and IVIG have been used in refractory cases or in nonsurgical candidates (ASFA category II).[18]

Phytanic Acid Storage Disease (Refsum Disease)

Refsum disease is an inherited deficiency of the enzyme that metabolizes phytanic acid, resulting in phytanic acid accumulation and neurologic deficits. Phytanic acid is a branched-chain fatty acid derived from dietary sources, and the mainstay of therapy is dietary control.[19] TPE has been used to remove phytanic acid in severe disease and/or exacerbations (ASFA category II).

MISCELLANEOUS
Pediatric Autoimmune Neuropsychiatric Disorder Associated with Group A Streptococci and Syndenham Chorea

Pediatric autoimmune neuropsychiatric disorder associated with streptococcal infections (PANDAS) and Syndenham chorea (SC) are postinfectious autoimmune neuropsychiatric disorders. The cause is thought to be due to a cross-reactive antibody against CNS epitopes and group A Streptococci.[20] One randomized controlled trial of 29 patients with PANDAS showed that both TPE and IVIG were significantly more effective than placebo.[21] Another randomized controlled pilot trial suggested that TPE and IVIG may be effective in treating SC.[22] PANDAS and SC are both ASFA category I indications.

Renal

Focal segmental glomerulosclerosis

Focal segmental glomerulosclerosis (FSGS) is a major cause of nephrotic syndrome in children. Idiopathic or primary FSGS is thought to be due to a circulating factor that increases glomerular permeability. Other causes of FSGS include genetic abnormalities in the podocyte foot-process proteins. Following renal transplant, disease recurs in at least one-fourth of children. Immunosuppressive pharmacotherapy is the mainstay of FSGS treatment, although no specific drug regimen has been shown to slow progression consistently in native kidneys or decrease recurrence posttransplant. TPE has been explored as adjunct treatment in the setting of disease recurrence posttransplant. Small retrospective studies of pediatric patients with FSGS who received renal transplant suggest that preemptive TPE does not decrease recurrence rates posttransplantation but may be beneficial in treating recurrent disease (ASFA category I).[23]

Vasculitides

Henoch Schönlein purpura (HSP) and Kawasaki disease account for most childhood vasculitis. HSP is a leukocytoclastic vasculitis predominantly affecting small blood vessels resulting in lower extremity purpura, arthralgias, abdominal pain, and/or renal involvement. Therapy for HSP is primarily supportive, although steroids may be used in more severe disease. TPE (with or without more potent immunosuppressants) has been performed in life-threatening cases of HSP or those resulting in renal failure.[24]

The antineutrophil cytoplasmic antibodies (ANCA) -associated vasculitides are characterized by small and/or medium vessel inflammation and multiorgan involvement in the presence of circulating ANCA antibodies. The 3 classic ANCA-associated vasculitides are granulomatosis with polyangitis (formerly known as Wegener granulomatosis), microscopic polyangiitis, and Churg-Strauss syndrome. Severe cases may involve pulmonary hemorrhage and respiratory failure and/or rapidly progressive glomerular nephritis (RPGN) and renal failure. Children are more likely to have more severe disease. Standard induction therapy includes steroids and cyclophosphamide. A randomized controlled trial in adult patients showed that TPE may benefit those with elevated creatinine (>5.7 mg/dL) and dialysis dependence.[25] TPE is performed in severe cases, such as diffuse alveolar hemorrhage or acute renal failure concerning for progression to dialysis. ANCA-associated RPGN resulting in diffuse alveolar hemorrhage or dialysis dependence is an ASFA I category indication for TPE. Dialysis-independent RPGN is a category III indication.

Systemic lupus erythematosus

Systemic lupus erythematosus (SLE) is a chronic autoimmune disorder affecting multiple organ systems. Circulating autoantibodies, immune complexes, and complement activation lead to tissue injury. Randomized controlled trials in adults have not demonstrated benefit of TPE in lupus, including lupus nephritis.[26] Retrospective reviews, case series, or anecdotal case reports have suggested a possible role for rare but severe manifestations of SLE, such as lupus cerebritis, diffuse alveolar hemorrhage, lupus-associated thrombotic thrombocytopenic purpura (TTP), lupus-associated catastrophic antiphospholipid antibody syndrome (CAPS), hyperviscosity, and cryoglobulinemia.[27] One retrospective study of TPE in children with SLE suggests that TPE may be useful as adjunctive therapy in refractory or severe cases.[28] Severe manifestations of lupus (ie, cerebritis, diffuse alveolar hemorrhage) are an ASFA category II designation and nephritis is a category IV indication.

Antiphospholipid antibody syndrome

Antiphospholipid antibody syndrome is characterized by recurrent arterial or venous thrombosis in the setting of antiphospholipid antibodies. In CAPS, systemic coagulation leads to multiorgan involvement. A retrospective review of 31 adults with CAPS suggested that refractory cases may respond to TPE.[29] A review of the CAPS Registry showed that most patients received multiple treatments with recovery being strongly associated with the use of anticoagulants. Multimodal therapy with anticoagulants, steroids, and TPE and/or IVIG was associated with the best outcome.[30]

Miscellaneous

Goodpasture syndrome (GS) is characterized by pulmonary hemorrhage and/or renal involvement, and the presence of an autoantibody to the $\alpha3$ chain of type IV collagen. It is rare in the pediatric population. The standard treatment of GS is immunosuppression and TPE. One randomized controlled trial of 17 patients showed that TPE in addition to immunosuppression may decrease progression to ESRD.[31] Initiating TPE early in the disease process may help prevent permanent renal damage. Dialysis-independent GS or GS with pulmonary hemorrhage are ASFA category I indications. Dialysis-dependent GS is a category IV indication.

Solid Organ Transplant

TPE and ECP have been used as adjunct therapy in preventing and treating solid organ transplant rejection.

Renal

In renal transplantation, hyperacute and acute antibody-mediated rejection (AMR) are caused by recipient anti-A or anti-B isohemagglutinins and donor-specific HLA antibodies, respectively. TPE has been used to remove circulating antibodies during desensitization pretransplant and posttransplant for both ABO-incompatible and HLA-incompatible renal transplants. A recent longitudinal study demonstrated a survival benefit of renal transplantation facilitated by densensitization versus remaining on dialysis or waiting for a compatible organ.[32] Desensitization for incompatible, living donor kidney is a category II indication, whereas high PRA and cadaveric donor is category III. TPE has also been used to treat AMR, typically along with IVIG treatment. It is difficult to assess the specific contribution of TPE from most reports but retrospective case series and one small randomized controlled trial[33] suggest that TPE as a component of a multimodal regimen may have a role in treating AMR. AMR is an ASFA category I indication.

Cardiac

Cardiac allograft rejection may be hyperacute or acute antibody-mediated, acute cellular, or chronic. Desensitization pretransplant is typically impractical due to timing of organ availability. Intraoperative TPE has been used with risk stratification by the C1q-SAB assay.[34] Pre transplantation and posttransplantation TPE in conjunction with immunosuppressive therapy in one group of sensitized pediatric cardiac transplant patients resulted in survival comparable to those nonsensitized.[35] TPE has also used in ABO-incompatible heart transplants, both pretransplantation and posttransplant, to remove antibodies to the ABO antigens on the cardiac endothelium.[36] TPE for treatment of AMR is a category III indication. ECP has been explored in preventing cardiac rejection. A randomized controlled trial of 60 adult cardiac transplant recipients showed that although pretransplant ECP decreased the number of acute rejections, there was no significant difference in survival.[37] ECP for prophylaxis and treatment of cardiac rejection has been given ASFA category I and II designations, respectively.

Pulmonary

Chronic rejection manifests as bronchiolitis obliterans syndrome, resulting in airflow obstruction. ECP may slow the decline of lung function in and stabilize FEV1 in refractory bronchiolitis obliterans syndrome.[38] Lung allograft rejection is an ASFA category II indication for ECP.

Liver

Although ABO compatibility is not a prerequisite for liver transplantation, incompatibility increases the risk of AMR and may decrease graft survival. Several groups have reported using TPE in addition to immunosuppression in patients receiving ABO-incompatible transplants, although successful outcomes have been reported without posttransplant TPE.[39]

Familial Hypercholesterolemia

Familial hypercholesterolemia (FH) is an inherited disorder resulting in elevated levels of LDL-cholesterol (LDL-C) and premature coronary artery disease. Patients with persistent LDL-C elevations despite maximal drug therapy may undergo LDL removal by TPE or LDL apheresis. LDL apheresis has the advantage of selectively removing apoB100-containing lipoproteins LDL and lipoprotein (a). A single lipid apheresis procedure can result in an immediate 60% to 65% reduction in LDL-C with return to baseline levels 1 to 2 weeks postprocedure. Some studies have found that LDL apheresis improves angiographic findings and reduces coronary events[40] in patients with FH. ASFA has given LDL apheresis category I and II designations for homozygous and heterozygous FH, respectively.

Infection

Malaria and babesiosis

Malaria and babesiosis are vector-borne parasites that infect red cells causing intravascular hemolysis, tissue hypoxia, and inflammatory cytokine release. RBC exchange had been thought a promising approach to rapidly reduce parasitemia. Although RBC exchange in severe malaria is an ASFA category II indication, surveillance data and comparative studies demonstrate no benefit and the CDC does not recommend it.[41] The efficacy of RBC exchange in severe babesiosis has not been rigorously analyzed but are extrapolated from case reports. Those recommendations suggest performing RBC exchange for parasitemia ≥10% and/or acute respiratory failure, disseminated intravascular coagulation, congestive heart failure, hemolytic anemia, and acute liver or renal failure.

Bordetella pertussis

Hyperleukocytosis secondary to *Bordetella pertussis* infection is seen in severe disease, and with white counts greater than 100,000 cells/μL, is associated with increased mortality. A few case studies and one case series have described using either leukapheresis or exchange transfusion in the setting of severe pertussis with clinical improvement. One retrospective study using historical controls showed that either leukodepletion or double volume exchange transfusion improved mortality from 90% to 55%.[42]

Sepsis

TPE has been proposed as an adjunctive treatment in sepsis to remove toxic and inflammatory molecules. Two randomized trials of TPE and one trial of continuous plasma filtration in sepsis show mixed results. One study of TPE in 10 children showed improved organ severity scores and improved treatment survival.[43] Sepsis with multi-organ failure is an ASFA category III indication.

REFERENCES

1. Kim HC. Therapeutic apheresis in pediatric patients. In: McLeod BC, Weinstein R, Winters JL, et al, editors. Apheresis: principles and practice. 3rd edition. Bethesda (MD): AABB Press; 2010. p. 445–64.
2. Bolan CD, Yau YY, Cullis HC, et al. Pediatric large-volume leukapheresis: a single institution experience with heparin versus citrate-based anticoagulant regimens. Transfusion 2004;44(2):229–38.
3. Szczepiorkowski ZM, Winters JL, Bandarenko N, et al. Guidelines on the use of therapeutic apheresis in clinical practice–evidence-based approach from the Apheresis Applications Committee of the American Society for Apheresis. J Clin Apher 2010;25(3):83–177.
4. Kim HC, Dugan NP, Silber JH, et al. Erythrocytapheresis therapy to reduce iron overload in chronically transfused patients with sickle cell disease. Blood 1994; 83(4):1136–42.
5. Wahl SK, Garcia A, Hagar W, et al. Lower alloimmunization rates in pediatric sickle cell patients on chronic erythrocytapheresis compared to chronic simple transfusions. Transfusion 2012;52(12):2671–6.
6. Swerdlow PS. Red cell exchange in sickle cell disease. Hematology Am Soc Hematol Educ Program 2006;48–53.
7. Abboud MR, Yim E, Musallam KM, et al. Discontinuing prophylactic transfusions increases the risk of silent brain infarction in children with sickle cell disease: data from STOP II. Blood 2011;118(4):894–8.
8. Neumayr L, Koshy M, Haberkern C, et al. Surgery in patients with hemoglobin SC disease. Preoperative Transfusion in Sickle Cell Disease Study Group. Am J Hematol 1998;57(2):101–8.
9. Bandarenko N, Lockhart E. Therapeutic leukocyte and platelet depletion. In: McLeod BC, Szczepiorkowski ZM, Weinstein R, et al, editors. Apheresis: principles and practice. 3rd edition. Bethesda (MD): AABB Press; 2010. p. 251–67.
10. Ganzel C, Becker J, Mintz PD, et al. Hyperleukocytosis, leukostasis and leukapheresis: practice management. Blood Rev 2012;26(3):117–22.
11. Gatza E, Rogers CE, Clouthier SG, et al. Extracorporeal photopheresis reverses experimental graft-versus-host disease through regulatory T cells. Blood 2008; 112(4):1515–21.
12. Plasmapheresis and acute Guillain-Barre syndrome. The Guillain-Barre syndrome Study Group. Neurology 1985;35(8):1096–104.
13. Hicks CW, Kay B, Worley SE, et al. A clinical picture of Guillain-Barre syndrome in children in the United States. J Child Neurol 2010;25(12):1504–10.
14. Hahn AF, Bolton CF, Pillay N, et al. Plasma-exchange therapy in chronic inflammatory demyelinating polyneuropathy. A double-blind, sham-controlled, cross-over study. Brain 1996;119(Pt 4):1055–66.
15. Dyck PJ, Litchy WJ, Kratz KM, et al. A plasma exchange versus immune globulin infusion trial in chronic inflammatory demyelinating polyradiculoneuropathy. Ann Neurol 1994;36(6):838–45.
16. Weinshenker BG, O'Brien PC, Petterson TM, et al. A randomized trial of plasma exchange in acute central nervous system inflammatory demyelinating disease. Ann Neurol 1999;46(6):878–86.

17. Keegan M, Pineda AA, McClelland RL, et al. Plasma exchange for severe attacks of CNS demyelination: predictors of response. Neurology 2002;58(1):143–6.
18. Andrews PI, Dichter MA, Berkovic SF, et al. Plasmapheresis in rasmussen's encephalitis. Neurology 1996;46(1):242–6.
19. Baldwin EJ, Gibberd FB, Harley C, et al. The effectiveness of long-term dietary therapy in the treatment of adult Refsum disease. J Neurol Neurosurg Psychiatr 2010;81(9):954–7.
20. Yaddanapudi K, Hornig M, Serge R, et al. Passive transfer of streptococcus-induced antibodies reproduces behavioral disturbances in a mouse model of pediatric autoimmune neuropsychiatric disorders associated with streptococcal infection. Mol Psychiatry 2010;15(7):712–26.
21. Perlmutter SJ, Leitman SF, Garvey MA, et al. Therapeutic plasma exchange and intravenous immunoglobulin for obsessive-compulsive disorder and tic disorders in childhood. Lancet 1999;354(9185):1153–8.
22. Garvey MA, Snider LA, Leitman SF, et al. Treatment of Sydenham's chorea with intravenous immunoglobulin, plasma exchange, or prednisone. J Child Neurol 2005;20(5):424–9.
23. Garcia CD, Bittencourt VB, Tumelero A, et al. Plasmapheresis for recurrent post-transplant focal segmental glomerulosclerosis. Transplant Proc 2006;38(6):1904–5.
24. Kawasaki Y, Suzuki J, Murai M, et al. Plasmapheresis therapy for rapidly progressive Henoch-Schonlein nephritis. Pediatr Nephrol 2004;19(8):920–3.
25. Jayne DR, Gaskin G, Rasmussen N, et al. Randomized trial of plasma exchange or high-dosage methylprednisolone as adjunctive therapy for severe renal vasculitis. J Am Soc Nephrol 2007;18(7):2180–8.
26. Lewis EJ, Hunsicker LG, Lan SP, et al. A controlled trial of plasmapheresis therapy in severe lupus nephritis. The Lupus Nephritis Collaborative Study Group. N Engl J Med 1992;326(21):1373–9.
27. Pagnoux C, Korach JM, Guillevin L. Indications for plasma exchange in systemic lupus erythematosus in 2005. Lupus 2005;14(11):871–7.
28. Wright EC, Tullus K, Dillon MJ. Retrospective study of plasma exchange in children with systemic lupus erythematosus. Pediatr Nephrol 2004;19(10):1108–14.
29. Asherson RA, Piette JC. The catastrophic antiphospholipid syndrome 1996: acute multi-organ failure associated with antiphospholipid antibodies: a review of 31 patients. Lupus 1996;5(5):414–7.
30. Bucciarelli S, Espinosa G, Cervera R, et al. Mortality in the catastrophic antiphospholipid syndrome: causes of death and prognostic factors in a series of 250 patients. Arthritis Rheum 2006;54(8):2568–76.
31. Johnson JP, Moore J Jr, Austin HA 3rd, et al. Therapy of anti-glomerular basement membrane antibody disease: analysis of prognostic significance of clinical, pathologic and treatment factors. Medicine (Baltimore) 1985;64(4):219–27.
32. Montgomery RA, Lonze BE, King KE, et al. Desensitization in HLA-incompatible kidney recipients and survival. N Engl J Med 2011;365(4):318–26.
33. Bonomini V, Vangelista A, Frasca GM, et al. Effects of plasmapheresis in renal transplant rejection. A controlled study. Trans Am Soc Artif Intern Organs 1985;31:698–703.
34. Chin C, Chen G, Sequeria F, et al. Clinical usefulness of a novel C1q assay to detect immunoglobulin G antibodies capable of fixing complement in sensitized pediatric heart transplant patients. J Heart Lung Transplant 2011;30(2):158–63.
35. Holt DB, Lublin DM, Phelan DL, et al. Mortality and morbidity in pre-sensitized pediatric heart transplant recipients with a positive donor crossmatch utilizing

peri-operative plasmapheresis and cytolytic therapy. J Heart Lung Transplant 2007;26(9):876–82.

36. Gambino A, Torregrossa G, Cozzi E, et al. ABO-incompatible heart transplantation: crossing the immunological barrier. J Cardiovasc Med (Hagerstown) 2008; 9(8):854–7.

37. Barr ML, Meiser BM, Eisen HJ, et al. Photopheresis for the prevention of rejection in cardiac transplantation. Photopheresis Transplantation Study Group. N Engl J Med 1998;339(24):1744–51.

38. Jaksch P, Scheed A, Keplinger M, et al. A prospective interventional study on the use of extracorporeal photopheresis in patients with bronchiolitis obliterans syndrome after lung transplantation. J Heart Lung Transplant 2012;31(9):950–7.

39. Heffron T, Welch D, Pillen T, et al. Successful ABO-incompatible pediatric liver transplantation utilizing standard immunosuppression with selective postoperative plasmapheresis. Liver Transpl 2006;12(6):972–8.

40. Koziolek MJ, Hennig U, Zapf A, et al. Retrospective analysis of long-term lipid apheresis at a single center. Ther Apher Dial 2010;14(2):143–52.

41. Tan KR, Wiegand RE, Arguin PM. Exchange transfusion for severe malaria: evidence base and literature review. Clin Infect Dis 2013;57(7):923–8.

42. Rowlands HE, Goldman AP, Harrington K, et al. Impact of rapid leukodepletion on the outcome of severe clinical pertussis in young infants. Pediatrics 2010;126(4): e816–27.

43. Nguyen TC, Han YY, Kiss JE, et al. Intensive plasma exchange increases a disintegrin and metalloprotease with thrombospondin motifs-13 activity and reverses organ dysfunction in children with thrombocytopenia-associated multiple organ failure. Crit Care Med 2008;36(10):2878–87.

Index

Note: Page numbers of article titles are in **boldface** type.

Pediatr Clin N Am 60 (2013) 1581–1596
http://dx.doi.org/10.1016/S0031-3955(13)00172-7
0031-3955/13/$ – see front matter © 2013 Elsevier Inc. All rights reserved.

pediatric.theclinics.com

Moving?

Make sure your subscription moves with you!

To notify us of your new address, find your **Clinics Account Number** (located on your mailing label above your name), and contact customer service at:

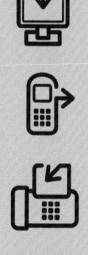

Email: journalscustomerservice-usa@elsevier.com

800-654-2452 (subscribers in the U.S. & Canada)
314-447-8871 (subscribers outside of the U.S. & Canada)

Fax number: 314-447-8029

Elsevier Health Sciences Division
Subscription Customer Service
3251 Riverport Lane
Maryland Heights, MO 63043

*To ensure uninterrupted delivery of your subscription, please notify us at least 4 weeks in advance of move.

Printed and bound by CPI Group (UK) Ltd, Croydon, CR0 4YY

03/10/2024

01040409-0013